CURABLE AND INCURABLE NEUROTICS

*Problems of "Neurotic"
versus
"Malignant" Psychic Masochism*

Books by Edmund Bergler, M.D.

FRIGIDITY IN WOMEN (in collaboration with
   E. Hitschmann)
TALLEYRAND–NAPOLEON–STENDHAL–GRABBE
PSYCHIC IMPOTENCE IN MEN
UNHAPPY MARRIAGE AND DIVORCE
DIVORCE WON'T HELP
THE BATTLE OF THE CONSCIENCE
CONFLICT IN MARRIAGE
THE BASIC NEUROSIS
THE WRITER AND PSYCHOANALYSIS
MONEY AND EMOTIONAL CONFLICTS
COUNTERFEIT-SEX
THE SUPEREGO
FASHION AND THE UNCONSCIOUS
KINSEY'S MYTH OF FEMALE SEXUALITY (in
   collaboration with W. S. Kroger)
THE REVOLT OF THE MIDDLE-AGED MAN
HOMOSEXUALITY: DISEASE OR WAY OF LIFE?
LAUGHTER AND THE SENSE OF HUMOR
PSYCHOLOGY OF GAMBLING
ONE THOUSAND HOMOSEXUALS
PRINCIPLES OF SELF-DAMAGE
TENSIONS CAN BE REDUCED TO NUISANCES
CURABLE AND INCURABLE NEUROTICS
JUSTICE AND INJUSTICE (in collaboration with
   J.A.M. Meerloo)
PARENTS NOT GUILTY!
SELECTED PAPERS OF EDMUND BERGLER, M.D.:
   (1933-1961)

CURABLE
AND
INCURABLE NEUROTICS

Problems of "Neurotic"
versus
"Malignant" Psychic Masochism

by
EDMUND BERGLER, M.D.

INTERNATIONAL UNIVERSITIES PRESS, INC.
Madison, Connecticut

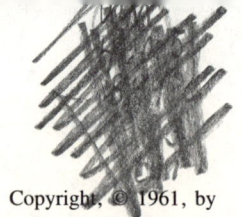

Copyright, © 1961, by
EDMUND BERGLER

First Published 1961
LIVERIGHT PUBLISHING CORPORATION

Copyright Renewed 1989
THE ESTATE OF EDMUND BERGLER

Introduction to the 1993 Printing by Dr. M. L. Iscove
Copyright 1993

EDMUND and MARIANNE BERGLER
PSYCHIATRIC FOUNDATION

All rights reserved. No part of this book may be reproduced by any means, nor translated into a machine language, without the written permission of the publisher.

Library of Congress Cataloging in Publication Data

Bergler, Edmund, 1899-1962
    Curable and incurable neurotics : problems of ''neurotic'' versus ''malignant'' psychic masochism / by Edmund Bergler.
       p. cm.
    Originally published: New York : Liveright, 1961.
    Includes bibliographical references and index.
    ISBN 0-8236-1092-6
    1. Neuroses. 2. Masochism. 3. Self-defeating behavior.
4. Resistance (Psychoanalysis) I. Title.
    [DNLM: 1. Neurotic Disorders. 2. Masochism. 3. Psychoanalytic Therapy. 4. Psychoanalytic Interpretation. WM 460.5.P5 B498c 1961a]
RC530.B398 1993
616.85'2—dc20
DNLM/DLC
for Library of Congress   93-18828
                                                                CIP

Manufactured in the United States of America

CONTENTS

INTRODUCTION TO THE 1993 PRINTING   *xiii*

FOREWORD   **15**

    Differentiation between neurotics and "not-too-neurotic" people, the latter euphemistically called "normal"—Definition of "cure"—Manageable and unmanageable neurotic traits—The decisive importance of "psychic masochism"—After adequate psychoanalytic treatment an ex-neurotic is better off than his allegedly healthy confrere—Conservatism in science—Importance of the neglected visual drive—Deep masochistic pleasures in neurosis—The infantile debacle—Neurotics unconsciously want improvement of their neurotic pleasure—Rescue stations of libidinous and pseudo-aggressive nature, covering the masochistic substructure—Two types of psychotherapies—Gratitude of uncured neurotics—The basic neurosis—Differentiation between neurotic and malignant types of psychic masochism—The "lifeblood of neurosis."

1. **THE CRUCIAL QUESTION IN PSYCHOANALYTIC THERAPY: "NEUROTIC" OR "MALIGNANT" PSYCHIC MASOCHISM?**   **23**

    The dynamic unconscious—Neurotic manifestations—Popular misconceptions—The basic neurosis—Description of the "psychic apparatus"—The alleged happiness of the child—Psychic bookkeeping of the infant—Infantile megalomania—Misconceptions concerning food intake—Two dreams of schizoid people—"Septet of baby fears"—Adaptation to reality and progression of infantile fears—Consequences in later life—The "genetic picture" in psychic masochism—Universality of that reaction—Development of "department of don'ts and great expectations" ("ego-ideal")—Development of the "department of torture" ("daimonion")—The mutual interactions of both "departments" constituting the superego—Guilt and superego—Twenty-one "rules of torture"—Infantile aggression divided into four parts—"Clinical picture" in psychic masochism—The psychic masochist's life is a "rat race" for ever

CONTENTS

increasing stakes in order to "prove" to the superego that he does not enjoy his self-created defeats—"The only pleasure one can derive from displeasure is to make pleasure out of displeasure"—The fantasy of being "passively victimized" traced from the oral, through anal, to phallic phases—"Positive" and "negative" Oedipus—Summary of passive defeats and aggressive countermeasures on three genetic levels—Differentiation between relatively harmless "neurotic," and dangerous "malignant," psychic masochism—Schizoid personalities and "malignant" psychic masochism—The dread of being manipulated in complete helplessness by the giantess of the nursery—Neurotic masochism already an inner defense in schizoids—Reasons for therapeutic inaccessibility of schizoid people—Early and late diagnosis—Phenomenology of schizoids—Clinical example—Loss of beneficial effects of protective fear—Incurable neurotics characterized as mostly schizoid personalities detected too late—Should schizoids be treated?—Dreary consequences of misunderstandings of neurotic structure—"Success because of unconscious fear."

2. *WHAT IS BEHIND THE CONTROVERSY OVER THE ALLEGED EXAGGERATED EMPHASIS ON PSYCHIC MASOCHISM?* 56

Sequence of analytic discoveries vs. sequence of the child's actual development—Confusion in "analytic geology"—Difficulties in acceptance of deeper layers, especially orally based psychic masochism—Confusion between guilt and psychic masochism—"Pet theories" on psychic masochism—Incurability of neurotics if psychic masochism overlooked in treatment—Differential diagnosis between normal and neurotic aggression—Confusion between parasitic tendencies and defensive misuse in neurosis—Minimizing of the role of the superego—The argument of "exaggerated claims"—Three-layers vs. five-layer structure in neurotic manifestations—Only the "defense against the defense" is observable, and not a volcanic eruption of repressed wishes—Prevailing opinions and Freud's statement, "It seems necessary to retract the generality of the statement that the Oedipus complex constitutes the kernel of neurosis"—"Footnote attitude" towards deeper layers—The pre-history of the Oedipus complex—"The pleasure-in-displeasure pattern" as basic neurosis—"Every neurosis dramatizes in an unconscious innuendo (either actively or passively) a libidinous and/or pseudoaggressive

CONTENTS

denial of some aspect of the masochistic theme 'I'm the innocently refused and fearfully mistreated child and have learned to enjoy it' "—"Admission of the lesser intrapsychic crime"—Conspicuous first line of defense vs. inconspicuous "inner fortress"—The lifelong battle with basic psychic masochism and the piled up libidinous-pseudoaggressive camouflages—Recent curability of homosexuality—Typical homosexual traits—The homosexual is a psychic masochist-plus; the plus consists of "reduplication of his own defense mechanism" and handing over of the "power to torture" from the mother-image to man—Clinical pictures in homosexuality—The baby-mother situation in homosexuality—"Bisexuality," a popular misnomer, vs. biological meaning of term—"Statistically induced homosexuality"—Spurious homosexuality—Therapeutic problems in homosexuality.

3. WHAT DOES PSYCHOANALYTIC THERAPY ACCOMPLISH? 79

Every neurotic is a person who lost his individual "battle of the conscience"—Shortchanging of torture emanating from the inner conscience (superego) into masochistic pleasure—"Taking the blame for the lesser intrapsychic crime"—Increase of self-created torture bribes—"Throwing a monkey wrench into the machinery of neurosis"—Unproductivity of the neurotic solution and learning to fight back—The unconscious exchange rate: every ounce of unconscious pleasure is paid for with tons of conscious unhappiness—Analytic technique—Differences concerning deeper layers—Successful analysis (provided the basic scourge of psychic masochism is analyzed in transference and resistance situations) provides patient with new energy to fight inner conscience—The source of that new energy: retrieving the original aggression from the masochistic amalgam—Three longer cases histories as paradigm—Summary of changes in successful analyses; strengthening the unconscious ego by partial de-masochization, and at the same time humanization of the ego ideal—Neurotic vs. schizoid cases.

4. ARE THE LIMITATIONS OF ANALYTIC THERAPY INHERENT IN THE MATERIAL, THE TECHNIQUE, THE PATIENT, OR THE THERAPIST? 125

Analysis no cure-all—Medical applicability to neuroses exclusively—Progress constantly being made, though the more becomes known, the greater complexities arise—Examples of neurotic disease entities presented by the author—Conserva-

CONTENTS

tism in science unjustified—Six factors influencing the patient's curability—Every neurotic should be given a chance to face his real problem—Objections against concentration on superficial layers—Fourteen technical errors in clinical analysis in our transitional period—Unconscious "pseudomoral connotation" as dangerous prop in neurosis—if not detected—"Two-way immobilization trick"—Clinical examples of "pseudomoral connotation"—Rationalization—Other hurdles at which many an analysis falters: misuse of free associations—Specific technique in orally regressed masochistic cases—Handling of "regret depressions" because of missed masochistic opportunities—Scale of therapeutic successes: excellent results; middle-of-the-road improvements; half-losers; failures; schizoid personalities.

5. HOW DOES NEUROTIC ESCAPISM IN TREATMENT MANIFEST ITSELF?   146

Interruption of treatment—"Lost souls"—Naive transference-"improvements"—Giving up some of the trimmings while maintaining neurosis—Pseudo-success because of unconscious fear—Flight into "love" with an outsider—Psychology of tender love—Projection of one's ego ideal on the beloved—Love is a powerful weapon against guilt—Normal love vs. transference (counterfeit-love)—Real love is an episode in the great battle of the conscience—Postanalytic misuse of preanalytic symptoms—Minimum and maximum program in analysis—"Reopening of insoluble problems"—Premature resignation—Shifting of psychic masochism to points unrecognizable to the patient—Intellectualization—Pathological lies about the analyst—Three clinical examples of such cases—"Acting out" by misuse of the transference—Neurotics who never enter treatment.

6. ARE THERE NEUROSES OF THE "GRAND DESIGN" TYPE?   180

Two ways of learning something new for the analyst—Neurotics dominated by one, and only one, climactic unconscious fantasy—The basic unconscious motivation of these neurotics: reducing mother to absurdity by total masochistic submission via pseudo-identification and/or "outdoing" the mother-image—Impossibility of analyzing future possibilities not yet materialized—The neurosis treated and the "grand design" never identical—Three case histories of "grand design" neuroses—"Amazing changes" and total inapproachability are

CONTENTS

encountered—Even guessing that such a peculiar neurosis is involved, helps sometimes (not the patient) but the mate—Occult nature of the "grand design" neurosis: the material is latent and has not been lived out–yet—Impossibility of analyzing of conflict not yet materialized—The analyst cannot be suspicious enough with latent masochistic possibilities.

7. HOW DOES THE VISUAL DRIVE, THE LEAST EXPLORED CHAPTER IN PSYCHOPATHOLOGY, CONTRIBUTE TO THERAPEUTIC FAILURES?   193

Neurotic elaborations of voyeurism and exhibitionism, subsumed under "visual neuroses"—Only voyeurism original drive, whereas exhibitionism is a later defense—Parity between the two spurious—Exhibitionism contains "confessional elements," the admission that one has actually passively seen (or imagined seeing, or wished to see) what one now (in active repetition) exhibitionistically repeats, frequently in exaggerated caricature and on one's own substitutive organs—"Confessional elements" as guilt-diminishers and invitation to punishment—Meeting point with infiltrating psychic masochism—Looking as "proof" of having been denied sight, masochistically exploited—Every neurosis connected with the visual drive and its defensive derivatives is based on the masochistic elaboration of the infantile peeping conflict—Two basic elaborations of peeping interdictions in infancy—Genetic and clinical pictures in the visual sphere—The voyeuristic-exhibitionistic exchange mechanism—Activity and passivity—Some neurotics are more severe in visual affairs than their educators actually were—Problems of privacy—Twenty-two clinical pictures in neurotic elaboration of the visual sphere—Therapeutic dangers in overlooking or misunderstanding visual components in neuroses—Development of voyeurism and its transformations—The voyeuristic-exhibitionistic (and vice versa in the clinical picture) exchanges in different neurotic entities—"In the battle for the breast every child is the loser"—The boy's attempts at reparation, and seeking a substitutive organ on his own body—Tragic consequences of reality factors—The parallel development in the girl, and the differences—Consequences in intercourse—Eleven specific features in the defense: exhibitionism—Normal, half-neurotic and neurotic elaborations of the visual component—The "mechanism of stubborn reparation"—"Sublimation with renunciations"—"Sublimation on probation"—"Incognito exhibitionism"—Stendhal's visual

CONTENTS

problems and the literary elaboration—Neurotic elaborations—Exhibitionism in the service of the "pseudomoral connotation" of neurotic manifestations—Two types in the exhibitionistic defense—Shyness—Non-analytic material: the religious explanation—The theory of protection—The theory of guarding against disturbance by rivals—The domestication theory—The disgust theory—The evil spirit theory—The woman as property theory—The olfactory theory—The anti-incest theory—Non-analytic theories on shame contrasted with a genetic interpretation—Problems of the uncanny—The psychology of clothes—The condition of the forbidden and its consequences—Four reasons for man's insistence of female "modesty" in clothing and attitude—Blushing—Fear of confined places—Street fear—Fear of heights—Fear of examinations—Jealousy, pathological curiosity and logorrhea—Writer's block (painter's, sculptor's, composer's block)—Block in scientific, photographic, journalistic endeavors—Depersonalization—Stage fright—Boredom (alysosis)—"Negative exhibitionism"—"Thinking block"—Lack of imagination in perceiving external phenomena and lack of "business acumen"—Success hunter—Guideposts for judging success and failure—Temper tantrums—General inhibition in reproducing verbally or graphically what has been seen or heard—Coprohemia (active and passive utterance of obscene words)—The demonstration character of neurotic and psychosomatic manifestations—"Sham-shame" and the fear of "being found out"—Difference between guilt and shame—Perversion voyeurism—Psychodynamics of perversions—The "Mechanism of Criminosis"—Perversion exhibitionism—Problems of "magic gesture"—The unsuspected importance of the visual drive—Romantic love—Literary examples, pointing to intuitive understanding in some writers.

8. *HOW CAN ONE PROVE THAT THE SUPEREGO IS THE REAL MASTER OF THE PERSONALITY?*   374

The real troublemaker, and "boss", of the personality is the superego—To prove the point, 13 *purposely* unconnected reactions are scrutinized: A new approach to the old problem of masturbation—The universal, though underestimated, importance of passive beating fantasies covering deeper fears—The multiple meaning of psychogenic phenomena—"Mortgaging one's future through indignant reproaches"—The inner identity of "refusing" and "giving under impossible conditions"

CONTENTS

—The danger of "caricaturistic relationships"—Tears of anticipation—The greatest compliment: "I never thought of that"—Errors in judgment when faced with an "affront"—"Nowhere to hide"; the problem of weak identifications—The clinical importance of "Rumpelstiltskin" anti-male manifesto—The use and misuse of yawning in the "battle of the conscience"—Proof of brilliance before defeat.

9. IS THERE A BRIGHT OUTLOOK FOR THE FUTURE? 434

The technique of offsetting scientific limitations of the present by envisioning bright, interminable vistas of "future research"—Future of psychoanalysis—Hopeful sign in growing cooperation between different branches of medicine—Psychiatric "Pointers" for the general practitioner and internist treating psychosomatic diseases—Another example of cooperation between branches of medicine: psychiatric-obstetrical cooperation in post-partum depression—Zigzag of "progress."

NOTES 455

INDEX 461

INTRODUCTION TO THE 1993 PRINTING

> I like your advice [in *The Basic Neurosis*[1]], which seems to me ironic, to take [masochistic neurotics] one at a time . . . . It seems to me that in this part of the world there are no other sorts of neuroses.[2]
>
> —George Wilbur, Editor
> *American Imago*

> One cannot escape the impression that analysis of psychic masochism is the destruction of an infantile house of cards in which each card is a carefully guarded illusion. The amount of resistance put up by the patient cannot be overestimated.
> —Bergler, *The Superego*[3]

Every patient entering psychotherapy, and especially psychoanalysis, believes to some extent that the process will create "a different person." This corresponds to a complicated inner defense mechanism of the guilt-ridden unconscious ego: "It's not true that I like to suffer; I want nothing to do with suffering." The unconscious resistance which appears soon enough in all patients makes it clear that their conscious eagerness for sweeping changes in no way reflects the totality of their deepest *unconscious* motives in entering therapy.

Other patients, such as those with features of the impostor-psychopath, want circumscribed changes only, such as removal of superficial symptoms like headaches or insomnia, while leaving their deeper pathology undisturbed. This we cannot do; the "troublesome" symptoms are a direct outgrowth of the same masochistic difficulties the patient does not want treated.

Artistically creative individuals seeking treatment to increase their productivity and decrease their misery often anticipate creating great masterpieces after treatment. These same patients, however, frequently fear that probing inner conflicts to reduce their suffering will rob them altogether of their creative ability.

Paradoxically, when analysis tries to reach the deeper layers of the personality and patients realize that fundamental changes are necessary, they balk. Envisioning that they will be "bored and boring" if cured, they defend the very traits that drive them to despair. Then at other times, discouraged because "nothing has changed," they fear they will be stuck with their problem.

Freud was well aware of the unrealistic expectations (and fears) of analyzands. Chicago analyst Roy R. Grinker, Jr., wrote in *Medical World News* in 1973 about his analysis with Freud in Vienna in the 30's; he told Freud he was concerned that his transformation would deprive him of his healthy assertiveness and ambition. Freud's response to his American patient was gently ironic: "Your friends will recognize you when you get back."

On the other hand, many psychotherapists, including analysts, avoid talking or writing about "cure." They downplay the fact that treating a neurosis means treating a serious, sometimes life-threatening, condition. They speak of the patient being "in therapy," without acknowledging therapy's intended goal: identifying, treating, and overcoming an illness.

To further complicate a complicated situation, naive therapists fail to recognize the full extent of a particular patient's pathology. Mistaking severe personality disorders for mild cases of symptomatic neurosis, they commend themselves on the disappearance of a symptom or two after several months of treatment. The illusion is shattered when the "cured" patient returns later with a new symptom, a major depression, or a disastrous entanglement—all stemming from the unrecognized underlying pathology.

It has become taboo to call neurosis an illness; the word "cure," which implies illness, is also taboo. This comes as no surprise in the age of

INTRODUCTION TO THE 1993 PRINTING

euphemisms, when there are no more "janitors," only "maintenance engineers," and "insane asylums" have given way to "mental health centers." If only the name change could eliminate the grim reality of psychosis, or the problems of treating it! Neurosis, although "milder," affects more people, and incapacitates more insidiously; it is also a major problem which does not disappear by changing labels. At the turn of the century, Freud compared neurotic dysfunction to that resulting from a heart condition; he also said neurosis is no less dangerous to the population than tuberculosis. In 1914 he pointed out, in "Recollection, Repetition, and Working Through," that a change must occur in the patient's attitude toward his illness—from disowning it to regarding it as "an enemy worthy of his mettle" (*Collected Papers,* Vol. II, p. 372). Reinforcing the patients' whitewashing tactics means unwittingly condoning their unwillingness to face the reality of their problems.

Leaving aside patients' exaggerated hopes and impossible demands, and therapists' unwarranted pessimism or false optimism, the question remains: Realistically, what can and should be achieved in psychoanalytic treatment? Also, is there such a thing as "cure," and, if so, how is it defined? What about the concept of incurable neurosis? Are their patients who, though "only" neurotic, do not "take to" psychoanalysis, and what determines whether they will or will not? Are there in fact others who, though not psychotic, are in some fundamental way different from neurotics, remaining unresponsive to the same treatment that can cure neurotics? How can this be explained? And what can be done for such patients?

These are the questions taken up by Edmund Bergler in this 1961 volume, the twenty-second and last published in his lifetime. The Vienna-born and trained psychoanalyst, a leading authority in this field, was at one time the Assistant Director of the Psychoanalytic Freud-Clinic in Vienna, and later a lecturer at the New York Psychoanalytic Institute. In approximately 300 papers and twenty-one books published in twelve countries, beginning in 1929, he reported an increasing number of neurotic entities (listed on pp. 125-6) rendered accessible to psychoanalytic treatment specifically as a result of his theoretical and technical contributions. On the basis of thirty-five years of psychoanalytic practice (in Vienna to 1938, then in New York), he gives his conclusions about how much psychoanalysis can offer neurotics. In addition, he considers the obstacles to achieving the optimum result that qualifies as "cure."

This volume contains for the first time his thorough description of the incurable neurotic, in extension of his observations and conclusions stated in the 1961 paper, "Psychopathic Personalities are Unconsciously Propelled by a Defense against a Specific Type of Psychic Masochism—'Malignant Masochism' " (*Archives of Criminal Psychodynamics*). Malignant masochism is distinguished from the more benign neurotic psychic masochism which Bergler investigated and described over many years. Bergler indicates the clinical importance of the malignant form of masochism; it is easily confused with the neurotic form which it resembles only superficially. The dynamics and the problems of management are quite different.

We are reminded that psychoanalysis does not provide magical solutions; only children and neurotics believe in magic—and are rewarded with disappointment. Bergler does point out that psychoanalysis can do more for suitable patients than is generally realized. It should be understood that when Bergler refers to the therapeutic potential of psychoanalysis he is talking about *psychoanalysis as he practiced it,* i.e., incorporating his own key findings and methodology. He writes unequivocally of the limitations and deficiencies of psychoanalysis which fails to take cognizance of these additional findings. From his personal experience he asserts that it is "the deepest and most successful therapeutic tool in helping neurotics." People generally are still unaware of this fact; for psychological reasons, the negative results in psychiatry achieve more publicity and a more enthusiastic reception than the positive.

Bergler considers here why even dynamically correct interpretations, correctly applied, do not cure the schizoid. His conclusion: "Psychoanalysis is exclusively a therapy for neurotics; we can do little for schizoid personalities, except in cases where neurotic admixtures are extensive." (Bergler's "schizoid" corresponds to elements of the DSM-IIIR's borderline, narcissistic, antisocial, and paranoid personality disorders. It should not be confused with DSM-IIIR's "schizoid personality," a severe condition representing in some cases the pre-psychotic stage of schizophrenia.)

Even many neurotics are unable to achieve optimum inner change. Bergler cautions the outside observer, uninformed of the depth of the patient's pathology, and the degree of resistance, to keep in mind that a particular patient may be beyond help; knowing this might prevent unwarranted negative conclusions about the analyst's competence, or the validity and effectiveness of the therapy. Sometimes one hears the provocative

INTRODUCTION TO THE 1993 PRINTING　　　　　　　　　　　　xvii

statement: "X told me that he was once a patient of yours; if *he* is an example of a cure, I am not impressed." A correct response would be: "Did X tell you what his problem was, or what he was like before treatment, or how he responded to treatment?" Neurotic patients deemed incapable of progressing further after a reasonable attempt at analysis may still achieve what Bergler labeled the "minimum program" (see pp. 157-8). And certain incurable patients may nevertheless be "monitored" for years in analysis, deriving some stabilizing benefits from their knowledge of unconscious mechanisms, without which knowledge they would suffer and hurt themselves more.

The psychoanalytic definition of cure presented in this book agrees considerably with the layperson's, namely, that *neurotic symptoms should be removed, negative behavior discontinued, personality distortions diminished, resulting in a more realistic, well-adjusted person.* Bergler acknowledges that living means dealing with a constant stream of potential disturbances, both from within oneself and from other people; the latter, because neurotic tendencies are ubiquitous, tend to make trouble because of their own neuroses. Psychotherapy must reduce internal malfunctioning that interferes with the ability to deal effectively with life's burdens.

In a case summary, Bergler states the aim of analysis: ". . . to help you to make your acquaintance with your own self." *This is what analysis is really about.* No one knows his or her own unconscious. Patients are surprised to find out they now are perpetuating harmful inner "solutions" manufactured in early life, and deriving forbidden unconscious masochistic pleasure in the process. Once that interpretation—including all the details of their individual cases—penetrates beyond the intellectual level to the unconscious emotional core, change occurs, as they replace self-damaging unconscious defenses with healthier ones. The individual cured of sexual promiscuity understands emotionally the reasons for this behavior and the related lack of satisfaction, no longer wants or needs the old pattern, and unconsciously discards it; the cured gambler has no desire to gamble; and so on for each specific symptom or trait.

Bergler reiterates his clinical conclusion that all neurotic difficulties are based on inner masochism developed in the "oral" (pre-Oedipal) stage—the earliest stage of unconscious psychic development. Chapter 2 summarizes the known facts of psychic masochism, "the basic neurosis," as worked out theoretically and applied clinically by Bergler. (Chapter IX in *Principles of Self-Damage*[4] contains a synopsis of the sequence in which these facts were discovered, along with a more comprehensive review of basic theory.)

The deep-seated but hidden attachment to pleasure in suffering clarifies why early maladaptive, self-defeating attitudes and behavior patterns are carried into adult life even though logic and experience dictate they should be altered, or dropped entirely. Once established, the inner masochistic pattern functions like a cancer, in this case encroaching more and more on the personality. As Bergler puts it, ". . . the greatest stress on [psychic] masochism is still an understatement. It is *THE BASIS* of all neurotic troubles." This pattern persists despite all opposition, and opposition there is—from the inner conscience, the superego. Unconscious psychic masochism appears consciously as working against oneself; the self-created disappointments, defeats, rejection, and failure provide inner masochistic pleasure. The therapeutic difficulty starts at this point; "no human being wants to renounce unconscious pleasure" (foreword); however, keeping it means paying with conscious unhappiness in symptoms, personality distortions, and neurotic repetitive conflicts.

Throughout the book, Bergler draws attention to the hostility toward psychoanalytic findings. What is its cause? Psychoanalytic science, like all science, deals impersonally with impersonal facts; but, whereas the findings of other sciences are viewed more or less objectively, people take the impersonal findings of psychoanalysis very personally. "We do not deal much in facts when we are contemplating ourselves," wrote Mark Twain. Freud's discovery of the existence of the unconscious created an unintentional furor in the scientific and non-scientific worlds. By demonstrating that our conscious thoughts, feelings and actions are determined and directed by inner motivations, infantile in origin, over which we have no conscious control, he "hit a raw nerve."

At first Freud was puzzled and dismayed when fellow scientists rejected his new findings; he assumed that his clinically applicable observations and deductions would be as well received as his previous research in neurology. He later understood that the negative reaction was impersonal and emotional, and accepted it with ironic good humor. In a voice recording made shortly before his death, he summarized his career: "I started . . . as a neurologist trying to bring relief to my neurotic patients. I discovered some important new facts about the unconscious. . . . Out of these findings grew a new science, psychoanalysis . . . and a new method of treatment of the neuroses. *I had to pay heavily for this bit of good luck . . .*" (emphasis added).[5] Some ten years later Bergler, encountering the same opposition to his discoveries, adopted a similar tone in *The Basic Neurosis:* "I have been *unfortunate* enough to find 'something' which every human being . . . harbors unconsciously" (emphasis added).

Freud and his early adherents, seeking to establish the basic facts of the unconscious, left us a formidable body of knowledge about the internal mental world, initiating some understanding of the irrational factor in human experience. As the founder and head of psychoanalysis Freud continually uncovered deeper tributaries behind the less deeply repressed layers. His work included some preliminary investigation of how inner masochism developed, but he died before fully determining the content and significance of the deepest (oral) unconscious layer.

As an active member of Freud's Psychoanalytic Clinic and the Vienna Psychoanalytic Society, Bergler played a key role in continuing these investigations. He had the ideal combination of inner qualities and external circumstances for success in this: the intellectual capacity, the opportunity to study and work in an academic and clinical setting still enriched by Freud's living presence, plus the necessary inner psychological makeup to enable his research to produce specific answers to many questions still unanswered at Freud's death. We are particularly indebted to Bergler for discovering the enormous clinical significance of unconscious psychic masochism (which he recognized and appreciated early in his career), for working out its connection with the oral phase, and for persisting with the task of studying this subject despite great internal and external obstacles. (See, for instance, footnote 48 on Jung's role in 1932—working for the Nazis and proclaiming their ideology—in the rejection of Bergler's major paper on agoraphobia. It was later published in America.)

A major breakthrough, Bergler tells us in *Principles of Self-Damage,* came in 1932 when he realized that "the oral pessimist does not aim for the *fulfillment* of official wishes dating from childhood (such as the wish to be loved), but for the *denial* of these very wishes" (p. 329). This bold formulation, completely new in psychoanalytic theory, led ultimately to the theoretical and clinical conclusion that *the central unconscious neurotic wish is the repressed masochistic wish to be refused by the "bad mother" of earliest infantile fantasy; all other repressed wishes inwardly camouflage that deepest masochistic wish.* Mother is "bad and refusing" from the standpoint of the baby's omnipotence fantasy which is insatiable in the real world. Neurotic suffering is not an unfortunate by-product of maintaining inner wishes, but an integral part of the whole neurotic process. External reality is then misused for masochistic purposes, as an arena for repeating repressed conflict throughout life. The internal superimposed pattern clouds the actual reality of external situations, which cannot be seen and dealt with effectively for what they are.

Bergler's work in effect uncovered and helped place in perspective the deepest unconscious layer, the foundation underlying the phenomena studied and described by earlier analysts. He also clarified the role of the previously discovered superficial layers. They represent the defenses against deep inner masochism—defenses developed after establishing the masochistic solution, to shield the now masochistic ego from superego counteraction (see the superego's twenty-one rules of torture, pp. 34 ff.). In this sense, all inner defenses are created to appease the superego. Freud wrote in "The Economic Problem in Masochism" (1924) that "the sadism of the superego and the masochism of the ego supplement each other" (*Collected Papers,* Vol. II, p. 267). But it was Bergler who clarified and emphasized the cruel irrationality of this inner department, its specific connection with psychic masochism, and how these inner events are to be interpreted clinically. (For details of Bergler's findings on the unsuspected significance of the inner conscience, see *The Superego.*) In Chapter 8, Bergler provides a summation, plus new illustrations of the superego's domination of the personality, and the inner ego's desperate but masochistic countermeasures. After verifying his facts during decades of clinical work, Bergler asserted: "a complete overhauling of our thinking concerning the structure of neurosis is necessary" (p. 63).

Unconscious psychic masochism, unhappily present in everyone, is also everyone's darkest secret. The conscious personality knows nothing of this "hidden treasure," only the defenses dictated by the unconscious ego to cover up the fact. The first line of defense consists of unconscious and conscious denial: "I am not a masochist"; this is reinforced by: "there is no such thing as masochism." For this reason, the scientific fact of inner masochism, much less subsequent discussion of specific masochistic mechanisms in the personality, cannot be accepted by anyone on the conscious

INTRODUCTION TO THE 1993 PRINTING   xxi

level—even intellectually—strictly on its own merits. *What an irony! The universal central fact of human existence—unconscious psychic masochism—is universally unknown, with an inner psychological mechanism universally in place to see that it remains so.* Any hint at psychic masochism's existence leads automatically to the inner reaction: "Not true!" *This emotional response can be predicted and explained; but it cannot be prevented.*

The defensive denial applies equally to colleagues attending lectures and case presentations on psychic masochism and to readers of books on the subject. Such discussion and writing, respectively, simply violate the inner taboo. Books like the present one can do no more than state these inner facts, bringing them to the reader's awareness. Outside of clinical analysis, which can convince by revealing one's own unconscious psychic masochism in operation, no means exists to engender deep emotional benefit from these facts. *As a result, the material in this book, revolutionary in its own time, remains "new" to many colleagues today.* And what was never fully assimilated into psychoanalytic thinking cannot be dismissed, as one sometimes hears, with the argument that it represents "old" theory from the 1940's and 50's. As this volume shows, Bergler warned vigorously against sterile analytic conservatism. He describes his own personal, protracted, but ultimately successful struggle against inner obstacles which constantly threatened to block his research on masochism. Neither can this material be watered down or prettied up to make it more palatable. Nor does the material lend itself to easy incorporation into an "eclectic" system alongside other psychological theories, any more than Copernicus' discovery of a sun-centered planetary system could be "incorporated" into the older idea of an earth-centered one. It goes beyond, and is therefore at odds with, earlier theories and their derivatives.

Bergler's scientific output—in a life twenty years shorter than Freud's—emulates his predecessor's in magnitude and depth of perception. There is even a parallel with Freud's cancer: for his twenty last years—fully half his adult life—Bergler labored in the shadow of a cardiovascular illness which overtook him, in a fatal heart attack, at age 62. In the final five years, after publishing *Homosexuality: Disease or Way of Life?*,[6] he worked longer hours again, including Saturdays, to accommodate the scores of desperate homosexuals who "inundated" him (Mrs. Bergler) with letters and telephone calls from all over the United States and Canada requesting analytic help. In a 1958 letter to a colleague he indicated that in two years since the book's publication he had seen almost 300 homosexuals in consultation! Mrs. Bergler pointed out that this selfless effort was undertaken out of compassion for the large number of homosexuals who read his book and wanted this form of analysis, but had trouble finding therapists trained to provide it. As a result, many more cases were treated and cured by Bergler and like-minded colleagues. From what became a spontaneous vast clinical study, Bergler produced a second major book, *One Thousand Homosexuals*,[7] documenting his further clinical experience and conclusions; that book's foreword describes the overwhelming positive response to Bergler's first book on the subject.

This volume summarizes much of Bergler's important contribution on the unconscious origins of homosexuality and the possibilities for analytic treatment where the patient wants to change, an aspect of his work which is regularly misquoted, misrepresented and even maligned in newer books on the subject. Objectors overlook that Bergler's clinical experience showed homosexuality to be one of many possible elaborations of all humanity's basic inner masochistic conflict; analyzing that basis can help every masochistic neurosis, be it agoraphobia, overeating, psychosomatic illnesses, or whatnot. Bergler's pioneering work on homosexuality ranks with his work on gambling and writer's block as a prime example of how psychoanalysis can change, in certain cases, what many still believe unchangeable altogether. (See pp. 65-78, 159-64, 346-8, 408-9, and a longer case history condensed from *One Thousand Homosexuals*, pp. 105-21. The discussion includes Bergler's warnings about Kinsey's erroneous statistics, antedating by thirty years the exposure of the actual facts of Kinsey's devious aims and nefarious methods; these are now revealed in such works as Reisman and Eichel's *Kinsey, Sex, and Fraud: the Indoctrination of a People*.[8])

Chapter 3 offers two other long case histories demonstrating results achievable in treating masochistic neurosis. In studying these cases the reader should remember that the analyst's energy is directed against a dangerous self-damaging illness in the patient, *not against the patient;* that the analyst, in order to help, must bring the patient face to face with unpleasant facts about himself; and that the process is vindicated by the successful result. Analysis freed all three patients from severe self-damage and enabled them to achieve greater productivity and contentment in life.

INTRODUCTION TO THE 1993 PRINTING

In Chapter 2 Bergler cites a key obstacle preventing therapists from recognizing the central role of inner masochism: "the ability to see psychic masochism in the patient presupposes that one's own masochism has been thoroughly 'aired' in one's own analysis and (at least partially) made ineffective." Failing this, the therapist is as much "in the dark" as the patient with regard to this deepest layer of the patient's problem, and as much emotionally disinclined to believe that masochism even exists. The consequences for therapy are serious. One cannot explore and treat an unknown aspect of the problem. It is one thing to treat symptoms, and the more superficial unconscious defenses which appear to be the patient's hidden "wishes"; another to identify, treat and attempt to cure the underlying illness by undermining its basis. Bergler puts it plainly: "Without analyzing the basic masochistic substructure the neurotic cannot be changed" (p. 64). Also, the therapist whose masochism has been analyzed gains immunity against countertransference, which is invariably a masochistic reaction whatever its superficial appearance.

Instead of time wearing down the resistance to Freud's basic discoveries about the unconscious, resistance has increased in many quarters. Those retreating from psychoanalysis' disturbing conclusions about the human being's deep inner attachment to self-damage reinforce each other's resistance via identification, often producing vociferous propaganda against the fundamentals of psychoanalysis. There have been many attempts to replace or "improve" psychoanalysis with various theories that bypass the painful issue of unconscious motivations, especially inner masochism. But the dynamic unconscious, with its superabundance of masochistic baggage, does not go away when ignored.

Paradoxically, this has complicated the task for therapists instead of easing it. Unprepared for the strong unconscious resistance put up by patients when their deeper motives are even hinted at, therapists fear that *they* have upset the patient. Their patient is fighting against help (on the unconscious level—which they no longer acknowledge), but these therapists take at face value the patient's conscious assertions of wanting help. Their own system leaves the therapists with only themselves to blame if things do not go smoothly in the therapy. Eager for their patients to like them and feel good in therapy, these therapists take the safer route of "telling them what they want to hear." This amounts to reinforcing superficial defenses, including patients' all-pervasive unconscious defense: "if only everyone (past and present) treated me better, everything would be all right." In "supportive therapy," patients' innumerable conflicts with their environment cannot be traced to the patients' inner unconscious pattern, i.e., patients' masochistic provocations or misuse of reality factors. As an enraged or self-pitying patient rants and rails against the alleged meanness of everyone else, the therapist is forced to listen helplessly, with an occasional interjection to the effect that the patient is really well-meaning but misunderstood. Therapy pushed and guided by the patient's resistance may not upset the patient, but it will not change the patient's inner masochistic problem, unknown and unrecognized by patient and therapist alike.

Today everyone is a "therapist." Non-psychoanalytic related professionals undertake to treat the kind of complex emotional conflicts described throughout this book. In the process, they discard hard-won knowledge whose value their background does not allow them to appreciate. Many non-professionals use the designation "counselor," further confusing the issue, since counseling and therapy are not the same thing, nor are either the equivalent of analysis. In many instances "therapists" are laypersons, whose only claim to familiarity with the problems they presume to treat, e.g., substance abuse, or eating disorders, comes from having themselves been treated for the problem, often by equally untrained "therapists" utilizing the flimsiest of unconfirmed, trendy "therapies."

The ignorance of these would-be therapists is surpassed only by their arrogance in assuming that simplistic explanations and methods—often no more than "pop psychology"—can be applied effectively to neurosis. They unknowingly become the dupes of their own and their patients' unconscious. Even professionals have been caught up in this. In an authoritative article in *The American Scholar,* Paul R. McHugh, Professor and Director of Psychiatry at Johns Hopkins University, speaks of "the power of cultural fashion to lead psychiatric thought and practice off in false, even disastrous directions."[9] He cites "multiple personality disorder" as an "example of misidentified hysterical behavior . . . bolstered by an invented view of its cause ['forgotten sexual mistreatment in childhood'] that fits a cultural fashion."[10]

Interviewing self-styled, non-analytic therapists, and treating them in analysis, one observes the high personal price they pay for their self-bestowed titles, in the form of irritability, anxiety, depression, self-doubt,

INTRODUCTION TO THE 1993 PRINTING

and helplessness even to the point of suicidal thoughts. This self-punitive ransom unconsciously represents the fee to the superego, which charges the ego with incompetence; the guilt-ridden ego cannot come up with a better defense to refute the charge. *All of this does nothing for deeply self-damaging neurotics except help them feel better temporarily, while their dangerous inner pattern of self-damage continues producing deleterious effects, and even worsens.*

The situation described by Bergler in this book still exists thirty years later. One repeatedly sees patients who have had one, five, even ten years of "therapy," without ever hearing of "masochism." The situation is comparable to offering only reassurance and support to someone who has an activated time bomb in the basement of his home—instead of finding and dismantling the bomb. The fellow may calm down and even feel good after soothing words of encouragement, but this does not protect him from the bomb, which will go off—eventually. Pleasant talk does not defuse bombs. In this analogy, "upstairs" represents the conscious, and the person talking with the therapist corresponds to the conscious ego; the basement represents the unconscious, and the bomb the dangerous inner self-damaging pattern.

The topic of resistance forms a major focus of concern in this book. It is not only encountered in the analysis of every patient; it pervades the analytic experience, and analyzing it occupies our energy to a degree unfathomable to the outsider. Here is an incident which conveys the essentials:

A young patient, after a visit in which he felt the impact of analysis, returned several days later for his next appointment. On the way from the waiting room to the consultation room for his appointment, he unthinkingly removed his coat from the coat rack. Stopping himself in mid action, he muttered "What am I doing?" and replaced the coat. I suggested analyzing this reaction. "It's as if I were trying to leave, rather than come in," he said. "That's what you want," I said, "*unconsciously. Without knowing it consciously,* you are fighting against further help. *You yourself have just proved it by your own action.* And in the waiting room you were thinking just the opposite, weren't you—that you were impatient for your appointment to *begin*?" He grinned an embarrassed grin, and confirmed that analytic assumption.

Sometimes a patient's resistance shows up in a strange "error," amounting to a devaluation of the very concept of "cure." In referring to this book, the patient reverses the order in the title, calling it *"Incurable and Curable Neurotics."* Why the switch, and why the emphasis on incurability? The reader's superego misuses Bergler's word "curable" as a pretext to reproach the guilt-ridden ego: "See, *you* could be cured too, but you don't want it." The masochistic ego fights back—masochistically—by discounting the possibility of improvement. "There's no such thing as cure," runs the argument, "so how can I be guilty of masochism in not seeking it? On the contrary, I'm just being realistic, as I should be; I don't chase after something that doesn't exist. I am what I am, and I accept my fate."

Many people unconsciously use this neurotic defense to justify not seeking psychological help at all. In analysis, all patients produce this argument at some time. Applying Bergler's theory we can remind them: "Why come here to be changed, then try to prove change is impossible? You are defeating your own aim. Besides, you are the one who labeled yourself 'not well'; you have voluntarily consulted a psychiatrist, hoping to achieve a change that you inwardly require to decrease your own inner guilt. Now your superego accuses you of not wanting cure; why don't you show your superego that you do want it—by letting the analysis cure you—instead of attacking the idea of cure? *This is a pseudo-aggressive defense that leaves you with nothing."*

Sometimes the skeptical patient treats analysis as a con artist's crooked scheme. Bergler's case of Mr. B. who feared he was being tricked is a prime example. "How many of your patients were *really* cured?" taunts the typical doubter, the antagonism barely concealed behind the facade of "seeking information." The inner message reads: "Admit that you're a big fake; no one can be changed, and you know it!" Under analytic scrutiny the faking turns out to be a projection—of the patient's own "fraudulent" inner defense: "I *want* to change, but I *can't* and I can't help it." By projective shift, they conclude therapy "can't" help anyone!

Bergler devotes an entire chapter to "neurotic escapism," a more serious degree of resistance than the typical "fight between the couch and the door" (the phenomenon applies equally to psychoanalysis with the patient using the chair rather than the couch). His catalogue of twelve escapist techniques gives a good indication of the devious "weapons" employed

INTRODUCTION TO THE 1993 PRINTING   xxvii

by patients to block analysis altogether. Three of them—"flight into love," "intellectualization," and "pathological lies about the analyst"—warrant addenda to Bergler's important observations:

Every masochistic patient unconsciously uses the "search for love" as a defense to cover masochism. As soon as one understands that the basic unconscious repetition of the masochist is "I want to be *refused* (deprived, hurt, mistreated, disappointed)," one can appreciate the strength of the universal inner defense: "I don't want to be *refused,* I want to *get* (food, sex, love, success, money, etc.)." *In the last few decades an entire branch of psychoanalysis was built around that neurotic defense, taking it at face value and offering patients "empathic understanding"—rather than interpretation and analysis of their deeper masochism—as the road to health.* Bergler explains how patients unconsciously resist analysis of their deepest masochistic layer by hiding behind the defense of seeking "love." *Masochistic neurotics, unless analytically helped, are incapable of love: instead they play out a masochistic attachment in their relationships.* The same applies to these liaisons begun before therapy, or shortly after starting. Attempts to show the patient the masochistic basis of their particular romance often lead to the accusation that analysis is "against love." If a sick marriage is involved, and the partner rejects help, we are accused of "marriage-wrecking"—by the same person who suffers intensely and complains bitterly about the self-created hopeless relationship.

"Intellectualizers" are another problem: they treat analysis as an academic course in psychology. Why do they seek treatment? "To understand why I feel the way I do," they tell us. This must be countered with: "Is there something about yourself which you can no longer live with, and feel you *must change*?" If the patient replies: "No, I'm not *that* bad," this may be a face-saving tactic covering a deeper despair which will emerge under pressure of questioning. If it reflects a *stable inner masochistic balance,* as Bergler explains, the patient is not ready for analysis. Such patients, if accepted, may make an intellectual game of it, reducing the mother-image to absurdity in the transference. Later they turn the tables on the analyst, complaining: "I understand everything, so how come nothing has changed?" Freud warned about "patients whose habitual [maneuver] it is to shirk analysis by sheering off into the intellectual, and who speculate much and often with great wisdom over their condition, thereby sparing themselves from taking steps to overcome it" (*Collected Papers*, Vol. II, p. 332).

Bergler explains that resistance expressed in pathological lies about analysis to outsiders often indicates schizoid or malignant masochism. Such patients don't want treatment; usually they are trying to further some impostor scheme by convincing parents, fiance(e) or spouse of "good intentions." Bergler describes cases in which the lies are fed to the person around whom the original conflict centered; the personal clinical experience of the present writer has been that *these lies are also typically fed to the person who referred the patient for analysis, especially if it is the spouse*. Ironically, the spouse, also in analysis and usually more favorably disposed to it, immediately doubts the veracity of the accounts, which serve only to inform the spouse that his or her partner is inwardly rejecting therapy.

Some of the falsehoods are so blatant because the deceiver is inwardly begging to be caught and "punished," in these cases via divorce. One patient, for instance, fought the interpretation of her masochism and made little progress, complaining to her husband for months that analysis was not helping. She then discontinued treatment, telling her husband that *I* had said she was cured. Her husband quite rightly asked her how I could have proclaimed her cured when she still had the incapacitating psychosomatic symptoms that led her to consult me.

As Bergler has pointed out, this is not atypical of such patients. In unfavorable cases the transference repetitions and projections are not emotionally understood and corrected by the patients. They retain their neurotic distorted views, now largely shifted into the relation to the therapist, whom they continue to see inwardly as the villainous "bad mother" of their repressed infantile fantasy. Inwardly guilty about their resistance, they defend themselves against superego reproaches by projecting responsibility onto the therapist and the therapy. This negative reaction cannot be foreseen in individual cases, because we don't know which patients will complete their analyses successfully. *Often the hatred and vindictiveness of uncured patients are inversely proportional to the satisfaction of cured patients. This is the paradox: the only way we have of achieving the favorable outcome is to analyze fully, thereby risking the unfavorable outcome.* Bergler describes the course of events:

INTRODUCTION TO THE 1993 PRINTING

xxix

> Exactly the incurable patient and those who run away from analysis during a resistance-phase, are the loudest propagandists against us; they need confirmation from the ignorant environment [i.e., ignorant of psychoanalysis] how "stupid" and "dangerous" analysis is. The cured impotent man or frigid woman keeps the secret of the artificially acquired potency—that is understandable; not less than the silence of the cured drinker or homosexual. The uncured or runaway patient, however, talks—and loudly, for that matter. (*The Basic Neurosis*, p. 334)

Sometimes these uncured runaways are themselves psychotherapists who wanted to enhance their professional work by learning Bergler's approach, but could not take the analysis of their own masochism. Unable to see the project through because of their own resistance, they are beset with superego reproaches, and blame the failure on the analyst and the method. I have encountered this reaction in physicians (including psychiatrists and analytic candidates), psychologists, social workers, and students leaning toward these professions. Occasionally we find that the fantasy of becoming a therapist conceals questionable motives, including impostor features covered with a magic gesture (see pp. 361 ff.). These individuals are inwardly furious at being understood, and resent the recommendation to repair their own personality before undertaking to help others. Some are malignant masochists, incapable of changing.

One example involved an intelligent social work student, daughter of a chronic schizophrenic mother to whom she was masochistically attached. She was shocked to discover, from the emergence of her own repressed material, that her ambition to help severely disturbed patients was a rationalization of a severely neurotic aim. Fantasies of "saving" hopeless patients covered, first, her unconscious antagonism toward them ("sick mother"), and, more deeply repressed, a masochistic wish to be murdered by one of the psychotics she would attempt to treat. She had fantasized this happening; in addition, her defenses against this deep masochism included strong hostile impulses toward strangers in the street. She produced a fantasy of throwing a bomb at the analyst's office building after hours. Despite considerable analysis and working through, her inner masochistic attitude remained unchanged. When it was suggested she reconsider her future plans, she left in anger, never returned, and began to disparage the analyst to a schizoid friend, even though she had once lauded the same analyst to that friend, and had convinced the friend to come to me for analysis!

More serious are cases in which schizoid masochists act out by lodging false complaints of mistreatment with disciplinary bodies. These patients are really lost souls, often somewhat paranoid, who project their own pathology on the therapist and blame the therapist for their own failure to respond to analysis. Unconsciously they cannot and will not accept the analysis of their masochism; usually it has not been their idea to come for help, and they deeply resent their family's suggestion that they need treatment. Every effort to assist them is misconstrued as malicious attack and misrepresentation of their motives, and taken as proof of "conspiracy" between the analyst and the referring source. In acting out their resistance, they reverse the roles as they see them, maliciously attacking the therapist as "crazy." This mechanism utilizes the pathological lying technique combined with some of the other acting out techniques described under section 12 of the "escapism" chapter—all built upon a preexisting foundation of unconscious antagonism to doctors specifically, present to some extent in everyone (see pp. 441 ff.). The best protection against this danger is to be as judicious as possible in the selection of cases for treatment, to be constantly on the lookout for warning signs of greater impairment than was at first evident, and to keep a thorough and detailed record of the sessions particularly where it appears the patient may have this tendency.

The last group of escapists is the largest: neurotics who never enter treatment. Only a relatively small number of neurotics come for analytic treatment and persevere to a successful conclusion. Bergler explains that there are certain unconscious prerequisites for a workable analytic patient. Speaking practically, this means that many more people need psychological help than are unconsciously willing and able to receive it. As a result, it is difficult to estimate how many incurable (unchangeable) neurotics and schizoid personalities there are in the general population, but it is safe to say that a very large number go undetected because they judiciously avoid treatment. *The fact that someone has never gone for help does not prove his or her psychic health; often it is the opposite. Because of this, statistics on mental illness automatically understate the problem.*

People who pride themselves on never having voluntarily consulted a psychiatrist forget with whom they share that "honor": the most severely

INTRODUCTION TO THE 1993 PRINTING   xxxi

impaired psychiatric patients—psychotics and serious criminals—who typically have no conscious awareness that they are emotionally ill. A sad epidemiological fact of psychopathology, an almost weekly occurrence reported in our newspapers, involves the mass killing of innocent people in public places by the "nice quiet boy who kept to himself and never gave anyone any trouble," or "the angry, belligerent, vengeful loner who wanted to get back at society for 'injustices' done to him" etc. These murders often end with the suicide of the killer. These most masochistic of masochists, with their defense of murderous pseudo-aggression, also did not think they needed the services of a psychiatrist.

In Chapter 4 Bergler considers the essential ingredients of successful therapy. Further to Bergler's comments, an additional pitfall might be noted here: *some therapists underestimate the necessity of full analysis for achieving permanent resolution of inner conflict.* Some confusion exists about the difference between psychoanalysis and psychoanalytic psychotherapy; the latter often signifies the limited application of psychoanalytic theory and interpretation in the course of an ongoing discussion about day to day problems. The active analytic exploration aimed at discovering the origin and individual meaning of the patient's difficulties is omitted. This short cut tends to become a kind of intellectual exercise in the appreciation of psychoanalytic theory; the patient uses analytic terminology, but does not learn emotionally. Playing intellectually with abstract, generalized analytic concepts, or applying them to oneself mechanically, does as much toward solving neurosis as looking at fire extinguishers does for putting out fires. The great danger is that the patient deals with the unconscious as if it were an outside force and never realizes: "my unconscious is *me*; *I'm* doing things to hurt *myself!*" Without seeing and digesting that fact, no emotional change occurs; the patient, unaware of what is missing, mistakenly believes consciously that the problem has been identified and solved. Unconsciously the patient knows, and is grateful for, what remains unchanged.

I have seen such patients in continuing analysis (begun with other therapists) who are happy to deal with the unconscious "at arm's length" only. Some are malignant masochists camouflaged as neurotics and seeking therapy for alibi purposes only, but some are genuine neurotics capable of changing. That they have not been adequately helped is evident from the fact that they still have difficulties, and are looking for something more.

They are shaken when shown in their new analysis that the unconscious masochistic wishes are actually *their own* deepest motivations. "But *I* don't want that," they protest. "It's my unconscious! I have no control over my unconscious!" They want to continue their old pattern of playing "innocent victim of outside forces," calling the latter by a new name: "the unconscious." This error is understandable, since neurotic repression itself treats internal psychic material as if it were foreign to the ego. *Reinforcing neurotic repression, however, does not cure neurosis.* This process must be clarified with the patient, by showing that the material is located within the patient, and the repressed conflict must be understood and resolved. (Bergler summarizes the process on pp. 79-81.)

It is particularly ironic that the psychotherapist using psychoanalytic theory expects such therapy, a half-measure at best, to achieve results the same as or better than actual psychoanalysis. *I have seen cases where that half-measure was diligently applied for twenty years, with minimal results, where analysis might have cured the patient, if a suitable candidate, in less than a quarter of that time.* At the very least, a trial analysis could have determined the patient's suitability for major change, sparing a lot of futile effort if the answer were in the negative. Bergler's case illustrations indicate that results in analysis come from first selecting suitable cases, then analyzing correctly and thoroughly.

Bergler provides examples of incomplete understanding, neurotic oversights, and errors in thinking which show that *the resulting schematic application of the theory of psychic masochism leads to erroneous conclusions and unnecessary therapeutic failure.* In Chapter 8 he emphasizes that the specific meaning of the problem must be puzzled out in each new case, citing an example where the same symptom meant different things in two cases (p. 397 ff.). The preliminary impression can turn out to be the opposite of the actual unconscious dynamics.

A striking illustration of this problem was provided some years ago when the parents of a teen-age girl, recently in analysis with a colleague, asked me to continue her analysis. The case is instructive because it permits a comparison of two analyses applying the same basic theory differently, with different results. Here is a summary:

The patient, now sixteen, had been studying gymnastics, with a view to entering the Olympics, when she developed peculiar pains in her left thigh and knee. Walking had become difficult; gymnastics were out of the

INTRODUCTION TO THE 1993 PRINTING xxxiii

question. Thorough medical investigation could find no organic basis for the pains.

In the previous analysis, she had been introduced to the concept of masochism, and her physical symptom had been discussed. The explanation offered (she showed me the notes taken in sessions with the colleague) was as follows: she was unconsciously masochistically producing the pains in order to defeat her aim of pursuing a career in gymnastics to the Olympic level. According to this interpretation, her masochism was being satisfied by her having to forgo achieving her lifelong ambition. This interpretation, diligently applied over a period of months, had made no impact on the pains.

A review of her history revealed that the symptom began two years earlier, around the time she started having second thoughts about an Olympic career. She became upset after reading that a world-famous gymnast, a former Olympic medalist, was anorexic. Looking around her, she suddenly realized to her horror that "they're all like that!" as well as being workaholics whose life revolved totally around exercise regimens, dieting, and competitions. She began to think about withdrawing from the training program. But here was the difficulty; she felt she couldn't approach her parents about it.

"I thought they would kill me," she said, "after all the time and money they poured into my training."

"But surely at fourteen a girl is entitled to change her mind about a career."

"You don't know my parents!" she replied. "They were very aware of the sacrifices they made for me. Besides, my dad has a terrible temper. When he gets angry I'm still afraid of him."

Additional material emerged and it became possible to construct a hypothesis. I told her:

"By creating your pain you made it *physically* impossible to continue in gymnastics. You're out of the sport, without even having to tell your parents you changed your mind about it, and they can't be angry at you. Now the story reads '*I don't want to say no to my parents' wishes and get in trouble; I'm sick, so I can't compete, and I can't help it.*' "

"Well, that means I'm getting my way and avoiding trouble. But this doesn't sound like masochism to me. According to this treatment, I'm an unconscious masochist. This is getting confusing. Where's the masochism?"

"It's not that hard to find, provided you are looking for it, and recognize it. Aren't we talking here about *inwardly self-created pain?* Didn't you tell me the pain is with you all the time, and often incapacitating? Isn't it spoiling your modern dance classes, and dramatics, which you *do* enjoy? Even walking is difficult for you, you told me. Look at the price in suffering you are paying for your defense mechanism! Not a very good bargain on that score."

"I was concentrating on the fact that I got out of gymnastics, and overlooking the pain I got stuck with."

"You mean, stuck yourself with—unconsciously. But there's more masochism in this. All of this presupposes that your parents would have been furious at your change of heart. They would 'kill you'; those were your words. Surely you don't really mean they would become violent? This exaggeration stems from inner masochistic fantasies of the 'bad mother.' Did they ever hit you or even threaten you?"

"Other than a spanking or two—when I was really being an impossible brat—they never laid a finger on me."

"So you *assumed* they would react violently, and on that basis you have put yourself in constant torment. And look at the injustice you collected against your parents: 'I have to be in agony before they let me do what *I* want!' Isn't it masochistic to put yourself through all this on the basis of an unproven assumption? And aren't you also masochistically anticipating another spanking anyway, acting out the pain of it beforehand?"

The interpretation "clicked." Her pain subsided; she provided more confirming material, especially about her masochistic fears, by now attached to her father. These centered around the baby fear of being devoured, and, as suspected, had nothing to do with reality. She had developed a "peculiar feeling" about eating the dark meat of chicken, after being frightened on hearing Prokofiev's "Peter and the Wolf." She remembered the entire ending particularly, where the duck, swallowed alive, was heard still quacking plaintively inside the wolf's belly.

"What part of the chicken is the dark meat?" I asked her.

"The leg," she answered. "*Now* what are you getting at?"

"How about connecting that with your thigh and knee pain?" I replied. "Unconsciously you identified masochistically with the innocent little duck, and now in your pain you act out, *in anticipatory masochism,* the accusation: '*cruel mother is eating me up and it is killing me!*' The earlier complaint was shifted later from mother to father. This also reveals the deeper infantile precursor behind the punishment fantasy of being spanked. The triggering factor reviving your old fantasy was your fear of your father's terrible anger if you dropped out of training.''

"That's amazing! But wait till you hear what just came into my head: my father's nickname on his baseball team! He's a big guy, and they call him—'The Bear.' This masochism thing is really something!"

The pains decreased further and soon virtually disappeared. She told her parents about her changed view of gymnastic competition, and was only a little surprised to find that they were not angry at all. They actually admitted that they had made similar observations about the lifestyle of the professional athlete, and doubted the wisdom of continuing her program. They hadn't said anything though, because they were certain she had her heart set on it!

We have in this a demonstration that acknowledging and explaining masochism are not enough. The specific masochistic mechanism must be identified and interpreted in each individual case, and for each situation within that case. This girl was told in her first analysis that in her self-created pains she was masochistically spoiling her own aim to do gymnastics. In actual fact, as the second analysis revealed, she felt that it was her parents who expected her to do the gymnastics, and she inwardly created her pains because she did *not* want that career. Both interpretations were plausible, but only the latter was correct, and unfortunately incorrect interpretations do not bring lasting results in analysis.

It was even possible, as a kind of postscript, to speculate why the first analyst overlooked that children sometimes pursue careers they do not want but which are forced on them by parents. A colleague who knew the first analyst told me recently that he had never wanted to study medicine, but his poverty-conscious father encouraged him to enter this field, "because he could be self-supporting." He later tried to convince himself that he really "loved" medical-psychiatric work. Apparently his own inner defense mechanism against masochistic submission—"I do medicine because I want to"—created a blind spot, resulting in his false and misleading assumption that gymnastics was *the girl's choice!*

Among other technical reasons for therapeutic failure, Bergler makes an important point about the "silent analyst." Citing discussions with Federn and Jekels, he suggests that this *misconception* of Freud's technique may have originated in an ironic misunderstanding of Freud's relative silence in his later years. (That silence was based on two factors, neither of which had anything to do with a deliberate technical device.) Bergler already pointed out in his 1945 paper " 'Working Through' in Psychoanalysis" (*Psychoanalytic Review,* Vol. 32, No. 4) that some colleagues seem to believe that the patient's verbally and emotionally expressing the neurotic conflict in analysis is curative in and of itself. This line of thinking would see interpreting these repetitions as somehow redundant. Bergler discounted this notion, which he labeled the "cafeteria idea" of analysis (i.e., self-help in the presence of the inactive analyst) and explained why it is both erroneous and ineffective.

This is important because one still encounters evidence that this silent approach remains the standard one. Patients who have previously had "classical analysis" are still often unable to say how the analyst explained their problem. We hear such comments as: "I did all the talking, he just listened." A young colleague recently told me of a psychiatric supervisor who informed his trainees that months may go by in his analyses of patients during which he says nothing, but merely "mirrors the patient" and offers "unconditional positive regard"; he then played a tape for them from his own practice, in which the patient was heard yelling at the unresponsive doctor. The supervisor said it went on like that in the therapy *for two years*—an approach which he upheld as correct therapeutic technique.

In contrast to this, as Grinker points out in the article already quoted, Freud himself spoke at length. Grinker puts it (ironically?): "As has frequently been said, *Freud was not really Freudian. In other words, he did not stick to the rules and regulations his followers advised for psychoanalysis.* His sessions were quite informal. . . . American analysts very literally adopted the notion that the psychoanalyst is solely a mirror and doesn't do anything on his own. Not Freud. . . . He would joke or tell stories. In fact, *relating pointed stories was a technical device Freud used to accent his interpretations.* The number of stories seemed endless . . ." (emphasis added).

Where the subject of interpretation comes up at psychotherapy seminars—even psychoanalytically-oriented ones—one hears the following suggested as "interpretation": "I can tell that you have some strong feelings about that"; "you seem to be really angry now," etc. Bergler emphasizes that interpretation in analysis refers to the analyst presenting the decoded *unconscious* contents of the patient's conflict to the patient. *Superficial statements about the patient's conscious feelings, or withholding comment altogether, cannot be expected to change the patient's inner structure.* The trouble with this kind of pseudo analysis is that it helps neither the patients nor the reputation of psychoanalysis as a serious branch of medical science.

Bergler reminds us that analysis of transference and resistance are the pillars of analytic treatment (p. 136), and recalls the central role played by the "bad mother" transference during the neurotic's entire lifetime. It is this masochistic transference, and not "falling in love with the analyst," that we see and interpret in analyzing masochistic neurotics; the so-called erotic transference is really pseudo-erotic, camouflaging masochism. Recognizing and analyzing transference remains central to psychoanalysis, yet this subject is still misunderstood. Freud first described and defined the phenomenon; he pointed out in "The Dynamics of the Transference" (1912) that "[it] is not a fact that transference emerges with greater intensity and lack of restraint during psychoanalysis than outside it . . . these characteristics of transference are therefore to be attributed not to psychoanalysis but to neurosis itself" (*Standard Edition,* 12:101). Later, in "Recollection, Repetition, and Working Through" (1914) he added that this reaction takes place in non-analytic treatment, e.g., in institutions, where it is not recognized as such, and occurs with neurotics in all their relationships. The instance with the analyst differs only in that we can use it to show the patient the repressed emotional conflict (*Collected Papers,* Vol. II, pp. 370-1, 374). For many this distinction has been lost; transference has been wrongly thought to be unique to the analytic situation—in fact, as an artifact created by the analytic situation. Bergler reminds us that "transference . . . is not a prerogative of the analytic situation. It occurs on and off the analytic couch" (p. 441).

Bergler also considers a little-known phenomenon—the "grand design" neurosis—that accounts for some perplexing surprises after an apparently successful analysis. The "grand design" concept helps to explain those patients who show improvement, only to return years later with a new conflict totally foreign to the neurosis previously treated. Most significant is Bergler's observation that these patients use analysis to achieve limited changes, only to live out later an even more self-damaging aspect of their neurosis. This mechanism represents one option in the "future masochistic potential" of the patient; knowing about it makes it possible to suspect the presence of a grand design the first time around, and follow up hints pointing in that direction.

Chapter 7 concerns the visual drive—"looking and showing off . . . *the stepchildren of psychiatric-psychoanalytic investigations.*" It presents a comprehensive textbook—a "book within a book"—on this complicated subject, which occupied Bergler's attention throughout his psychoanalytic career and resulted in a large number of major published papers. As early as 1951, Dr. Theodore Branfman wrote to ask Bergler if he had considered writing a book on this. Bergler's answer: "I have been thinking time and again about a monograph on scopophilia; the enormity of material and the many unclarified spots were the impediment." The result of his deliberations fits aptly in this book, since this is a major area in which inadequate understanding has led to therapeutic failure.

Divided into four subsections, the third and largest of these, with twenty-two clinical pictures of "visual neuroses," parallels Chapter 6 of *The Basic Neurosis*, "Twenty-Seven Clinical Pictures of Oral Regression." Several of the twenty-two, already presented in the former book, are updated here with newer theoretical deductions based on further clinical material. Now, thirty years later, this aspect of neurosis and its psychoanalytic treatment remain generally unknown and misunderstood; yet, as Bergler emphasizes, the visual drive is a subdivision of the oral libidinous drive, so some disturbance of voyeurism-exhibitionism is evident in practically every orally-regressed neurotic. Bergler's extensive knowledge of the masochistic component meant that he could add the consideration of that otherwise neglected dimension to his pioneering study of problems in the visual sphere.

This chapter offers a wealth of fundamental theory and clinical application to introduce both the general and the professional reader to this subject. Via the application of his essential work on masochism, complex clinical problems in the area of voyeurism-exhibitionism, all built upon a masochistic base, became clinically accessible. Bergler's conclusions on pathological blushing, blocked creativity, stage fright, and voyeuristic block in

INTRODUCTION TO THE 1993 PRINTING   xxxix

business, scientific research, journalism and photography—all have widespread practical applications. How many graduate students, experiencing an agonizing block trying to work out and write M.A. or Ph.D. theses, know they could be helped analytically? Their problem, though not the same as creative writing block, is related, and carries an excellent prognosis.

Bergler's lifelong interest in artistic creativity and its neurotic inhibition led to his theory and method of treatment of "writer's block," presented in 1950 in *The Writer and Psychoanalysis*.[11] That book—based on thirty-six cured cases—brought Bergler's work to the attention of the entire creative community; the response from that group is indicated by the new total reported here—over seventy blocked writers cured. In 1987, one radio and television writer successfully treated by Bergler presented recollections of his analysis to a meeting of trustees of the Edmund and Marianne Bergler Psychiatric Foundation in New York. He remembered telling Bergler that writing was difficult for him, "like giving blood." Bergler explained that, once unblocked, writing should be "like turning on a faucet." "Well, it never got to be like turning on a faucet," mused the former patient, "but it was a lot easier to 'give blood.' "

The discussion of "fear of examinations" relates to the broader problem of pseudo mental deficiency, or "neurotic learning-block," on which Bergler first wrote in 1932. Psychoanalysis has revealed that much of what passes in daily life for "stupidity" has less to do with weak intelligence than with unconscious masochistic provocation by "playing dumb"; the negative repercussions affect both the possessor of this mechanism and his or her "victims." Bergler undertook a separate investigation of this complex subdivision of neurosis, in *The Talent for Stupidity*.[12] It will be the first previously unpublished Bergler book to appear since *Parents Not Guilty!*[13] in 1964, and will follow the present volume from International Universities Press.

Bergler shows that lack of original observation in "scientific block" stems from a voyeuristic inhibition. Studying scientists' impairment made it possible, as with creative writer's block, to explain the unconscious psychology of scientific activity. As was typical of Bergler, his comments here represent a mere summary of his thinking on this subject. His amplified ideas survive in an incomplete manuscript bearing the title *The Making of a Scientist*.[14] It is of interest to note that Bergler directed his scientific inquiry toward every facet of human experience, including his own personal sublimation, the phenomenon of scientific inquiry itself.

His concern with anticipating and predicting future expressions of masochism (see pp. 436 ff.) was followed up in a manuscript outline dating from the same period. In the foreword to *The Pursuit of Happiness and the Pursuit of Unhappiness: The Masochistic Potential*,[15] he states his theme: "the question [of] whether *totally unforeseen, never realized* masochistic potentialities can be dealt with—*preventively*. Should this prove possible, an enormous amount of suffering could be avoided, even lives saved." One chapter contains a significant postscript to the present volume's "Mortgaging One's Future through Indignant Reproaches." It reads: "I admit that I was frankly surprised at that reaction. [My experience led me to conclude] that in every case of divorce of the parents [from the] time the child is small till [the child is] pre-adolescent, the bitter accusation, later masochistically tinged, is present, regardless of whether or not the patient knows or admits it [consciously]" (editing added).

This volume, filled with original theoretical and clinical advances, concludes with a reminder that we still need "to find out more and more about the unconscious and to give help to those in mental distress." As Bergler shows, however, the double challenge of having to master complicated intellectual material and also achieve a higher degree of personal emotional development, before even beginning the quest for further answers, explains why many feel intimidated and withdraw. Not everyone has, or can develop, the necessary unconscious sublimations for doing this kind of work. Nor does every aspirant have the needed stamina to follow through for years, treating patients and writing up the results of ongoing clinical research.

Curable and Incurable Neurotics is above all a psychoanalytic textbook, written not only to inform but also and primarily to teach. Its success may be measured by the fact that it remained continuously in print for thirty years on the basis of public demand. Unlike psychiatric books which present a kind of "thinking out loud," the ideas expressed by Bergler in this book are neither hypotheses nor speculation. In *Principles of Self-Damage,* Bergler described his inwardly self-imposed pattern of self-criticism, a kind of strict self-censorship. *As a result, the observations and opinions in this book represent carefully established and verified conclusions based on first developing a theory and then testing that theory over*

INTRODUCTION TO THE 1993 PRINTING xli

a period of years by applying it clinically in dozens of cases to solve specific clinical problems. Certainly considerable weight can be given to an explanation such as that of the mechanism of writer's block previously cited, which is based on successful application to almost eighty blocked writers, restoring their artistic creativity. This was in effect the test standard to which Bergler submitted all his ideas before publishing his conclusions.

Newcomers to psychoanalysis will find in this book an excellent introduction to the world of the unconscious, and an unexpected view of neurosis and its treatment. Prospective patients can obtain a general idea of their problem, and what this form of analysis might provide for them. Analysts reacquainting themselves with Bergler's work can discover concepts, theoretical explanations, and clinical applications that throw light on clinical stumbling blocks. Even analysts already working with Bergler's theory and technique can re-read this work after years of clinical experience and notice additional details and connections that have greater impact with each reexamination or that suggest further applications and areas for investigation.

The picture conveyed in this book contrasts sharply with the current practice of training psychiatric residents to "establish warm rapport," or "display non-judgmental empathy" in a general way. Even a cursory reading of the dialogue from Bergler's analytic sessions conveys the therapeutic impact of making the patient confront unconscious masochistic motives. Analysis is hard work: neurotics are not as eager as they think they are to give up their suffering. This book underscores Bergler's point: *the chief reason for therapeutic failure remains the lack of emphasis on inner psychic masochism, the "pleasure in displeasure pattern."* As he put it: " . . . not all neurotics in treatment are capable of renouncing their 'hide-outs,' but *they should be given a chance* to face their real problem."

Melvyn L. Iscove, M.D., F.R.C.P.(C)

Toronto, October 1992

NOTES AND REFERENCES

1. *The Basic Neurosis* (1949). Reprinted by Grune and Stratton, New York, 1977, with a new preface.
2. 1949 letter to Bergler.
3. *The Superego: Unconscious Conscience—The Key to the Theory and Therapy of Neurosis* (1952), Grune and Stratton, New York. Reprinted by International Universities Press, Madison, Connecticut, 1989, with a new Foreword.
4. *Principles of Self-Damage* (1959), Philosophical Library, New York. Reprinted by International Universities Press, Madison, Connecticut, 1992, with a new Introduction.
5. A copy of the recording is on file at the Michigan State University Voice Library.
6. *Homosexuality: Disease or Way of Life?* (1956), Hill and Wang, New York.
7. *One Thousand Homosexuals* (1959), Pageant Books, Inc., Paterson, New Jersey.
8. Reisman, J. and Eichel, E., *Kinsey, Sex, and Fraud: The Indoctrination of a People* (1990), Lochinvar-Huntington House, Lafayette, Louisiana.
9. McHugh, Paul R., Psychiatric Misadventures, *The American Scholar*, Vol. 61, No. 4, Autumn 1992, p. 498.
10. Ibid., pp. 505-506.
11. *The Writer and Psychoanalysis, Second Edition* (1954), Robert Brunner Psychiatric Books, New York. Reprinted by International Universities Press, Madison, Connecticut, 1986, with a new Foreword.
12. *The Talent for Stupidity*. Unpublished manuscript. To be published by International Universities Press.
13. *Parents Not Guilty! of their Children's Neuroses* (1964), Liveright Publishing Corp., New York.
14. Archives of the Edmund and Marianne Bergler Psychiatric Foundation.
15. Ibid.

There exists no stronger impression of the resistances during analytic work than that of a force defending itself by every means against recovery and wanting absolutely to cling to illness and suffering. . . . Looking over the whole picture, with the added phenomena of immanent masochism in so many people, . . . and the inner guilt of neurotics, one can no longer hold to the belief that psychic life is exclusively ruled by the pursuit of pleasure.

—Freud, ANALYSIS, TERMINABLE AND INTERMINABLE (1937)

FOREWORD

NEUROSIS is a disease of the unconscious. That souvenir of childhood is universal; only the quantity varies. A small amount is called a "neurotic tendency" or "peculiarity," approaching "normality," a pompous word covering *not-too-neurotic* personalities. For larger doses of the identical "stuff" the term *neurosis* is applicable. Thus the difference between the emotionally "healthy" and the emotionally "sick" is quantitative, not qualitative. Still, as an eighteenth-century philosopher correctly observed, there is a point where quantity changes into quality.

Having discarded the pompous words "normality" and "emotional health" as unwarranted exaggerations, one is immediately confronted with their hopeful sister under the skin, "cure." The latter pomposity simply denotes the removal of too conspicuous neurotic symptoms and personality distortions, which gives the afflicted person the possibility of living in relative peace with himself and others. The decisive factor is the amount of unconscious self-torture emanating from the inner conscience and its masochistic or not-too-masochistic inner elaboration by the unconscious ego.

The quantity of these self-damaging, psychic-masochistic tendencies represents the great divide between manageable and unmanageable neurotic traits. Modern psychiatric-psychoanalytic medical methods provide—in certain cases—the possibility of changing unmanageable neurotic traits into manageable ones. The transition from the former into the latter state is imprecisely designated in popular parlance as "cure."

"Improvement of the neurotic trade balance," a term preferable to "cure," includes two further advantages. First, the automatic and unavoidable progression of neurosis is stopped; left to itself neurosis is a progressive, not a self-limiting disease. Secondly, the ex-neurotic is provided with a new, effective, weapon to fight his inner enemy, thus rendering the latter less powerful. *After adequate psychoanalytic treatment an ex-neurotic is better off than his allegedly healthy confrere.*

Psychoanalysis, based on Freud's brilliant studies, is still a science in an early stage of development. It is naive to believe that everything is known in this field. Quite the contrary; so far the surface has only been scratched. Nothing is more dangerous, even ludicrous, than to apply conservatism in a young science. Those who do, and rest on the laurels of material discovered by the pioneers and confirmed by their successors, are in for disagreeable surprises, provided tax-free by the present and future research of live minds.

Conservatism in psychoanalytic psychiatry looks with a jaundiced eye (if it does not close both eyes) at the grave, though legitimate, differences of opinion in our field, already recorded. These center around the primary role of the "pleasure-in-displeasure pattern" (psychic masochism, injustice-collecting), the three-layer versus five-layer structure in neurotic symptoms and in sublimation, the question whether neurotic aggression is pseudoaggression or "true" aggression, the importance and clinical contents of the deeper layers, and so forth. Since I am responsible for stressing these questions I shall elaborate in the text. The convenient and complacent principle of *quieta non movere* is inapplicable to a fluid situation.

Added to the unwillingess to face (sometimes even fear of facing) new and bothersome problems is the fact that some aspects of the unconscious are still little explored, and these contribute heavily to therapeutic failures. Among them is the whole orbit of the *visual drive*. In the present volume twenty-two disease entities belonging to this orbit are discussed.

The question arises: What do neurotics really want from psychotherapy? Consciously the answer is simple: They want help for their suffering. *Unconsciously* the story is much more complicated and the answer by no means simple. In their various neuroses neurotics *unconsciously enjoy deep masochistic pleasures,* camouflaged by the various defenses that constitute their symptoms and personality quirks. These are attached to different "rescue stations" of libidinous or pseudoaggressive nature, depending on what level of infantile development they finally reached. What it practically amounts to is that penance is paid, in the form of symptoms, inhibitions, personality distortions causing conscious unhappiness, for the underlying and hidden unconscious happiness. That "happiness" does not rest on living out instinctual drives but on maintaining the neurotic balance by multiple defense mechanisms achieved vis-a-vis the torturing inner conscience. Hence the neurotic fights for his inner defenses, especially his masochistic defense. Every neurotic rescued "something" from the *infantile debacle,* and to that "something" he holds on for dear life.

No human being wants to renounce unconscious pleasure. Consciously, of course, neurotics cannot tell us this fact because they are consciously unaware of their secret treasure. But unconsciously they know very well what is going on, as is visible in their unavoidable "resistance" in therapy. In short, they want to maintain their hidden pleasure but, at the same time, to get rid of the automatic penance in the form of painful symptoms. *Inwardly what neurotics want is not "cure" but improvement of their neurotic pleasures*—an impossible proposition. They want permanent domicile in the neurotic paradise without paying the usurious entrance fee.

If a neurotic considers psychiatric treatment he is confronted with two possibilities. One type of psychotherapy—let's call it a *psychotherapy aiming at destruction of neurosis*—attempts to attack the variegated and damaging unconscious defenses. The other—let's call it a *psychotherapy aiming at temporary conscious improvement of the patient's suffering*—will leave the edifice of the neurosis intact, though it may increase the patient's conscious well-being—*temporarily*. Therefore the patient's behavior will be quite different during the two procedures, whatever labels one attaches to these two types of therapy. I have been repeatedly struck by statements of patients who, before entering deep analysis, were treated by adherents of different schools of the second type of psychotherapy, or by analysts who did not go beyond the superficial layers of the unconscious. They spoke with amazing friendliness and benevolence about their therapists, giving them credit for trying to do their best, acknowledging short-lived improvements, etc. When, however, these patients were for even a short time in an analysis that really attempted to reach the essentials (some of them did not finish, terminating it by running away) none of this kindness and benevolence was discernible. They mercilessly attacked the analysts with anger and contempt. The question arose: why the benevolence and why the malice?

I have been forced to conclude that the benevolence and gratitude pertained to the fact that the neuroses were not even touched. That is less paradoxical than it sounds at the first moment. The patient who enters psychotherapeutic treatment unconsciously expects a *day of judgment*. Therefore, if nothing of that tragic expectation materializes he is unconsciously grateful. This does not cure him, but his feeling of benevolence is thus explainable.

Assuming that the prospective patient is informed about the superficial and deeper forms of psychotherapy and chooses psychoanalysis with a medical man, a psychiatrist well trained in psychoanalysis and belonging to one of the accredited societies, can he be sure that his "deepest layers" will be penetrated? The answer is no, simply because of the differences of psychoanalytic opinion as to what constitutes these deepest layers. Some colleagues analyse as though the year were still 1910; some have progressed to 1926; and so on.

Personally, *I believe that there exists only* ONE *basic neurosis, acquired in the first eighteen months of life: psychic masochism. All later neurotic manifestations of libidinous-pseudoagrressive nature are only rescue stations* to hide the basic conflict. I have elaborated on this contention in my books THE BASIC NEUROSIS (1949), COUNTERFEIT-SEX (1951), THE SUPEREGO (1952), and PRINCIPLES OF SELF-DAMAGE (1959).

It is naive to assume that an analyzed person, even if his psychic masochism has been thoroughly dissected in treatment, will be immune to all conflicts all his future life. Such total immunization does not exist and cannot exist. What successful therapy achieves is diminution of that scourge by forcing it out of truly dangerous deposits. It also makes clear to the patient that whatever happens to him later *he will have to fight to the end of his earthly days with one basic and a series of camouflaging conflicts* (rear-guard retreat symptoms, rescue stations).

FOREWORD

The basic conflict will always be the same: psychic masochism. The camouflaging libidinous-pseudoaggressive conflicts will be manifold. Although it is improbable (though not impossible) that he will produce symptoms again, the chances are that depressive moods will be discernible at times. In such situations the patient is advised to distinguish between basic masochistic conflict and the camouflaging package-wrapping, stressing the former and debunking the latter. Experience proves that when those rare postanalytic attacks of the unconscious come they can be disposed of by the ex-patient alone in a few minutes. If worst comes to worst he should call again on the analyst, having been told that no future conflict can confront him that cannot be solved in a few appointments.

The general human conflict of masochistic injustice-collecting can be diminished, never fully eradicated; analysis cannot make a person healthier than the healthiest person is.

It is obvious that this division between basic masochistic conflict and camouflaging libidinous-pseudoaggressive retreat symptoms can be made exclusively by analysts who accept the above-mentioned theory and use it. Those who don't are confronted with painful surprises when patients, after being "cured," become "recidivists." Lost in the maze of libidinous and pseudoaggressive superficial layers (the latter confused with real aggression to boot), they don't even understand what hit the patient: *a new, desperate attempt to run away from the basic, and untouched, masochistic conflict.*

In recent years one of the typical complaints of psychoanalysts has been that most of their patients are not neurotics but "schizoid borderline" cases. These are not neurotics and still not psychotics—yet (a later progression to psychosis may or may not occur). The situation has been ambiguous. Some masochistic neurotics these colleagues did not know how to handle (psychic masochism is still an enigma to many) were unjustifiably subsumed under that classification, whereas in other cases the complaint was totally justified. *Psychoanalysis is exclusively a therapy for neurotics;* we can do little for schizoid personalities, except in cases where neurotic admixtures are extensive. *This volume presents for the first time a distinction between neurotic and schizoid (malignant) masochism.*

The decisive point in psychoanalytic therapy is whether we are dealing with *harmless-neurotic psychic masochism or malignant-schizoid psychic masochism*. Some cases are immediately recognizable to the experienced psychiatrist. Unfortunately, in many other cases this differentiation can be made only in the course of treatment. Most incurable neurotics are undetected, or unavoidably too late detected, schizoids. In those cases where little or nothing can be achieved the physician is blamed by ignorant outsiders for incompetence, fakery, and what not.

I reiterate my conviction that Freudian psychoanalysis is the deepest and most successful therapeutic tool in helping neurotics. I believe, however, that our science is still in a developmental stage and that conservatism—holding on to early assumptions that have later been modified or, needing modification, should be brought up to date—is wholly indefensible. I also reiterate my conviction that psychic masochism is THE universal neurotic early infantile difficulty constituting the "life-blood" of neurosis, and all later libidinous-pseudo-aggressive "rescue stations" are only camouflages and "hide-outs" from the basic infantile human conflict.

Edmund Bergler, M.D.

New York City, January, 1961

CURABLE AND INCURABLE NEUROTICS

Problems of "Neurotic"
versus
"Malignant" Psychic Masochism

CHAPTER 1

THE CRUCIAL QUESTION IN PSYCHO-
ANALYTIC THERAPY: "NEUROTIC" OR
"MALIGNANT" PSYCHIC MASOCHISM?

TODAY the basic analytic tenet, "neurosis is a disease of the dynamic unconscious," is more or less accepted. The disease manifests itself in neurotic symptoms (e.g., impotence, frigidity, homosexuality, pathological gambling, street fear, hypochondria, depression, anxiety, psychosomatic manifestations) or personality distortions (e.g., repetitive choice of wrong mates, spoiling one's chances, chronic provocations, constantly being taken advantage of, feeling left out and excluded, etc.), or a combination of the two.

Before the advent of modern psychoanalysis, founded on Freud's basic studies, the neurotic was considered a medical nuisance and had no status other than that of a pariah. Psychoanalysis rehabilitated the neurotic sufferer and took him seriously as a legitimate patient. It even distinguished him by offering him a couch, instead of the usual chair.

The sympathy was by no means mutual. Even today, nearly seventy years after the creation of psychoanalysis, many ignorant neurotics are bitterly opposed to our science and never enter treatment. This rule of thumb applies: if you meet an *enraged* enemy of psychoanalytic therapy he is betrayed by his emotionalism as a neurotic who unconsciously prefers to remain unchanged.

The trouble is that every layman considers himself a specialist in psychiatry—a naivete matched by profound ignorance. Whereas the average layman would not pronounce judgment or give a "considered opinion" on atomic or electronic research, his reticence vanishes where psychoanalysis is concerned; the "cocktail-party analysis" is a familiar and ludicrous phenomenon.

Seldom in the history of science has so much nonsense been uttered by even otherwise intelligent people as on the subject of psychoanalysis. P. W. Bridgman was perhaps right when he stated (in a different connection): "There is no adequate defense against the impact of a new idea except stupidity."

Such "stupidity" is frequently only pseudo stupidity, emotionally conditioned. Something in every person objects to acknowledging the fact that he is not even "master in his own house" (Freud).

The unconscious is un-conscious, and there's no bargaining on that score. The whole analytic therapy is based on the principle of making the unconscious conscious through an emotional therapeutic process, thus changing the unfavorable inner structure. All the misconceptions current about "self-analysis" via book knowledge are empty talk; self-analysis is a fancy word for arriving at wrong conclusions about one's own wonderful self. A psychiatric guide is needed for the descent into one's "inner hell."

Psychoanalysis has always had the distinction of presenting unpalatable ideas. This fact is not based on some peculiar predilection of analysts but is inherent in analytic discoveries. Since our science deals with psychic material typically repressed (expelled from consciousness because too painful and shameful to remain conscious) the reaction of the conscious ego is an indignant "no." Facts, however, do not change by simple denial of them.

It took the world fifty years to accept as fact the concept of the Oedipus complex; popular acceptance is always miles behind. In the meantime new discoveries have been produced by Freud and his pupils. Obviously the acceptance of these has to wait for your children's grandchildren.

As a matter of fact, analytic discussions in the last decades have centered around the precursors of the Oedipus and the complicated mechanism of defense against these early experiences and fantasies. The alleged "pansexualism" of analysis is old hat; as early as the twenties Freud accepted repressed libido and repressed aggression as equal partners in the unconscious. Analytic discussions also gravitate around the paramount importance of the "superego" (the unconscious part of conscience).

I am personally responsible for having stressed one specific aspect of the unconscious: PSYCHIC MASOCHISM. In my opinion that particular defense mechanism is THE BASIC NEUROSIS and is the cause of most of the mental misery encountered in human beings.

I hasten to add that the concept of the "pleasure-in-displeasure pattern" is even more repugnant to our contemporaries, scientist and layman alike, than anything else a psychoanalyst ever presented. The rejection of, and distaste for, this concept is based on fear, pure and simple. It is a terrifying idea, unfortunately very real, because it applies to everybody.

In the following pages a description of the "psychic apparatus" (Freud) is presented as I see it and as I have learned it from clinical experience, elaborated on in thirty-some years of practice and in 21 books and 271 scientific studies, published in 12 countries.

A tenaciously maintained legend has it that the infant, the baby, and the small child are the only happy inhabitants of this globe. The legend was certainly not created by babies; nobody asks these star witnesses. It was invented and is propagandized and perpetuated by adults, who use "common sense" of the it-stands-to-reason variety in arriving at their astounding conclusion. They compare the infinitesimal number of restrictions imposed on children, and their freedom from obligation to work, with their own lot. It is a glorification in retrospect, created by dissatisfied people who, having repressed their own past, nostalgically pursue lost years, hopes not materialized, shattered illusions, now projected in their original shape on their children.

The nursery, where the alleged happiness is supposed to blossom, is the place that holds the world record for mutual misunderstandings. Adults misconstrue their children's feelings and children those of adults. Verbal communication being yet impossible, intuition and empathy are supposed to bridge the lack of speech. Unfortunately child and mother are tuned to different wave lengths.

The mother's viewpoint is understandable; sacrificially and lovingly she cares for the baby, and she expects love and gratitude in return.

The baby's "viewpoint" is less "logical" and more complex. First of all, the baby acts as though everything *"good"* that happens to him were *self-bestowed* and treats everything *"bad"* as *stemming from outside*. This peculiar psychic bookkeeping at first absolves the very young child of exactly those emotions his mother logically expects: gratitude, love, acknowledgment of kindness received.

The wherewithal of this fantastic first bookkeeping system of the baby is understandable when the baby's limited experiences are scrutinized. What are the experiences he can draw on to explain the world that surrounds him? In the womb all effort was superfluous; oxygen and foodstuff were conveniently pumped into his blood vessels via the mother's circulatory system. Not even breathing and swallowing were required; after birth these two functions became obligatory but again were conveniently made easy by inborn reflexes. In their intuitive understanding mothers try to imitate in the first weeks of the child's life the prenatal conditions in order to soften the postnatal shock. The baby is left undisturbed in nearly continuous sleep in a darkened and noiseless room, warm milk is provided the moment he wakes up and gives the hunger sign by crying, excretions are removed to keep him dry and comfortable.

All this contributes to the first unwarranted assumption that the newcomer to this world makes: he is an omnipotent sorcerer, and everything he wishes is available just for the asking—either by his magic power or at his slightest sign.

This unwarranted assumption—technically called "infantile megalomania" (Freud, Ferenczi)—is the first of many abstruse and unrealistic theories built by the child in rapid succession. All these faulty theories have one common denominator: the outer world does not exist, or if it does it has only one purpose, to be the subservient and executive organ of the baby's omnipotence.

The next step is disturbing to the baby. He finds out that these "non-existent" slaves seem to have a life of their own and are not always at his beck and call; in short, they are unreliable and disappointing. They seem to have some peculiar notions, totally incomprehensible to His Majesty in swaddling clothes. For instance, they let him wait when he "gives a command." They are apparently addicts of cleanliness and bathing, and in washing him they stretch his body "cruelly," though they seem to be as tender as they can. Most disappointing, they constantly endanger his fantasy of omnipotence; they are stronger than His Majesty.

The baby's aversion to being forced to do the bidding of the "bad" outer world (actually the giantess of the nursery that he is later taught to call Mother) starts with the harmless and necessary act of sucking. Certainly nothing sinister and dangerous is hidden in this necessity. Still, there are children who are poor eaters or go on hunger strikes. A baby who was consistent on that score—refusing to give an inch of infantile megalomania—would die of starvation. In one of the many variants of the Greek legend of Narcissus, the youth, enamored of and preoccupied with his own image seen in a brook, does die of starvation. But it seems that the universal early infantile aversion to being forced (meaning: being pushed into the passive position) is counteracted by a more powerful force, the newly discovered oral pleasure of sucking, helped by the *vis a tergo* of hunger.

In any case, even sucking is not the process naive adults make of it: "It's natural to eat." Natural functions also carry a psychological superstructure. If the natural function conflicts with an offense to "infantile megalomania" the outcome is by no means certain, unless a new allure of libidinous nature is added. In the case of eating there is fortunately such an allure—oral libidinous pleasure.

Of course the whole idea that a baby could misconstrue the act of being fed as "unwarranted malicious intrusion and penetration" by nipple or bottle seems ridiculous to an adult. Since the average adult has no longer any conscious recollection of his own repressed megalomaniacal yardstick he is prone to frown at analytical "fantasies."

Here are two examples of dreams of schizoid people. The first patient, analyzed twenty-five years ago, dreamt that he was suspended from the ceiling by his feet ("like a reversed fixture") and that, to his helpless horror, an enormous ball or stone was forced into his mouth. No associations were forthcoming, and I did not divulge my suspicion that he represented the act of being fed as torture, exaggerating the half-reclining position of the baby at the breast. A few days later the patient reported this incident: He had entered the room of his elderly landlady (having knocked and received no answer) to find her daughter nursing her baby. His immediate thought was: "She will smother the baby with her enormous breast." After this he was willing to accept the interpretation of his dream.

The second patient dreamt that he bought an olive. Before putting it into his mouth he looked at it and saw that a bee was coming out of it and was about to sting him; he dropped the olive in horror. No associations were elicited. I asked the patient whether he could name an organ of the body faintly resembling an olive. He went through the whole anatomy (including the ovary)—he was obviously making fun—and rejected as "far-fetched" the possibility of a nipple. A few days later he informed me of a "peculiar item" pointing to his mother's involvement in the dream. He had written down the dream in half-slumber during the night, and when he reread it he noticed that he had misspelled the word "bee"; he had written "bea." His mother's name was Beatrice, and she was called, by him and others, Bea!

Once again the dangerous mother with the dangerous nutritional apparatus!

The "threatening intrusion" of the mother's nipple is followed by a long series of misconceptions on the part of the baby, who misinterprets all his mother's harmless actions as dangers intended to destroy him. I have suggested calling these faulty baby theories the "septet of baby fears." As will be seen, in each successive "theory" the baby makes some slight concession to newly observed realistic facts. He reformulates previous misconceptions into new ones and seems to take his cue from William James's dictum "Some people think they are thinking, while they are only rearranging their prejudices."

The dismal procession starts with

Fear of starvation. The adult neurotic, simply because he is alive, proves that this fear was delusive and unwarranted. Mothers ordinarily do not let their babies starve. The "starvation" here is an offense to the infant's megalomania, which exaggerates the hardship of waiting even a few seconds for breast or bottle and resents any delay as an insult.

Fear of being devoured. This grotesque fear has been clarified by the English school of psychoanalysis as a projection of the child's *own* aggressive designs upon the nipple (bottle). It is formulated: "I don't want to bite; mother wants to devour me."

Fear of being poisoned. Sooner or later even the child who claims that his mother is "starving" him must admit that he is being fed. He preserves the essence of his grievance by shifting it: "Mother does feed me, but the food is poisonous and harmful."

Fear of being choked. This fear involves fantasies that have to do with being choked by the mother's breast or body. They are *not* set in operation by the disproportion of the mother's body and child's, nor by the clumsiness of mother or nurse in pushing the nutritional instrument into the baby's mouth too forcibly.

Fear of being chopped to pieces. At the root of this fear is the baby's failure to understand the mother's harmless intentions in the routines of washing and cleaning. The baby translates these actions into a procrustean-bed fantasy. Again, the evil design is imputed to the mother by the child; the overforcefulness of the upbringers is not responsible.

Fear of being drained. This fear arises from the infant's "helplessness" against "propelling forces" in the elimination of urine and feces. The child feels that he is being forcibly "drained." He retaliates, secondarily, with megalomaniacal and aggressive ideas connected with both products.

Fear of castration. This fear is the climax of the septet. It is characterized by concessions to reality in the form of more or less rational disguises, and is most clearly visible during the oedipal phase.

Not all children have actually been threatened with "castration"; the fact that all children manifest this fear, whether or not threats have been made, has puzzled many analytic authors. In recent literature, however, it is agreed that the fear grows out of a series of nongenital precursors. The sheltered uterine existence vanished, the breast (bottle) was withdrawn, stool was "drained," later the milk teeth fell out. Thus groundwork was laid for the idea that "pleasure leads to the loss of the pleasure-giving organ" (F. Alexander).

The deepest reason is more complicated. It is identical with the fact that the septet of baby fears is still alive, although disguised by shifts to successive phases and organs. Much that is classified as "phallic castration fear" is at bottom undigested oral fear stemming from the septet.

It is clear that this septet of baby fears is characterized by a certain progression. Some of them, the fear of starvation, of being devoured, choked, or chopped to pieces, preserve infantile misconceptions. The others have "reformulated" the impossible but cling to the projected cruelty. The fear of being poisoned at least concedes that the mother gives food, even though imputing sinister designs to her. The fear of being drained or castrated at least acknowledges that only parts of the body, not the entire person, are the passive objects of destruction. These are, nevertheless, only halfhearted concessions. Moreover, the "reformulations" become more outspoken in later neurotic manifestations.

In later years, for example, the reproach of starvation is modified into that of being refused, and love, kindness, gifts, attention, etc., are substituted for food. After masochistic "stabilization on the rejection level" the game of "cruel mother refuses helpless child" is made permanent, its basis unconsciously self-chosen and self-initiated.

The fear of being devoured becomes visible in later years through animal phobias and unconscious fantasies. Fairy tales and dreams enshrine it.

The fear of being poisoned is the ancestor of the pathologic fear of impregnation, of neurotic intestinal disturbances and hypochondriacal complaints centering about food.

The fear of confined places, from true claustrophobia to neurotic fear of elevators, can be traced back to the infantile fear of being choked. Contributaries are visible in the psychological aspects of asthma.

Remnants of the fear of being chopped to pieces are apparent in neurotics who adduce the cutting of meat, fish, and fowl as proof positive that a woman is "capable of anything." In adulthood these remnants are subsumed into fear of operations and phallic castration fears.

One encounters the fear of being drained behind the adult's façade of miserliness in money, sex, and even words.

It would be erroneous to assume that the child takes all these fantastic fears—objectively fantastic but for the immature human being endowed with full "reality" value—without attempting countermeasures. The only countermeasure possible is—aggression; and the tragedy here lies in the inexpressibility of the baby's aggression, since his muscular apparatus is undeveloped. He can only cry, vomit, spit, make uncoordinated movements with hands and feet.

The sequence of events is always the same:

(1) offense to infantile megalomania;
(2) mobilization of fury, inexpressible fury;
(3) turning of the child's aggression against himself.

The last point requires some explanation.

Drives, Freud has taught us, are like rivers, more interested in discharge than in the direction of discharge. Imagine that a river flowing between high banks is dammed up by workmen in all directions; the result will be that the river eventually reverses its course. This is exactly what happens with undischargeable aggression; it turns against its originator. Sceptics who doubt this statement are invited to observe their own children. If a small child of one or one and a half is prevented from hitting a parent or nurse he will, in desperation, try to bang his own head against the wall. Is the child, as so many parents assume, "crazy"? By no means. Parents are just witnessing the basis for the scientific statement that "a drive is more interested in its discharge than in the direction of discharge." The show must go on.

Now being the object of "self-aggression" is painful and humiliating, to say the least. Every human being lives on the basis of the "pleasure principle." What pleasure, if any, can be derived from hitting oneself? Obviously none, unless one makes a pleasure out of displeasure. That is exactly what the future "psychic masochist" does. *The only pleasure one can derive from displeasure is to make pleasure out of displeasure ("psychic masochism").*

The psychic masochist is a genius: he solved an unsolvable problem, and at the age of four to eighteen months. No wonder every parent avers (if he is not ashamed to admit it) that his child is a prodigy. Parents don't even know how right they are; though they give the wrong reasons for their conviction, they are justified.

Thus we have to add a fourth point to the previous enumeration: (4) libidinization of the boomerang aggression by making it an *unconscious pleasure.*

Nobody can go through the protracted helplessness of childhood without acquiring some traces of this psychic poison. Psychic masochism is a universal human trait; to deny it is just as naive as to deny that every human being possesses an organ called a heart.

The genius of the infant, baby, small child solved one of the most complex problems of the psychic economy. It created the *"genetic picture"* in psychic masochism, dealt with in part by Freud. Unfortunately the process does not stop at that point.

The next development simply confirms the already established trouble. The aggression of the child is not directed against indifferent people; its targets are parents and their representatives, "people with a halo." Why exactly parents? They are "just around." Parents impress the moral dictum of holiness on the child, thus making it tough for him to discharge aggression. They invoke the "triad of retribution": punishment, moral reproach, guilt.

The problem of guilt is of decisive consequence. It acquires a double representation: mother (father) *and* the *inner conscience* (superego).

The origin of guilt dates from the earliest phase of development, when the inexpressible fury of frustration rebounds against the ego. The first results of this ricochet, a feeling of helplessness and unease and subsequent depression, are the pre-stages of guilt.

It is against the background of the inescapable accumulation of this rebounding aggression that we must view the child's pathetic attempts to cope with *external* troubles. His first inner expedient for dealing with the outer world was described by Freud as the *"ego ideal."*

In his frantic efforts to hold on to vestiges of his most cherished infantile fantasy—omnipotence, megalomania, autarchy—the child at two or two and a half discovers an ingenious device. It consists of identification with the prohibitions handed down by his mother and father. He thus substitutes an *inner* prohibition for the barrage of *external* prohibitions that have previously been so offensive. The effect is the same; the message is still "don't do it," the only change being the direction of the taboo. The child's new obedience, his acceptance of rules of his own "free will," saves face for him, saves punishment, even saves remnants of his illusion of omnipotence.

The ego ideal, therefore, is composed of the child's original and indestructible megalomania (later attenuated to narcissism and self-love) amalgamated with internalized parental prohibitions. In its introjected sectors, however, the ego ideal is *not* an exact copy of the parents. The precise formulation is "parents as the child perceived them." Since a good deal of the child's aggression was projected on the parents their images have already been colored and altered by a patina of this projected aggression.

The narcissistic sector, the larger ingredient of the mixture, has the purpose of protecting the ego from humiliation and maintaining the needed assurance of all-power. It contains the child's braggadocio, his boasting of what he can do, his grandiose promises for the future, his "dreams of glory," amusing to an adult sense of reality but utterly serious to the child. These high-pitched aims, created and advertised in childhood, later become one of the most fertile sources of self-torture.

Having established the ego ideal (the *"department of don'ts and great expectations"*), the child has solved an external conflict, but his *internal* conflict continues because of the backlog of undischarged aggression dating from infancy. Although he gradually gains increased muscular control and is capable of placing aggression outward in games and activities of various kinds, this ability does not come soon enough to save him from an inner usurper.

The accumulation of aggression directed inward (*"department of torture"*) was called by Jekels and myself *"daimonion."* This forbidding term was borrowed from Socrates, who held that every human being harbored a "daimoniacal something" within himself, an inner spirit. Socrates described his daimonion as a kind of voice that kept him from doing what he wished to do but never gave positive advice. It figures in a peculiarly fallacious argument in his provocative defense at his trial for his life (in which every point seems designed to defeat him in the eyes of his judges), the argument that since his accustomed "voice" was silent, death must be a desirable goal. Socrates refused efforts to save him and drank the hemlock; he wanted to die and achieved his aim through his "daimonion."

The daimonion, in psychoanalytical terms, is an inner malicious "something" (though Socrates subjectively mistook it for a benevolent guardian) that is each man's worst enemy. Every human being consciously wishes to be happy, but the fact is that there also exists in the human psyche an unconscious force that is averse to happiness, success, enjoyment of life, and whose aim is unhappiness, misery, and even self-destruction.

The ego ideal and the daimonion are the two constituents of the *superego*. These two impersonal departments work in this way: the daimonion uses the ego ideal for its campaign of torture. Constantly holding up to the ego its self-constructed ego ideal, the daimonion asks the searching if monotonous question, "Have you achieved all the aims you set for yourself in childhood? Have you fulfilled your promises?" If the answer is no, the result is guilt.

One cannot stress strongly enough that the superego's technique is *torture for torture's sake*. In previous books, especially PRINCIPLES of SELF-DAMAGE, I have attempted to codify the regulations by which the superego operates in its insidious attacks on the ego. Here are twenty-one *Rules of Torture:*

Rule 1. The superego (unconscious conscience) has nothing in common with conscious conscience except a badly fitting name. Most people fight a lifelong sham battle with "conscience," in which, if they seem to make peace, they have won nothing, because the superego is still beyond their conscious knowledge—and reach. Guilt feelings, depression, apprehensiveness, are not recognized by the conscious mind as results of *unconscious* torture, emanating from a hidden torture machine. On the contrary they are accounted for by rationalizations borrowed from conscious conscience. The average person is unaware of the superego and believes that he is battling the conscience he knows. When he first hears of the existence of an *unconscious* conscience he takes it for granted that it serves the same purpose. "The more conscience, the better," he thinks, ignorant of the superego's real function as a malicious internal tormentor.

Conscious conscience is a summary of conventional and necessary precepts of right and wrong, specific for specific societies. The

The Crucial Question in Psychoanalytic Therapy

effect of these rules is salutary. Everybody approves of them; nobody questions the need for them.

The superego is another story. Here illogic, anachronism, and cruelty of the most brutal variety are paramount, and the target is always the ego.

Rule 2. Anti-hedonistic principle predominant. The superego's attitude can be summarized in two words: *no pleasure.* The sentences pronounced by the superego are as severe as those meted out to an enemy of a dictator's regime in his "court of justice."

Rule 3. Mock rules of procedure. The superego is a court of last resort and there is no appeal from its judgment, but it follows strict "rules of procedure" with never varying routine. The defendant is reminded of the ambitions recorded in the ego ideal and is asked, "Is there any discrepancy between the actual achievement and the promises of childhood?" Any gap between present reality and past fantasy brings punishment in the form of dissatisfaction, depression, and guilt.

Rule 4. Formalism. The superego's rigid formalism is one of the few weak spots in an otherwise unassailable structure and can be used to defeat it. This is the method of the most successful slave revolts the ego is capable of: the revolt of the normal ego via tender love [1] and of the neurotic ego via hypocrisy and the pseudomoral connotation of neurotic symptoms (see pp. 130 ff.).

Rule 5. "Legalistic proofs." The superego is punctilious in "proving" beyond a doubt that the culprit really did harbor the forbidden wish or defense. But it is by no means difficult to find "proof," since the superego has direct connections with the department of repressed wishes and the factory of inner defenses, which represent the id and the unconscious ego, respectively.

Rule 6. The wish equals the deed. The superego admits no distinction between a forbidden wish and a forbidden act; thus opportunities for punishment are endless. Goethe, in saying that there was no crime he could not imagine himself committing, was speaking for all humanity.

Rule 7. Rejection of all excuses. Just as the superego makes no concessions for forbidden wishes not acted on, it makes none for even reasonable excuses (economic depressions, limited opportunities, personal inadequacies, etc.).

Rule 8. Cultural standards used as a blind for torture. Appearing to accept the standards of the particular environment, the superego uses them to disguise its cruelty. This has given rise to the mistaken belief that the individual is the product of his culture. The superego is in no way influenced by the culture or concerned with the validity of a specific prohibition; it is only interested in a handy excuse to catch a person out and pronounce sentence. As every culture has plenty of taboos, excuses are not lacking. The rule works both ways, however; the superego cannot impose punishment for an act or wish approved by the environment.

Rules 9 and 10. Both failure and success used as torture material. For any failure, whether self-arranged, accidental, or inevitable, the ego is held solely responsible. "If you had not been such a fool," the indictment reads, "you might have made it." Success also is contrary to the inner torturer's regulations and is paid for according to a long-range plan of devaluation in which it is discounted as piddling, insignificant, ineffective. The superego's motto throughout is "So what?"

A good example of the superego's technique in devaluating success is the dream of a masochistic patient in analysis, a brilliant industrialist and an ex-homosexual (the "ex" was analytically achieved), in the last stages of treatment. He had just had a highly impressive external success. He had bought "for a steal" two dozen chain stores in his specific field of endeavor. The success was a combination of cashing in on his reputation as a first-class specialist with a keen eye for future possibilities and simple luck. On the day the contract was signed he was elated. During the night he had two disturbing dreams:

(1) "I am in a delicatessen store with an acquaintance, an indifferent man. While he talks with the owner in the back of the store I take a piece of ham out of the refrigerator; I choose a slice from the middle, knowing that this is the juiciest part, and eat it. In leaving I am surprised that the owner of the store asks for payment. My acquaintance pays the few pennies but half-accuses

me of wanting to get away without paying. I ask him, 'Do you seriously think that I wanted to steal that little piece of ham?'

(2) "I am in the parking lot of one of my establishments. Only male colored people work there. I am looking for some piece of wire (or clay?) to make a brassiere I promised somebody. All at once I see that all the colored people have enormous breasts."

The associations of the patient to the first dream led to the pun "steal-deal." In other words, his superego does not give him credit for his smartness but reproaches him for the "steal." It also reproaches him for being a "ham," a despicable exhibitionist. (Other associations lead back to a religious interdiction: "What business has a Jewish boy to eat ham!") To top it all his superego calls him a penny-pincher. The allusion to the "middle" of the ham has, of course, a *defensive* sexual connotation: "I did not want to be refused (in the middle of the female body), I wanted to get."

The patient was at a loss to contribute anything in connection with the second dream, besides rectifying the fact that it was not only colored people that worked in this particular parking lot. The dream apparently begins with an attempt of the ego to defend itself against the devaluation of success. The superego seems to point out ironically that though he may have dozens of establishments (he has just acquired a new string of these in a field appealing to the taste buds) he will never get what he has always wanted, a breast. (The breast allusion is especially malicious. What a homosexual inwardly craves is not the breast but masochistic disappointment by the breast-bearer. Here the superego ironically inundates the ego with its own defenses: "You claim that you didn't want to be refused but wanted to get. Fine—you cannot get it!"—The weak rejoinder is that some men have an enormous penis, which is "better than breasts.") The fact that only colored people are employed is a twofold piece of snobbish malice on the part of the superego: allusions to past masochistic attachments to people "beneath his station" and irony in the vein of the popular phrase "to change one's luck" (denoting, in New Yorkese, to go with a colored prostitute). The implication seems to be, "Do you really think that kind of luck changes anything?" Finally, the allusion to "making a breast" is double-barreled. On the one hand the superego pokes fun at his attempts to make one ("wire," "brassiere"); on the other hand the ego asserts its megalomania: "Wasn't man made originally of clay? I can do likewise." But clay also alludes to the devaluation of success: "feet of clay." In the end the superego is victorious and has the last—torturing—word.

Not only is the superego no respector of success, it goes further in its malice and "hits the man who is down." In PRINCIPLES OF SELF-DAMAGE (pp. 58 ff.) I have collected a few dreams of dying men.

Rule 11. Killjoy treatment of happiness after success. There is also a short-range program of torture for successful achievement. This is the "bad mood" that frequently follows the first heady elation. Most people understand that depression tends to follow failure (though they explain it in terms of reality factors), but they are baffled by such an unpleasant postscript to success. The mystery can be solved by those who are aware of the torture-for-torture's-sake principle of the superego.

Rules 12 and 13. Immediacy of torture and the irony of delayed, over-severe punishment. Immediacy of torture is the predominant rule, but if followed too persistently the superego may suffer a reverse; the ego's "proofs" may sometimes be used for its own advantage. For example, as the superego turns the analyst's interpretations into instruments of torture, *one* of the reasons for producing recollections in analysis is to study this misuse by the inner tormenter. With its formal procedures the superego must first force the ego to provide proofs of forbidden acts or wishes (see Rule 4) by bringing to the surface what has been conveniently repressed. When the unconscious aim is correctly decoded the ego is strengthened by increased confidence in and identification with the analyst. Thus *correct* interpretations, and the working through of these interpretations,[2] lead to a strange and unexpected effect. Another result of the prodding of the superego in these situations consists of specific "dreams of refutation,"[3] a practically predictable phenomenon.

Ironically delayed torture is rarer. In this technique a trap is set, and later, when the victim is unsuspecting, even optimistic, the trap is sprung. Here is an example. A patient whose neurotic dislike of housework was being analyzed "forgot" an analytic appointment.

Thinking that it was a day when she did not go to the analyst, she spent the morning doing her otherwise hated household tasks, and with surprising good humor. Hours later she realized she had been fooled and sank into a deep depression.

Rules 14 and 15. Irrevocability of the ego's countermeasures and "incomprehensible depression." When the ego prepares a certain amount of defensive psychic masochism for a particular dangerous situation and the outcome is, unexpectedly, favorable, the masochism already mobilized cannot be put in storage but must be expended. This leads to depressions *post fortuito facto,* to "incomprehensible" mistakes, and—a grotesque result—"tears of happiness."

Rule 16. Enlargement on a mistake by invoking all past mistakes. When the ego sustains a failure or disappointment the superego disinters similar (or even unrelated) failures and mistakes from the victim's past. The "files are opened." In this way the specific minor failure is built up into generalized and all-embracing depreciation of the individual's achievements and undue magnification of his failures.

Rule 17. Acceptance of substitute crimes, within limits. Since the superego represents the peak of refined torture it seems contradictory that it should permit the ego to sidetrack reproaches by taking punishment for substitute crimes. This leads to the mechanism of "admission of a lesser crime" (see p. 63). But the technique of the substitute crime is a cornerstone of the neurotic structure. The explanation lies in the eagerness of the superego to produce suffering, and by the quickest means. Self-torture, even on a scale smaller than originally planned, deceives it for a time.

Sometimes, however, the superego, not satisfied for long with its "bargain," demands new and harsher terms. Clinical experience proves that inner defenses frequently lose their effectiveness and have to be replaced; also that the successive substitute crimes presented as bribes by the ego are increasingly self-damaging.

Rule 18. The simpler the trap, the greater the triumph. Mere torture, it seems, does not fully satisfy the superego. A brutal teaser, it frequently compounds suffering with an added ironic twist. The more primitive the trick, the better; after an unconsciously self-provoked defeat the ego increases its self-torture, whittling away at its narcissism: "How could I have been so stupid?" Sometimes the superego gets its way like a gangster by brandishing a gun that turns out after all to be only a disguised—cigarette lighter.

Rule 19. Encouragement of "repetitive mistakes." One of the unassailable platitudes concerns the illusion of learning from experience. When an unconscious pattern becomes dominant in a personality the same "mistake" is bound to recur again and again, apparently a victory for the specific set of stabilized defenses covering twice-filtered innuendos of unconscious wishes. But there is more to it.

The pattern of error is also licensed by silent consent of the superego, which encourages the victim to plunge once more into the same disastrous situation. Responding to the bribe of guaranteed suffering, the superego profits at the same time from a specific devaluation of conscious reasoning, overvalued by the victim, and from his humiliation at having failed to learn by experience, tellingly demonstrated by the foreseeable defeat.

Rule 20. The ego forced to supply the cathexis for its own torture. One of the typical ironic turns of the superego is a modification of the old, sadistic technique of making the naughty child go and fetch the switch. Here is the internal situation: the ego provides the cathexis for self-torture. This is indirectly visible in all defense mechanisms and directly observable in the torture of "first thoughts after awakening." These half-formulated, painful imaginings, including previews of the disagreeable events and duties of the day and possible dangers, present themselves as "bloodless schemes" lacking impetus and are put into full operation only secondarily by ego cathexis.[4]

Rule 21. The inner-torture principle makes neurosis a progressive, not a self-limiting disease. In the course of time even substitute defenses wear out, and the standard quota of self-torture is no longer enough. The self-torture, specifically, is psychic masochism. It was the component of self-torture in psychic masochism that originally led the superego to accept it, the inherent defensive purpose being a necessary concession in so good a bargain. Only later, and "behind the superego's back," is self-torture made pleasurable. An equivalent situation would be that of a jailer in a totalitarian prison confronted with a prisoner who spares him the trouble of torture by banging his

The Crucial Question in Psychoanalytic Therapy 41

own head against the wall. What if the jailer discovers that the "model" prisoner enjoys torture? The superego, the inner jailer, does in time discover that in the pleasure-in-displeasure pattern self-torture does not mean punishment. The ego can then appease it only by more frequent and more convincing alibis. As a result the "mistakes" made in later life are more far-reaching than those of earlier years. To prove innocence the psychic masochist takes greater risks and intensifies his provocations; his external defeats are accordingly intensified.

It would be erroneous to assume that all rebounding infantile aggression is changed into psychic masochism. To be exact, it is *divided into four parts:* one part accumulates in the *daimonion,* one is changed into *psychic masochism,* one is projected, and one, retained in its *original form, is the ego.* The varying distribution of that aggression determines the fate of the individual. The more neurotic the person is, the greater the shares of daimonion and masochism and the smaller the "normal" share of the ego.

The next step is that the superego begins to suspect the ingenious way the unconscious ego neutralizes punishment by shortchanging it into unconscious pleasure. This, in turn, leads to new defensive efforts of the poor ego, forcing it to progress from the genetic picture (see p. 18) and to create the *clinical picture in psychic masochism* (see p. 253). I was the first to describe the technique of this change. With train-schedule regularity, this happens:

1. Through their behavior, or the misuse of an external situation, neurotics unconsciously provoke disappointment, refusal, humiliation; they identify the outer world with the "refusing" pre-oedipal mother.

2. Repressing their initial provocation, they become *pseudo*aggressive, acting in righteous indignation and seemingly in self-defense.

3. Having received the rebuff or the retaliation unconsciously sought, they retire into the lachrymal corner, consciously indulging in endless self-pity of the "this can happen only to poor little me" variety, while their original masochistic capital yields compound interest.

The psychic masochist is one of the few mortals who can have his cake and eat it too. His real wish is to maintain the masochistic position—a difficult business, taking into consideration the savage objections of his inner conscience; the latter considers psychic masochism the "crime of crimes." To silence these objections (without sacrificing the masochistic solution) he presents himself as *the innocent victim of outside malice,* which he fights with a spurious show of aggression (pseudoaggression). Since his defensive battles are a sham he always loses, cashing in on secondary masochistic interests.

In its end effects the psychic masochist's life is a "rat race" for ever-increasing stakes in order to "prove" to the superego that he does not enjoy his self-created defeats. The greater the external self-damage, the better the alibying argument: "You can't accuse me of wanting that!" Better alibis but also greater self-damage and conscious misery.

The child's further development is influenced by two parallel processes: he discovers and has to deal with new experiences on higher levels (anal, urethral, phallic), and at the same time he is confronted with the "infiltration technique" of his ever-ready and ever-present psychic masochism. What it actually amounts to is that oral-masochistic experiences, and the defenses against them, are "reformulated" in the language of higher levels of development.

The connecting link between the oral phase and the succeeding phases is the feeling of being *passively victimized.* The child's life begins in complete dependence on his mother, and in his helplessness not only are her ministrations for his welfare misconstrued as acts of aggression but even the natural functions of his body are perceived by him as manifestations of some irresistible and malevolent force. His fantastic misconceptions, clearly shown in the septet of baby fears, are all the result of passive experiences, in which he feels himself a victim. Against his enforced surrender, in which, above all, his fantasy of omnipotence is constantly endangered by reality, aggressive and libidinous counter-devices are set in motion. This is the beginning of a continuous and desperate attempt to escape from passivity.

As the child grows older he gradually admits his mother's generosity and kindness, but without losing his fears or his resentment of her "cruelty." This recognition, however, which should lessen his conflict, only serves to increase it. His problem is now that of ambivalence, with friendly and inimical feelings for the same person at the same time battling within him, obviously an extremely disturbing situation.

The anal phase duplicates the passive oral experiences, with the addition of pseudoaggressive defenses. The child again feels overwhelmed by something more powerful than himself, which "drains" him and forces him to expel "parts of his body." His terror is only slightly lessened by the accompanying "anal elimination pleasure." The parallel is obvious with the earlier passive victimization in which his mouth was "pierced" by the nipple, an indignity only slightly mitigated by the libidinous gratification of sucking. The child's countermeasure on the anal level is the device of retention, which has aggressive connotations, strengthened later on by his realization that anal "stubbornness" is a way of infuriating his mother. In the late stages of his struggle against the passivity of being "drained" a defense is instituted: "I'm not drained at all; *I* produce the feces of my own free will; I like doing it and want to play with it." This defense, acted out, to the horror of adults, is also the basis for the unconscious fantasy of the "anal penis," an autarchic attempt to negate the dependence on the breast, and later on the paternal penis. In spite of pseudoaggressive defenses the anal opening, like the oral aperture, retains sizeable deposits of passivity.

The combination of fear and ambivalence in the pre-oedipal levels makes the child's situation unbearably difficult, and it is this that pushes him, at the age of one and a half or two, into the oedipal phase. The fight against, and the allurement of, passivity continue on this level too. In the Oedipus complex the active tendencies of the boy achieve a triumphant retaliation against the frightening "witch" of his babyhood by reducing her to his own former state of helplessness. The boy identifies with his father, wants to usurp his place and do all the "forbidden" things he imagines his father does with his mother; he "hates" his father as competitor and "loves" his mother. The Oedipus complex is frequently misunderstood to mean *only* that the boy desires his mother sexually, entirely disregarding the prehistory suffused with terror and massive passivity. Actually the boy's identification with his father's "cruelty" has one major purpose: to counteract passivity by demoting the giantess.[5] Thus, the oedipal phase is but a "rescue station" from unbearable pre-oedipal fears.

As we know from Freud, there exists also a negative, or inverted, Oedipus, in which the boy identifies with the oedipal mother, now overthrown as ruler of the nursery, and wants to replace her in his father's affections and to be sexually "mistreated" by him as he imagines his mother is (the pressure of castration fear is also a motive here). The negative Oedipus continues the history of enforced passivity and useless countermeasures that characterize all phases of the child's early development, just as the positive Oedipus represents one of the desperate attempts at rescue from that passivity via the tour de force of enhanced aggression.

Summarizing, one can state that there are passive defeats and aggressive countermeasures at all three genetic levels:

On the *oral* level, passive experiences include: fantasies of being pierced by breast (bottle); the aggressive countermeasures include: grasping breast (bottle), crying, spitting, vomiting.

On the *anal* level, passive experiences are connected with the fantasy of being pierced by feces; the corresponding aggressive countermeasures are fantasies of aggressive and autarchic use of feces.

On the *phallic* level, passivity is represented by feminine identification in the boy ("negative Oedipus"), and the aggressive countermeasure subsumed in masculine identification ("positive Oedipus").

The foregoing has been set forth in my previous books and studies, published during a quarter century. What is new and unpublished and of most recent origin is my conclusion that there exist *two forms of psychic masochism* which—though externally they may look alike—are completely different.

These two types of psychic masochism are the *"neurotic"* variety and the *"malignant"* variety.

The neurotic variety has been described above in the genetic and clinical pictures. In its end effects neurotic psychic masochism leads to humiliation, defeat, failure—unconsciously self-provoked, self-chosen, self-perpetuated.

Very much in contradistinction to the relatively "harmless" neurotic psychic masochism encountered in so-called normal as well as in neurotic people, "malignant" psychic masochism, visible in schizoid and schizophrenic personalities, entirely loses the quality of an amiable "game."

I agree with the prevailing opinion that schizophrenic and borderline cases (schizoid) have a—so far—unknown organic basis. This does not exclude a strong psychological overlay; only the latter is discussed here.

It is generally acknowledged that the most striking phenomenon in schizoid-schizophrenic personalities (whatever the superficial camouflage) is the dissociation of affect and thought (verbal expression or thought). Apparently something is missing: appropriateness, congruity, and fear of consequences. A schizoid patient discussed with me his plan to kill me as "an experiment." Knowing that the act would lead him to the electric chair, he was curious about the feelings (if any) he would have on the way from the death cell to the execution chamber. Observing himself while talking about this pleasant prospect, he confirmed the idea that he was "a cold fish"; no conscious fear appeared. The question arises: *where is the normal, protective fear in these people?*

I believe that these sick people are so "scared to death" of *one* specific feeling—their "malignant" brand of masochism—that they repress both it and all other feelings, including their deep terrors from the "septet of baby fears." *Inwardly* they are filled with those fears.

The absence of a warning signal of protective external fear is what makes their actions so unpredictable. They are capable of a sudden, unexpected outburst of murderous rage, or of suicide.

The decisive point seems to be that these schizoids live on the basis of a denial of their deep, terrifying, "malignant" masochism. This denial consists of coldness and pseudoaggression. Since protective external fear plays a key role in the avoidance of socially dangerous actions, the *primum movens* appears to be the necessity to furnish the specific defense.

Behind the defense of pseudoaggression (pseudo because it damages the ego and is just a vehicle for masochism) lies a truly overdimensional "malignant" masochism with paranoid connotations. The basic inner fear in malignant masochism seems to be directed against *the dread of being manipulated in complete helplessness by the giantess of the nursery*—a "something" the child later knows as "Mother." As adults, in the transference, these patients are highly suspicious; they are perpetually "discovering" some underhand trick. It is an amazing fact that the *transference repetitions,* though they do occur, *do not change anything.* The exact opposite happens in the treatment of neurotics, where changes take place when transference repetitions are explained and worked through. With schizoid patients the explanations are received with incredulity, and the aftermath is retirement to their inner "frozen fears." Consciously they show only ironic disbelief. In short, the deep "frozen fears" cannot be brought to the surface—at least in most cases.

One sometimes gathers the impression that the infantile megalomania of these people was so severely hit that the usual defense—neurotic psychic masochism—proved an insufficient shield. It is true that every neurotic psychic-masochistic action contains innuendos that ward off the fear of being passively manipulated by the mother. When the neurotic masochist provokes and finally achieves his desired defeat he unconsciously consoles himself with a trickle of megalomaniacal satisfaction: "That fellow thinks he kicked me, but he's wrong; *I,* by my provocation, *made him* kick me!" This defense seems to suffice in neurotic cases. Not so with the schizoids; *they hold on to the masochistic and provocative pseudoaggressive solution because in itself it is an active defense against a deeper danger, the total and absolute helplessness of being totally and absolutely manipulated by the mother. They cannot give up their "active" masochistic provoking defense because behind it lurks passivity of the near-catatonic type—exactly what I suggest calling "malignant" masochism.* Thus neurotic psychic masochism, with its pseudoaggressive antics, is already defensive.

I would not be surprised if future research sustained the suspicion that the *psychological* substratum of the various catatonic states is the ultimate unconscious, masochistic "joke" at the expense of the giantess of the nursery: "She wants me to be totally passive and subservient —an automaton!—and I am such an automaton! See what Mother did to me!"

Though neurotic and malignant-schizoid psychic masochism may look alike superficially, inwardly the two types are highly dissimilar.

We know from clinical experience that in the overwhelming majority of cases psychiatric and psychoanalytic treatment cannot "cure" a schizoid personality. (The exceptions are cases with very strong neurotic admixtures.) By some kind of protracted "guidance" we can—at least for a time—prevent many external troubles, provided the patient's family is willing to understand, to foot the bills, and to keep a good lawyer on call.

There are three reasons for the therapeutic inaccessibility of schizoid people. *The transference repetitions are ineffective; the absence of automatic preventive external fear leads to fantastic external self-damage; neurotic psychic masochism is indefinitely maintained because it represents in schizoids a shield and a pseudo-active defense against the deepest "malignant" masochism of pseudocatatonic type.* That triad accounts for therapeutic failure. The weightiest of the three reasons is the last; this point gives the schizoid the inner pseudo-aggressive illusion, "Instead of being passively manipulated by Mother, I actively manipulate her!"

Some schizoid personalities are recognizable by the experienced psychiatrist in a few minutes; some are unrecognizable even by the most experienced after months of treatment. Sometimes only the *negative reaction to therapy* gives the clue.

Schizoid personalities—a semantic battle royal is fought in the literature: "pseudoneurotic" (Hoch), "ambulatory schizophrenic" (Zilboorg), "latent schizophrenic" (Bychowski), etc.—can be subdivided phenomenologically into these groups:

(1) the undetected pseudoneurotic, later proving himself a schizoid personality;

(2) the cold, detached type;

(3) the "emotionally dead" personality constantly on the search for "sensation";

(4) the jovial, temporarily overenthusiastic variety;

(5) the seeming hypochondriac and worrier over "superficial," banal fears;

(6) the "petering out" type—all interests and professional endeavors end in lack of continuity, lack of perseverance, and quick change-over to another "interest," just as quickly abandoned;

(7) the megalomaniacal type—credit for future achievement is self-bestowed without corresponding hard work, reality and anticipatory fantasy are equated;

(8) the "psychopath," with or without criminal involvement.

It is obvious that transitions and different combinations occur in the actual clinical pictures.

The decisive point with these schizoids is the fact that *they cannot live without their constant pseudoaggressions*. In previous publications I have described the "empty bag" type of neurotic. This is a person, as I believed at one time,[6] "whose ego is so weak and empty that, bereft of its typical pseudoaggressive defense, it has nothing to offer and is incapable of finding a substitute." Later I described the case history of such a patient with "middle-age revolt,"[7] summarized here:

"A successful and solid advertising man" (his own estimate of himself), aged forty-nine, requested psychiatric help in solving a "messy situation—the old story of the man between two women." Business was O. K., he told me, ulcers included—at least they were golden ulcers. The two women were his "nagging, critical, and complaining" wife, to whom he had been married for twenty-four years, and a girl in his office. He wanted, he said, to marry the girl.

He undertook analysis ostensibly in the hope that it would remove his compunctions about divorcing his wife. It was weeks before his real reason came to light: he had heard that no vital decisions could be made during analysis, and he was using it as an excuse with his girl friend to postpone his problem.

His behavior was courteous and distant; he was constantly on his guard. When I gave him my impression that his cautious hyperpoliteness covered fear, his answer was, "I'm a polite person by nature. Are good manners suspect as a neurotic symptom?" When it was pointed out that his attitude towards me seemed to be a repetition of a childhood attitude in which he used detachment, coldness, and

The Crucial Question in Psychoanalytic Therapy 49

reticence as weapons against his "rather disagreeable, nagging" mother, he was politely incredulous.

This patient's technique was that of spurious stupidity in order to fend off *real* analysis. He refused to accept the idea of unconscious determinants in himself. At the same time he gradually came to the somewhat painful conscious realization that his actions in life were by no means as sensible as he maintained, with a certain mechanical grasp of the explanations presented. But his distrust continued:

"How can I help being suspicious of you when I feel that the whole deduction is only a trick to make me see that my relationship with my wife is a repetition also? You're luring me into dangerous territory."

Repeated interpretations—involving his *unconscious* wish to be mistreated by a governess (he had accepted this description of his wife's attitude with real enthusiasm) and his *conscious* complaints about such treatment, the inner guilt provoked by the repetition of his unconscious pattern and the wish for love and affection set up as an inner defense against this guilt—achieved nothing more than shocked disbelief.

The only change in him was that he now seemed to be obsessed with what he called his "mounting tensions," produced by his wife's "demanding and reproachful attitude," of which he gave many examples. For a while his mother became his scapegoat. These complaints continued, in spite of my warning that complaining would get him nowhere in analysis. To all interpretations his reaction was:

"Once more I'm responsible. Just pile it on me!"

"Not you but your unconscious elaboration."

"Mounting tensions" and furious but ineffective complaints were his guiding pattern. He was so absorbed in his mounting tensions that it was impossible to focus his attention on anything else. One could not avoid the impression that none of the knowledge acquired in analysis penetrated below the surface of his mind. He used analytic terminology, describing pre-analytic conflicts in analytic language, but it remained an intellectual, not an affective experience. I warned him:

"You just repeat the approximate words I have used, like a parrot. That's ineffective *lip service, not living reality.* If you continue to intellectualize you will remain faithful to the pleasure-in-displeasure pattern to the end of your days."

During the few weeks that followed this warning the patient's attitude towards me changed. He professed to like me and to regret his previous distrust. Of course this was just another means of avoiding the real issue, as I told him.

Then an interesting incident revealed his true feelings. At a party he met an old acquaintance, a millionaire with an ulcer of long standing. "When he complained to me I told him he needed an analysis; I even recommended you; he was scared; of course I had to admit that analysis is painful. But I told him it was worth while going through the aggravations of his symptoms that could arise during treatment because the total effect would be favorable."

I explained his pseudoaggressive action to him:

"Under the guise of helping your ulcer-ridden acquaintance and sending me a patient you teased both of us. I call it collecting ill will behind the mask of a good Samaritan."

The acquaintance was an important manufacturer and a possible advertising account, and the incident left the patient uneasy. He met the man a few days later and was given the cold treatment. I took this opportunity to point out the dangers of pseudoaggression, the cover for self-damaging tendencies:

"May I remind you that your alibi of *pseudo*—love for your girl friend is set up as a defense when your inner conscience accuses you of really wanting the seat behind the domestic eight ball. Your *pseudo*-aggression is a perfect parallel. To prove that you are not a passive weakling you maliciously play one person off against another. And it doesn't change anything. You are still being kicked, under the guise of doing the kicking yourself. Here is another proof that only masochism is solid in you."

My earlier impression returned: emotionally little or nothing had been achieved with this patient. He had the ability to throw off "disagreeable experiences" and behave as if nothing had happened. Some time later I told him:

"Take stock of your situation. Your monotonous story of *mounting tensions (masochistic tensions),* and I would add the monotonous defenses of *mounting pseudoaggressions,* seems to absorb all your

The Crucial Question in Psychoanalytic Therapy 51

inner energy. You act as if you were inwardly a balloon that would shrink and hang limp if these two ingredients were removed. If this suspicion is confirmed nothing can help you. You will solve neither your marital nor your emotional conflicts. Ask yourself whether your ego is really so completely stripped of any other contents."

It seems that schizoid people are the victims of a vicious circle based on their own defenses: having to repress their deepest masochistic fears of being "manipulated" by the ogre-mother of their baby fantasies, they unconsciously *lose the beneficial results of protective external fear*. Obviously they cannot have it both ways.

It has been said of schizoids that their threshold of fear is low. This statement pertains exclusively to their inner fears. For example, the patient with the "olive" dream reported on page 28, to whom I am indebted for having understood the basis of "malignant" masochism, was consciously not afraid of the dangers of arrest for his homosexual activities. When this danger was pointed out to him and he was shown that by frequenting a certain place he was courting arrest, he admitted the danger but said, "In such situations I *know* the danger, but I feel no fear. What am I to do? Am I to *imagine* how a normal fellow experiences fear?"

Attempts have been made to draw conclusions from the sex life of schizoids. In my experience this leads nowhere; the broad variety encountered ends only in blind alleys. Superficially almost every possibility is observable—from apparently normal performance to every form of impotence and frigidity, to homosexuality. It is true that if the masturbation fantasies are probed, very strong masochistic (or defensively pseudosadistic) components are found (beating fantasies).

Most of the difficulties of the schizoids are based on their defenses against malignant masochism. Their pseudoaggressions are the outward manifestations of their necessity to fight against "being manipulated" by the mother image. How easy it is to misunderstand that need is visible in this statement of otherwise excellent observers:

> The patient maintains a distance from reality, using the activity or person as a cushion—or as a convoy. Social, sexual, intellec-

tual, or aggressive activities may be involved. In those who feel apathetic, dead, or nonfunctioning, there is a tendency to reinforce emotional feeling, in order to feel more alive and functioning. *This may lead to provocative behavior and a display of aggression,* which often results in the other person retaliating in kind. For instance, one woman feels dead and empty, so she becomes aggressive and starts a quarrel, and others in her household respond accordingly. This makes for a difficult domestic situation, but it has given her the feeling of *being alive* for half an hour. (Paul H. Hoch and James P. Cattell, "The Diagnosis of Pseudoneurotic Schizophrenia." *The Psychiatric Quarterly,* 1959, pp. 18-43. The quotation is on page 34. Italics are mine.)

This "provocative behavior" is more than the attempt to live vicariously or "be alive." It is an integral part of existing at all— via unchangeable pseudoaggressions covering "malignant" masochism.

"Incurable neurotics" are mostly schizoid personalities detected too late. For practical purposes two groups can be distinguished among the "too late detected." One comprises those whose neurotic admixtures are extensive (in any case extensive enough to produce the mirage of neurosis), who make progress in analysis and after a few short years relapse into their old difficulties. They become the worst propagandists against their analysts, who, because of medical secrecy, cannot open their mouths.

The other group is made up of those who are totally resistant to the treatment from the start, barricaded behind a banal "neurotic" difficulty. The latter is tenaciously adhered to because it hides the schizoid totality. Here too the analyst is blamed as incompetent, if not a faker or charlatan.

Externally both types are bizarre because of their unchangeable pseudoaggression.

Should schizoid people whose diagnosis has been established before treatment starts be treated analytically? Definitely yes. But the aim of treatment is different: we cannot help them (as we can neurotic cases), but by some kind of "guiding, explanatory supervision" we can prevent them (frequently though not always) from getting into too extensive trouble. This presupposes three conditions: first a

The Crucial Question in Psychoanalytic Therapy

moneyed family with understanding of the real facts; second, willingness on the part of the psychotherapist to take the blame (before ignorant outsiders) of not having "cured" the patient "despite years of treatment"; third, collaboration with a lawyer versed in psychiatric facts, to be employed in the unavoidable entanglements the patient gets himself into with outsiders.

A special problem in the analyst's difficulties with schizoids is their inability to do sustained work. Frequently it is less expensive for the family to support them without insistence on work—their business ventures, masochistically conducted, are too costly.

On the lower level of income, where the schizoid has to support himself, he amounts to little and at best does mechanical, subordinate work.

There exists a curious parallel with the early years of analysis. In Freud's ON THE HISTORY OF THE PSYCHOANALYTICAL MOVEMENT this incident is recorded:

> A year later I had begun my medical career in Vienna as a lecturer in nervous diseases, and in everything relating to the etiology of neuroses I was still as ignorant and innocent as one could expect of a promising student trained at the University. One day I had a friendly message from Chrobak (the gynecologist at the University, perhaps the most eminent of all our Vienna physicians), asking me to take over a woman patient to whom he could not devote enough time, owing to his new appointment as professor and teacher at the University. I arrived at the patient's house before he did and found that she was suffering from attacks of meaningless anxiety, and could only be soothed by the most precise information about the whereabouts of her physician at every moment of the day. When Chrobak arrived, he took me aside and told me that the patient's anxiety was due to the fact that, although she had been married for years, she was still a virgin. The husband was absolutely impotent. In such cases, Chrobak said, there was nothing for a physician to do but to shield this domestic calamity with his own reputation, and put up with the reproach when people shrugged their shoulders and said of him, "He's no good if he cannot cure her after so many years." The only possible pre-

scription for such a disease, he added, is familiar enough to us, but we cannot order it. It runs:

> "℞ Penis normalis
> repetatur dosim"

(The prescription ordered: "A normal penis, plus repetition of the prescription.")
I had never heard of such a prescription, and felt inclined to shake my head over my benefactor's cynicism.

In the Victorian eighties the dark secret, to be kept at all costs, was impotence and frigidity. Today people are less reticent about sexual matters. Today's dark secret is—the patient's schizoid personality. Though the contents have changed, the physician must, by being silent, take the same blame before outsiders that Freud referred to: "He's no good if he cannot cure her (him) after so many years." Regrettable but true.

To return to neurotic cases, what happens if a masochistically regressed neurotic patient is given in analysis only interpretations pertaining to the defensive, "escape" layers, his pseudoaggression accepted as genuine aggression, his self-damage explained as guilt for repressed aggression, his masochistic "wish to be refused" misconstrued as the defensive ruse he inwardly tries to present—a parasitic "wish to get"—, his pre-oedipal regression seen as oedipal?
The answer is simple: the patient cannot be cured.
The Oedipus complex is discernible in *every* human being of our culture, hence can be demonstrated in *every* analysis. The problem is whether it is dynamically the reason for the specific neurosis, or—as in deeper neuroses—only a camouflage for the deeper layers.
Still, some improvements are achieved with superficial, even patently wrong interpretations. How is this possible?
Here a mechanism that I have suggested calling *"success because of unconscious fear"* enters the picture.
As this mechanism operates, the patient projects his own fantasies of omnipotence upon the analyst in the transference neurosis. He then sees the analyst as both all-powerful and all-knowing. Since this is the role the analyst plays in the patient's unconscious fantasy

the patient concedes that he will undoubtedly penetrate his "deepest" secrets. Although the patient is often far wide of the mark, he is frightened by his own inner prediction and "lightens ship," in other words, gives up a symptom in order to safeguard the basis of his neurosis.

Unfortunately such successes are short-lived. They resemble the story of the employee who had been for some time successfully stealing money from his boss's cash register. One morning the young man came to work looking tired and dissipated. His employer jokingly remarked on his evident enjoyment of night life and added, "You look pretty pale to me." Seeing this innocent remark as a hint that his theft had been discovered, the young man stopped stealing —for a time, till he found out that the boss was still ignorant of the theft. The point of the story is that the man stopped stealing only for a time, meaning that a mechanism of renunciation constructed *ad hoc* has no permanency.

These peculiar, short-lived, overnight "changes," so unlike the typical ups and downs of a painstaking and honest analytic success, are also characterized by the absence of any congruity with the material worked through in that specific phase of analysis. In short, they represent a preventive mechanism prompted by fear. Sooner or later the fear abates and the symptom recurs.

One cannot exactly claim that these pseudo successes can be confidently expected; nor, if they eventuate, can they be considered creditable analytic achievements. Their dubious value is thrown into even higher relief when one takes into account my impression that the vast majority of neurotics have a rendezvous with undigested orality.

CHAPTER 2

WHAT IS BEHIND THE CONTROVERSY OVER THE ALLEGED EXAGGERATED EMPHASIS ON PSYCHIC MASOCHISM?

IT is a recorded fact that the sequence of the analytic discoveries made by Freud is the exact opposite of the sequence of the "layers" and "stages" the child passes through in the course of his development. According to Freud, the child goes through the oral, anal, and phallic stages in just this order, whereas Freud's studies began with the phallic stage, progressed to the anal stage, and dealt with the oral stage last, in a rather sporadic and tangential way. Thus the analytic "geology" is slightly confusing, simply because the layers discovered first were more thoroughly stressed and had more "novelty" value than the "addenda." Unfortunately the deeper layers are dynamically more decisive than the superficial ones, especially since the more superficial only express in a new language the contents of the deeper layers.

One cannot prescribe to a psychological genius, which Freud undoubtedly was, the sequence of his discoveries. But one can state that the sequence he followed has produced among his pupils and generations of pupils of pupils a perpetual and perpetuated predilection for the superficial layers and a certain aversion and "footnote" attitude towards the deeper layers.

With all due respect for the historical facts in the development of our science, the pyramid must be set up as it belongs: basis on the bottom, apex on top, and not the other way around.

For decades after Freud began his brilliant observations on hys-

Emphasis on Psychic Masochism 57

terical (phallic) neurotics the Oedipus complex was the whole of analysis. Moreover, since the libidinous tendencies in the unconscious were discovered first, libido has been granted a preponderance out of proportion to its importance as apparently the sole motivating force. It is true that Freud later supplemented his genetic scheme by accepting aggressive tendencies as full partners in the unconscious, but many of his adherents still have, as its originator had, a sentimental affinity for libido. One sometimes has the impression that some colleagues treat everything "beyond Oedipus and libido" as unwelcome and bothersome intruders.

There are two difficulties involved in the unwillingness to acknowledge the vital importance of psychic masochism for the psychic economy. The first is an emotional problem in the analyst: the ability to see psychic masochism in the patient presupposes that one's own masochism has been thoroughly "aired" in one's own analysis and (at least partially) made ineffective. Since in most cases psychic masochism is not given the distinction of being analyzed, the analyst who did not hear of it in his own analysis does not transmit knowledge of it to his patients either. It is more than oversight; there is a deep emotional resistance of not wanting to see the *too* painful in oneself. Psychoanalysts are not exempt from the general trends in human nature.

Of course self-damaging tendencies in neurosis are so universal that no analyst can entirely ignore those. Here the second difficulty referred to above comes into play: the closeness of psychic masochism to inner guilt because of repressed aggression. Psychic masochism and guilt are by no means identical; psychic masochism is guilt *plus*. The *plus* is secondary libidinization of guilt. Since the genetic formula for psychic masochism consists of three closely related parts (aggression—rebounding against the ego, because of helplessness and guilt—secondary libidinization of guilt), the analyst can easily convince himself that when he analyzes guilt because of repressed aggression he also analyzes masochism.

We can call on an unimpeachable witness, Freud. Freud had originally approved the interpretation of a dream reported by the Dutch analyst Staercke, in which the dreamer saw a syphilitic chancre on the last phalanx of one of his fingers. As the German term for a primary syphilitic lesion is "Primaeraffect," Staercke concluded that an allusion to "prima affectio," first love, was meant. Freud revised his opinion by stating: "Another motive of opposite wish dreams lies so near that one easily runs the risk of overlooking it, *as had happened to me for a longer period of time . . . ,* the masochistic component." (GESAMMELTE SCHRIFTEN, III, p. 30; my italics.)

Numerous rearguard actions are recorded in our literature in the form of theories, all trying—as I put it in previous publications—to make a boa constrictor into a harmless pet. In PRINCIPLES OF SELF-DAMAGE I quoted, as a caution against "pet theories" on psychic masochism, a pertinent statement of G. K. Chesterton's: "If a man proves too clearly and convincingly to himself that a tiger is an optical illusion—well, he will find out he is wrong. The tiger will himself intervene in the discussion in a manner which will be in every sense conclusive."

The conclusive proof is the scores of analytic ex-patients who have been through protracted analyses with their psychic masochism unanalyzed and intact. One cannot call these people cured. The only result is that analysis gets a black eye; observers state that these patients are just as neurotic as before, though they themselves seem to harbor some illusions. Such illusions are frequently based on unconscious gratitude to their analysts for having left their basic problem untouched.

In some cases the patient's problem cannot be "solved" (even superficially) without analyzing masochism. These are the chronic analytic "wanderers," who travel from one analyst to another till they find one who does not overlook the masochistic scourge and cures them. I reported on many such cases in my recent books PRINCIPLES OF SELF-DAMAGE and HOMOSEXUALITY: DISEASE OR WAY OF LIFE?

Many analysts are so angry about the emphasis put on psychic masochism that the objection has been voiced that everything is neglected by me except my masochistic hobby horse. I have given my answer in THE SUPEREGO:

> Analysis of psychic masochism does *not* tend to invalidate the established rules of analysis (analysis of transference and resistance, use of free associations, analysis of dreams, "working

through," connecting "actual" conflicts with the repressed past, etc.). It merely adds another component (pp. 47-48).

Thoreau's statement is, unfortunately, quite accurate: "For telling the truth two people are necessary: one who tells it and another who listens."

The whole problem is intimately connected with another offense against analytic complacency of the "my learning days are over" variety: *the role of aggression in neurosis.* In my opinion the neurotic does not possess in his NEUROTIC sector any real aggression; what he displays is only PSEUDOaggression, covering psychic masochism. When the analyst follows the patient's unconscious lead, acknowledging his pseudoaggression as real aggression, he fosters the continuation of neurosis and acts about as wisely as a detective who follows false clues planted by the malefactor. The differences between normal and neurotic aggression are these:

1. Self-defense or pre-fabricated pattern?
   Normal aggression, is used only as self-defense Neurotic aggression (*"pseudoaggression"*) used indiscriminately when an infantile pattern is repeated with an innocent outsider.
2. Real or self-created enemy?
   In normal aggression, the object of aggression is a real enemy. In pseudoaggression, the object of aggression is a product of fantasy or an artificially created enemy (via provocation).
3. Presence or absence of unconscious guilt?
   In normal aggression, there is no accompanying unconscious feeling of guilt. In pseudoaggression, unconscious guilt is always present.
4. Discrepancy between provocation and counter-aggression?
   In normal aggression, the amount of aggression discharged corresponds to the provocation. In pseudoaggression, the "dose" of counter-aggression is paradoxical: the slightest provocation is answered with exorbitant pseudoaggression.
5. Inner intention of harming the enemy or oneself?
   Normal aggression is used to harm the enemy. In pseudoaggression, the procedure is often used to provoke "masochistic pleasure," unconsciously expected from the enemy's retaliation.

6. Waiting for the propitious moment possible or impossible?
   In normal aggression, the timing is rational: ability to wait until the enemy is vulnerable. In contradistinction, the timing in pseudo-aggression is faulty: inability to wait, since pseudo-aggression is used as inner defense mechanism against the reproach of the superego pertaining to psychic masochism.
7. Easy or difficult to provoke?
   The more normal person is not easily provoked; the neurotic is very easily provoked.
8. Presence or absence of masochistic excitement?
   In normal aggression, the element of infantile "game" is absent; no combination with masochistic-pseudo-sadistic unconscious fantasies discernible; the prevailing feeling is that a necessary though disagreeable job has to be performed. Quite the opposite can be analytically proved in pseudo-aggression: the element of infantile "game" unconsciously very much in evidence; that is combined with masochistic-pseudo-sadistic excitement, usually repressed.
9. Success or defeat sought?
   In normalcy, success is expected—consciously and unconsciously. In neurosis, unconsciously defeat is expected, though consciously the "best intentions" are asserted.

No less grotesque is the situation when orally based parasitism is explained as the "wish to get." Here the confusion lies in confounding the historical past with the clinical present. True enough, the baby was a "gimme." But the adult neurotic has gone through his typical masochistic vicissitudes and becomes masochistically fixated on the masochistic "wish to be refused." Secondarily he uses the wish to get as a defense against the wish to be refused.

To complicate the intricate process of naivete even further, the whole torturing role of the superego is minimized by many colleagues.

I am familiar with the typical objection of conservative colleagues to successes achieved by analyzing and putting in the center the problem of psychic masochism: what is achieved—runs this fal-

Emphasis on Psychic Masochism

lacious argument—is only a "quick transference phenomenon"; this is misunderstood and "exaggerated claims presented."[8] Different epitheta disornantia are attached to the procedure; even honest error is sometimes conceded.

The argument is naive. First of all, not analyzing psychic masochism themselves, these colleagues have obviously no conception what kind of transference one is confronted with when attacking that scourge. The transference phenomena are those of constant "injustice-collecting," hence clearly have nothing to do with the alleged "positive transference." This part of the argument is simply based on talking about things the critics have not checked by personal experience.

But perhaps "negative transference" is alluded to by the critics? Although this is unlikely, that possibility also does not exist clinically. General analytic experience teaches the unmistakable lesson that "negative transference" is not conducive to therapeutic successes on a "quick" basis.

What it practically amounts to is that these colleagues are presented with a new and untried (by them) fact which they cannot explain. In such emergencies old and inapplicable objections are raised.

I can understand the anger of colleagues enmeshed for years in cases of homosexuality or writer's block, severe cases of premature ejaculation, psychogenic oral aspermia, personality distortion, etc., without making any progress with these seemingly hopelessly recalcitrant patients, when they read (usually hear, sometimes even from patients) of my statements that these cases are not only curable but curable in eight to ten months. The resultant fury and indignation may be comical, but it is explainable. Analysts are human too.

All this leads to differences of opinion concerning the three-layer versus the five-layer structure in neurotic symptoms. In my opinion a neurotic symptom does not simply reproduce a defensively camouflaged unconscious wish but constitutes a DEFENSE AGAINST A DEFENSE.

The older, accepted formulation assumed that an unconscious wish (layer I) meeting with a superego veto (layer II) is then cloaked in a defense mechanism (layer III) and appears in consciousness in its new guise and covered by a rationalization. I believe that an unconscious wish can under no circumstances find so direct a path to the surface and emerge so thinly veiled. In my opinion the procedure has a five-layer structure: the inner wish (layer I) is warded off by a superego reproach (layer II), with the result that the unconscious ego institutes a defense (layer III). But this first defense, which invariably consists of changing the original wish to its opposite and in this way admitting performance of what intrapsychically ranks as a "lesser crime," is in its turn warded off by a second superego veto (layer IV), necessitating the creation of a second defense by the unconscious ego. Having pleaded guilty to a minor charge, the unconscious ego offers a denying alibi and accepts punishment for the lesser crime (layer V). Only the reverberations of this second defense (layer V) become visible in the neurotic symptom, sign, personality structure.

This necessitates a re-evaluation of the role of the Oedipus complex. The conclusion Freud came to in the statement he made on this point in 1931 has special significance:

> The pre-oedipal phase of the female reaches an importance which we did not previously attach to it. Since that phase has room for all fixations and repressions, to which we attribute the development of neuroses, it seems necessary to retract the generality of the statement that the Oedipus complex constitutes the kernel of neurosis. "On Female Sexuality," *Internationale Zeitschrift fuer Psychoanalyse,* 17:318, 1931.

Prevailing analytic opinion failed to accept that substructure *de facto* and relegated pre-oedipality to a footnote. But further study has convinced me that the Oedipus complex is exclusively a late "rescue station" from deeper and earlier infantile fears.

As I see it, the child's progression into the oedipal stage is to some extent due to the banal fact that he is learning to "digest" a reality situation; the more important factor, however, is his psychological situation. The father is present and proves to be a powerful contender for the mother's attention and love. Now a "new order" is set up—the triangle of mother, father, and child—supplanting the giantess-and-baby duality of the pre-oedipal phase. In this new situation the boy performs a magnificent tour de force. He manages to *demote the threatening and fear-inspiring "witch" of babyhood from her position of power*. The father is now the "big-shot," and by identifying with the father's strength the boy converts the giantess into a caricature and image of his own frightened and passive self. He now sees the mother as completely dominated by the father. He misconstrues the parents' sexual activity as a cruel act, in which the father is the conquering giant and the mother the passive victim. Identifying with the father's supposed cruelty, the boy finds the once frightening giantess of his infancy to be entirely "weak, passive, helpless," just as he had been in the past. The reversal of roles seems complete; poetic justice has been established via the unconscious repetition compulsion.

For thirty years it has been my gradually developed belief that—with all due regard for the historical reasons responsible for the present-day confusion—a complete overhauling of our thinking concerning the structure of neurosis is necessary.

It is my contention that the first and foremost conflict of the newborn, infant, baby, consists in the fact that he must come to terms with his inborn megalomania. That conflict invariably and without exception results in a masochistic solution, the "pleasure-in-displeasure pattern." This constitutes the "basic neurosis."

Every neurosis dramatizes in an unconscious innuendo—either actively or passively—a libidinous and/or pseudoaggressive denial of some aspect of the masochistic theme "I'm the innocently refused and fearfully mistreated child and have learned to enjoy it." Hence the masochistic pattern, starting in the first months of life and connected with the oral phase, is paramount; it is the universal end result of every infantile conflict, the *"basic neurosis."* The superficial libidinous and/or pseudoaggressive camouflaging conflict constitutes the *"admission of the lesser intrapsychic crime."* To repeat: the psychotherapist who takes the superficial defenses at face value, disregarding, or being uninformed of, the masochistic substructure, acts like the detective who falls for false clues planted by the criminal to confuse him and put him on the wrong track. Without analyzing the basic masochistic substructure the neurotic cannot be changed.

When the patient works through in the transference and resistance situation *both* parts of the problem—the masochistic substructure *and* the piled-up libidinous-pseudoaggressive camouflages—he is forced to make "concessions" to analysis. He is more willing, of course, to renounce the superficial camouflaging layers than the masochistic basis. Hence it is easier for the analyst to be "successful" in removing symptoms than in removing the underlying masochistic personality distortion.

The patient (provided the above-sketched priority list is adhered to) is more likely to allow the therapist to push him out of the *conspicuous* first line of defense—his symptoms—than to let him enter the *inconspicuous* inner fortress, his deep psychic masochism.

It is superfluous to mention that the secondary defenses, imbedded in symptoms, are not chosen by the patient at random. They correspond to very real wishes, secondarily established and inflated out of proportion in order to hide the inner fortress. It is the difference between "my main wish is" and "I also wish."

Two facts emerge. Many patients, having given up the more superficial symptoms, declare themselves "cured" and prevent the adequate analysis of their main—masochistic—trouble. These are the "most grateful" patients—grateful for the remnants of their psychic masochism. This, of course, presupposes that the analyst put "that damned masochism" in the center. This first fact is complemented by a second one, pertaining to cases in which the analyst failed to do exactly that. Having been fooled by the libidinous-pseudoaggressive camouflage and having mistaken the secondary defenses for the "real thing," he will find that the patient may lose his symptoms but not his underlying personality structure, permeated to capacity with psychic masochism. Though the therapist may be ignorant of what is really going on, the patient knows—unconsciously. Hence the host of objectively uncured patients produced by today's analysis.

The irony of the situation is extensive. The analyst believes that he helped the patient, and the patient is grateful for having his masochistic substructure left untouched. This gratitude does not make him any healthier.

One should also stress that masochism permeates the secondary defenses. In a situation of danger—when the analyst works on the libidinous content (the pseudoaggressive content is mostly misunderstood by him as "real aggression," to boot)—the infiltrating masochism is recalled into the "inner fortress." Thus, though the patient may lose a symptom his masochistic balance deteriorates. Sooner or later (rather sooner than later) the underlying psychic masochism plays havoc with his life by finding new, frequently more dangerous, depositions or reverting to the old ones.

Ironically, there are two types of "admission of the lesser intrapsychic crime." The *first type* is included in the libidinous-pseudoaggressive denial of the basic masochistic solution. The *second type* is included in different gradations in the secondary defense (e.g. exhibitionism a lesser crime than voyeurism, etc.).

Accused of overemphasizing psychic masochism, I can only answer that the greatest stress on masochism is still an understatement. It is THE BASIS of all neurotic troubles.

In recent years I have had the gratifying experience of seeing a specific "hopeless" disease, homosexuality,[9] become therapeutically accessible through the application of the theory of psychic masochism.

Ironically enough, homosexuality has little to do with sex proper (at best, it pertains to counterfeit-sex), but it has an intimate connection with psychic masochism.

To state this connection as briefly as possible:

Imagine a man who for some mysterious reason unconsciously wants to be mistreated by a woman, though consciously unaware of this wish. Imagine further that he inwardly fears his own wish but instead of giving up the wish itself gives up its alleged or imagined central figure, woman. Since there are only two sexes, this leaves him only one alternative in his frantic flight, man. Officially, and as a defense against his real inner wish, he turns to man in order to find peace, quiet, love, understanding, safety. But underneath these official aims his real, compelling need remains the need to be mistreated. His retreat to "another continent" does not alter the old, unofficial conflict. Sooner or later he will feel that the man with whom he has sought refuge mistreats him, misunderstands him, is unjust to him, deliberately tortures him by arousing his jealousy. Moreover, his flight in no way affects his sex glands. Since they are still working, it is inevitable that man, his antidote against the feared sex, woman, will secondarily be elevated to the status of a sexual attraction.

The homosexual, in short, is unconsciously a masochistic injustice collector who has shifted the power to mistreat from woman to man.

The personality structure of the injustice collector (psychic masochist) is, of course, not typical for the homosexual. It is the result of an unfavorable *unconscious* solution of a conflict that faces *every* infant, baby, small child when the objective reality of his life clashes with subjective magical notions. But two exaggerations of the universal troublemakers are typical. The homosexual's infantile fears, centered on the mother image, are greater than those of other neurotics and his masochistic elaboration more extensive. The homosexual is not merely an overdimensional psychic masochist but a psychic masochist *plus*. The *plus* consists of:

a) The application of infantile megalomania to the sex organ through the establishment of an autarchy: "I produce everything I need, my penis is the breast, and am independent of any else." But he is not sure of the permanency of his solution, and therefore in later life he looks for a "reduplication of his defense mechanism"; in the sex organ of his partner he recognizes as his own (penis-breast). This accounts for one of the most fantastic elements in the homosexual's pattern, disregard for the body of the partner and concentration on his sex organ, as observable in the impersonal relations taking place in urinals, etc. It also explains the enormously exaggerated narcissism of the homosexual. His megalomania was wounded at a very early age and he couldn't take it. Magically and compensatorily he "restored" and increased it as he grew older.

b) Moreover, the "power to torture" is transferred from the mother-image to—man.

The unconsciously propelled flight from the mother-image leads the homosexual to a quick succession of exchangeable men. In very rare cases of relationships of longer duration the homosexual will misjudge his jealousy, injustice collecting, suffering, as part and parcel of

Emphasis on Psychic Masochism

"love," without understanding the masochistic substructure of the pathological attachment.

A fuller explanation of the early development of the homosexual is included in the case history of Mr. C., pages 105 ff. See also examples in Chapter 5 (Mr. G., Mr. J., Mr. M.).

The pattern of injustice-collecting, with man as an antidote for the fear of women and secondarily elevated to the status of an attraction, is visible in any analytic discussion with a homosexual patient. The following excerpt is from the analysis of a fashion designer.

Analyst: "Time and again we've discussed your quarrels with your boy friends. Weren't they all reducible to one common denominator, 'someone is unjust to you'? And isn't it true, as we established in many of your conflicts, that these 'injustices' were unconsciously self-created?"

Patient: "That's what you claim."

Analyst: "That's what the record shows. Take your present friend as example. You told me that you met him at a party where he flirted with you; another friend warned you that he was promiscuous to the nth degree. You yourself observed this too. Still, you chose to have exactly this unreliable person for your friend. You go into tantrums every time the boy runs around with someone else. What reason did you have to assume that this psychopath was good material for a steady affair?"

Patient: "Everybody can make an error in judgment."

Analyst: "Make an error in judgment again and again? When this happens, the error is obviously part of a pattern, repeated *ad nauseam*."

The personality of the homosexual is a mixture of the following elements:

(1) masochistic provocation and injustice-collecting;

(2) defensive malice;

(3) flippancy covering depression and guilt;

(4) hypernarcissism and hypersuperciliousness;

(5) refusal to acknowledge accepted standards in non-sexual matters, on the assumption that the right to cut moral corners is due to him in compensation for his "suffering";

(6) general unreliability, also of a more or less psychopathic nature.

The most interesting feature of these traits is their universality. Regardless of the level of intelligence, culture, background, education, all homosexuals have them.

When confronted with the facts of injustice-collecting and self-damage implicit in their behavior, homosexuals react with incredulity, if not fury, and counter with confused misinformation and spurious arguments in defense of their "way of life." An intelligent young homosexual, sent to me by his parents, began by making his attitude crystal-clear.

"I have no intention of changing," he said. "I like my way of life. I'm happy. I promised my parents I would see you, and I have. Can I leave now?"

"Not before you get this information: Homosexuality is invariably connected with severe self-damaging tendencies that are fully unconscious and that must in time show up. You may not be able to see the connection at all, but it can be traced."

"Nonsense."

"Did you ever hear of an X-ray specialist's discovery of the existence of a dangerous internal cancerous growth, even though the patient himself has not yet experienced any symptoms?"

"You can scare children! I know what I want!"

"So you believe. But you are a puppet, and your unconscious is the puppet master."

"Tell that one to the Marines!"

"Provocations don't change facts. Please search in your memories, and tell me if happiness is the only emotion you experience in your homosexual contacts."

"It is!"

"And yet your parents told me that they had overheard telephone conversations in which you repeatedly reproached your assortment of boy friends for infidelity, and so on. Bitterness and jealousy don't make for happiness."

"Those sneaks! Now they've been listening in on the extension!"

"Why not say that you yourself masochistically staged this situation? Making those scenes on the telephone instead of face to face

Emphasis on Psychic Masochism 69

was an invitation to your parents to listen in. You provoked the disclosure yourself. Isn't this a good example of the psychic masochism I'm talking about?"

"I'll just have to move out and live alone."

"At whose expense? Your parents'?"

"To hell with their silly, antiquated notions!"

"These silly, antiquated notions are part of the reality you have to come to terms with. Your parents consider your homosexual perversion exactly as dangerous to you as an addiction to morphine or heroin would be, and they take it for granted that homosexuality, like drug addiction, has to be treated medically. Now you used your indignation over their attitude to sidestep the question I asked you a few minutes ago. Let's get back to it. How can you be so happy in your homosexuality if you are constantly embroiled in jealous or injustice-collecting conflicts with your successive boy friends?"

"Don't heterosexuals ever have lovers' spats?"

"Occasionally, not typically. Nor do they, if they are mature people, live so promiscuously."

"I've read your silly book on homosexuality and can only say that you totally misunderstand us. You don't even see the glamor, the excitement, the vitality that homosexuality promotes!"

"This 'glamor' is nothing but the allure of danger, which feeds your masochism. Objectively there is no more glamor in the disease of homosexuality than there is in a case of any other disease."

"That's ridiculous! And besides, you don't even mention the biological factor of inborn femininity. A homosexual has no choice. Nature made him that way."

"That theory is yellow with age, which wouldn't matter if it didn't contradict elementary logic. How can allegedly inborn femininity be responsible for the masculine homosexual? I will note that you cannot answer this objection. For your information, the biological 'anlage' cannot account for homosexuality simply because of cures in psychoanalytic treatment."

"What about Kinsey's statistics? If a third of all men have had homosexual contacts, how can homosexuality be classed as a perversion?"

"Kinsey's statistics are totally wrong. He mistook his neurotic volunteers to be a cross section of the U.S.A. And, being emotional in his rejection of dynamic psychiatry—and misunderstanding its basic tenets besides—he became the voluntary or involuntary dupe of the highly efficient homosexual propaganda machine.

"But Kinsey or no Kinsey, homosexuality is a disease with ramifications totally unknown to you. You say you don't want to change. Translate that: it means you haven't had enough punishment—so far. Wait till you find yourself faced with a good-sized and inexplicable depression, damage to your professional and social life, the demands of an extortionist, court actions, prospects of jail, venereal disease. The self-damage that is a part of homosexuality doesn't show itself immediately. It is a kind of time bomb, set to go off in a few years."

The clinical picture of homosexuality includes at least a dozen types:

1. *Puberal homosexuality.* Prepuberal and early puberal sex play among boys has always been analytically considered harmless and by no means indicative of future homosexuality. The analytical judgment has been obscured, however, as far as the layman is concerned, since the advent of Kinsey's fantasies on sex, adorned with his selective statistics derived from the statements of neurotic volunteers. These recollections from boyhood formed an important stepping stone to Kinsey's conclusion that homosexuality is widespread and consequently normal. He included these early experiences in the totals making up his estimate of homosexual incidence—without justification and for the purpose of proving what he was out to prove.

2 and 3. *Active and passive roles in full-fledged perversion.* A predilection for one of these roles is discernible in homosexuals, though the roles are occasionally exchanged.

Superficially the combination of active and passive homosexuals constitutes an imitation of the husband-wife relationship. On the *unconscious* level, however, *it is a re-enactment of the baby-mother situation.* The active partner plays the role of the mother, and the passive repeats the role of the baby. The scene is set for the combination "loving mother, loved baby." But so strong is the allure of masochistic displeasure that the characters, when they actually appear, are "refusing mother, innocently tantalized baby." For the situation has been constructed in such a way that the "cry for love" cannot be reciprocated; unconsciously reciprocation was never intended. As a defensive camouflage of the homosexual's real conflict the "ideal wish" to be loved is most useful.

4. *Homosexuality as an unconscious search for a duplicate of oneself as a boy.* This hypernarcissistic type is of great importance socially and legally. Homosexuals using this defensive camouflage are "specialized on minors" and thus are dangerous.

5 and 6. *The positive and negative magic-gesture types.* The positive magic gesture is the dramatization of a final inner alibi in which a person shows in his behavior how he wanted to be treated in childhood: kindly and lovingly. The beneficiary of the good deed that is the magic gesture is always an unimportant outsider; for the theme of the dramatization is the reproach: "You, bad Mother (Father), did not care for your own child. I care even for strangers." The more unimportant and undeserving the beneficiary, the greater the crop of injustice collected and masochistically enjoyed.

Positive magic gestures play an important part in some types of homosexuality. In the great stress placed on the giving of gifts, especially when one partner is older and financially well off, the donor refuses to recognize that his friend is simply a male prostitute supported in style. This is more than a matter of closing one's eyes to the intolerable; and because a magic gesture is involved it is especially painful for these homosexuals to be confronted with the naked facts. The masochistic substructure of the magic gesture always includes the veiled but bitter complaint "nobody loves me."

The negative magic gesture, denoting an unconscious dramatization of the theme "In my behavior I'll show you how I did *not* want to be treated," is frequently reserved for the last phase of an affair of some duration and explains the wild hatred of the ex-lovers.

7 and 8. *The protective type and the type seeking an older protector.* In the protective type the masochistic substructure is hidden in paternalistic attitudes, the official aim being to show that "Father loves his little boy." The disguise of the homosexual in search of a "protector" is that of a young boy wanting to be loved by his good

father, the repressed contents being "innocent victim wants to be mistreated by the bad mother." In both situations the unconscious wins out and the relationship is disrupted with "injustice" conflicts.

9. *Homosexuality combined with other perversions.* Homosexuality may be combined with sado-masochistic practices, with exhibitionism and peeping, with transvestitism, with urolagnistic and scatological acts, etc.

10. *"Bisexuality."* Some homosexuals are occasionally capable of lustless, mechanical sex with a woman. They tend to marry as a means of proving to themselves and especially to the environment that they are completely normal. The mirage of heterosexuality in "bisexuals" only too often makes them a poor possibility for therapy; they seldom come into treatment except as a result of strong outside influence. Inwardly, though they disclaim this, they know they are homosexuals at bottom. The fact that their wives so often discover their "secret" is their own doing—unconscious, of course. Masochism triumphs as usual.

The best proof that what is popularly called "bisexuality"—to be distinguished from the biological meaning of the term—is only a subdivision of homosexuality can be produced in cases in which there has been a switch from heterosexuality to homosexuality. A pertinent example is that of Oscar Wilde.

11. *Homosexuality in fantasy.* There are neurotics who never resort to overt homosexuality, though their masturbatory sex life is concentrated on homosexual fantasies. It is possible to distinguish between genuine and pseudo homosexuals in this group. A male homosexual is a person who predominantly uses the unconsciously based defense mechanism of man-man relationship to escape his repressed masochistic attachment to the mother and who predominantly exhibits the mechanism of injustice-collecting in his personality. These two elements are invariably combined in the homosexual. If the man's personality fits this yardstick he is a homosexual even though he uses only the fantasy outlet.

12. *Statistically induced homosexuality.* After the appearance of Kinsey's Volume I (1948) a new type of homosexual appeared. I have suggested for this type the name "statistically induced homosexual." Although Kinsey's fantastically exaggerated claims regarding

Emphasis on Psychic Masochism 73

the prevalence of homosexuality received only rare mentions in the press, his figure of 37 per cent was slyly put to use by the older, more experienced homosexual, who would ask a wavering youngster: "Who are you to argue with one-third of the male population? Do you know how many tens of millions are involved? So many good Americans can't be wrong!" Of course the argument did not produce new recruits among true homosexuals (they needed no arguments), but it was quite effective with some borderline cases of post-adolescents in their late teens or early twenties, in whom the decision to be a homosexual had been hanging in the balance. Only a certain percentage of these temporary, borderline cases are true homosexuals. Many are not. Their pseudo modernity and misplaced experimentation, growing out of the erroneous belief that homosexuality is "scientifically" approved and "normal," have the unhappy result of burdening them with damaging guilt and self-doubt. These burdens remain even after reversion to heterosexuality. The tragic and pitiful spectacle of these "statistically induced homosexuals" is due entirely to the failure to disseminate medical facts.

The types described above merely represent a series of elaborations on the homosexual's basic dilemma: "How can I show that I am mistreated by the image of my mother and still keep myself convinced that Mother had nothing to do with it and that I want love and not kicks?" The result is that a variety of camouflages are installed. Externally these give the impression of being types.

Spurious homosexuality. External behavior is an unreliable factor in identifying homosexuals. The behavior of the markedly effeminate homosexual, as has already been stated, is only a camouflage masking his real conflict. The similar behavior of the passive-feminine man often leads to his being taken for a homosexual, though he is not one. This confusion is related to an out-dated theory that mistakenly designated the negative Oedipus in men as "unconscious homosexuality," which, under conditions not clearly stated, bloomed into conscious homosexuality. The negative Oedipus, though it *never* leads to perversion homosexuality, does play a part in the development of the passive-feminine man. Children who carry too large a remnant of early pre-oedipal passivity into the rescue station of the oedipal phase express this passivity in *feminine identification.* Depending on the defenses secondarily installed, this leads to one of two neurotic types: the passive-feminine Milquetoast or the super-he-man. The wide disparity in personality in these two is caused only by the disparity in the strength of the defense.

Lesbianism. The genesis of female homosexuality is identical with that of male homosexuality: an unsolved masochistic conflict with the mother of earliest infancy. Here, for anatomical reasons (lack of penis), the paths of development divide. The incipient Lesbian goes through a series of complex vicissitudes with the mother. The striking feature in the development of Lesbians is that they cannot, like the male homosexual, flee to another sex, man. They remain with the first object of fear, without the flight to Ultima Thule.

When a child has a terrifying *masochistic attachment* and is incapable of shifting it, either partly or entirely, to other persons, the inner torture machine is certain to start its barrage of reproaches. What inevitably follows is the installation of an inner alibi, a defense mechanism. The inner lawyer (unconscious ego) always works on the "itinerary of the opposite": if the accusation is forbidden pleasure, the inner lawyer mobilizes derivatives of the opposite, hatred. Thus the child "hates" her mother as an inner alibi. The *pseudo* hatred is in turn vetoed, and the itinerary of opposites provides the next alibi, *pseudo* love. This alibi leads straight to Lesbianism.

Lesbianism is merely a specific subdivision (with slight modifications) of the general problem of homosexuality. It has the identical prognosis and treatment requirements.[10]

In December 1942 I delivered a lecture on homosexuality before the New York Psychoanalytic Society,[11] in the course of which I stated that the prognosis of analytical treatment of homosexuals is a favorable one provided the patient really wants to change, mistakes in the selection of cases are avoided, and treatment penetrates to the deep masochistic layers of the unconscious. This was a new thesis; at that time all analytic-psychiatric literature on the subject was permeated with unmitigated pessimism.

Not all homosexuals are suitable for treatment. Those who cannot live without their pseudoaggressive alibi, displayed in their view of themselves as fighters, despisers, flouters of established custom, have no intention of "changing over." The allegedly happy homosexual is not yet ready for treatment. His guilt is deposited in the never ending, always painful crises, both internal and external, produced by homosexuality. As long as he succeeds in striking an inner trade balance between his unconscious guilt and his self-created and unabsorbed external difficulties there will be no detectable "surplus" of guilt; therapy can work only with a detectable surplus.

Of the homosexuals who consult psychiatrists and want to change, some display therapeutically usable, others unusable guilt. Unhappily, the differentiation between usable and unusable guilt cannot be made in a few preliminary interviews. A trial treatment of four to six weeks is indispensable. During this period it is possible to test the patient against six key questions:

1. Can his inner guilt be detached from its spurious point of deposition and "mobilized" for analytic-therapeutic purposes?

2. What is the patient's reaction when, in treatment, he is constantly confronted with his psychic masochism?

3. What is the purely quantitative state of self-damage, as revealed in the patient's past history? (Reticence and shame invariably delay the full story.)

4. Is the patient's ego more or less stable or fully psychopathic?

5. Was his wish to change a mere fluke, or is there some stability behind it?

6. What external facts, in full detail, are responsible for propelling the patient into the desire to change?

The answers can be clearly indicated, if not fully outlined, during the trial period. It is then possible to tell the patient yes or no. The chances of cure for a favorable case are, statistically, 90 per cent.

The limited means of many patients, and/or their residence at a distance from New York, led me to attempt to fix the minimum requirement, in terms of time and appointments, for the effective analytic treatment of homosexuality. Experiences with these patients have produced the following conclusions:

The *optimum* situation calls for three appointments a week over a period of four months (including the trial treatment), after which the patient sees the analyst twice a week for another four months. This comes to eight months and approximately eighty to eighty-five appointments.

The *minimum of the minimum* is two appointments a week over a period of eight months. In some, by no means all, cases the minimum aggregate of about sixty-four appointments proved insufficient, and three appointments a week had to be scheduled during the first four months.

Certain additional measures must be taken in order to make this drastically curtailed treatment effective.

1. My experience has shown that, instead of allowing the patient to see a parallel between the cold, denying mother and the silent, "draining" analyst, the analyst must present a picture of the "generous, giving mother" by talking for long periods at the beginning of analysis (see specific technique in orally regressed cases, pp. 138 ff.).

2. It is essential to be selective about the material presented. The patient must be *constantly* confronted with his psychic masochism, whenever and wherever it shows up.

3. The homosexual's pseudoaggression must not be confused with "real" aggression. The patient's provocative technique must be shown for what it is: a means of achieving the unconsciously desired "kick in the teeth."

4. The analyst must consistently stress the fact that what consciously appears to the patient as *"homosexual tension"* is actually *"masochistic tension." This separation of the superficial from the deeper layer kills homosexuality.*

5. The analyst must be clear in his aims: curing homosexuality means destruction of a deep-seated masochistic neurosis and not "adaptation" to it. This presupposes the analyst's conviction that homosexuality is a severe illness and not "a way of life." It also means that the analyst must be *inwardly* capable of constantly singling out (as opposed to constantly overlooking) the masochistic component in the patient.

6. The analyst must remain *inwardly* unaffected by the homosexual patient's repeated attempts to force him into the role of "forbidding" authority. These patients needle the analyst endlessly in

Emphasis on Psychic Masochism

the hope of receiving an "order" to abstain from homosexuality. The analyst, however, imposes no restriction, unless it can be called a restriction to utter the obvious warning that analysis cannot be conducted in prison—the domicile the patient unconsciously desires.

Two specific complicating factors should be mentioned, which may prolong the treatment of some homosexuals beyond the typical limit of eight months and approximately eighty appointments. These are premature ejaculation during the first experiences of intercourse with women and too extensive inroads of masochistic traits into the total personality.

Whether in homosexuals or heterosexuals, premature ejaculation always represents a defense against masochistic attachment to the giantess of the nursery, which takes the form of pseudoaggression. To lend credence to his unconscious assertion that he does not want to be refused by the mother, the prematurist actively refuses pleasure to the mother substitute, the woman who is his sexual partner. The infantile aim makes use of an equally infantile symbolism. In external reality he is refusing her pleasure because of the brevity of his intercourse; in inner reality he is refusing her "milk" (which he equates unconsciously with sperm) by "spilling it before it can reach the mouth." In the same infantile symbolism the vagina represents the mouth, the penis the breast. The aggressive intent is as clear in an intercourse of four to six thrusts, as against the typical sixty or more, as it is when ejaculation takes place before penetration.

Prematurity in intercourse with women provides the partly changed homosexual with a new depository for his pseudoaggression. The same masochistic hatred of the mother that was at the root of his homosexuality now activates him in his prematurity. The new symptom must be worked through and perceived as just another unconscious delaying action that must be eliminated so that the patient can continue towards his cure.

Since the homosexual neurosis is masochistic in itself, masochism cannot but invade other sectors of the neurotic's life. The masochistic substratum of homosexuality can seldom if ever remain contained within the perversion. Though his disapproved sexual habits are his preferred way of satisfying his appetite for self-damage, they are by no means his only way. The quantity of masochistic involvement is decisive here. Sometimes, though homosexuality has already collapsed in a specific case, a few more months of treatment are indicated, just to be sure.

Experience has convinced me that the end of an analysis should never be fixed in advance, on a specific date, and this applies to homosexuals too. After the usual eight months of treatment have elapsed and the patient is no longer a homosexual, therapy should be continued at the rate of one visit a month—as long as the patient wishes to come.

CHAPTER 3

WHAT DOES PSYCHOANALYTIC THERAPY ACCOMPLISH?

EVERY neurotic is a person who lost his individual "battle of the conscience." Confronted with the torture emanating from his self-created Frankenstein's monster, he knows only one double-barreled unconscious technique of coping with the unbearable: officially he bows his head and accepts punishment, and unofficially he shortchanges that very punishment into masochistic pleasure.

Parallel with this goes the technique of "taking the blame for the lesser intrapsychic crime." Accused by his inner conscience of *felony A*, the neurotic admits to *misdemeanor B* and punishes himself for the admitted substitute crime, only to shortchange this punishment also into psychic masochism.

The upshot of the neurotic's strategem is that a good deal of psychic energy is expended to furnish suitable inner defenses to the accusing inner judge and executioner. The defendant's unspoken formula always reads, "Would you settle for *that?*"

The superego bids up its demand for torture. The result is that psychic masochists have to increase their *self-created torture-bribes*. Hence self-damaging stakes increase, and so does conscious unhappiness.

Psychoanalysis throws a monkey wrench into the machinery of neurosis. By clarifying the psychic "chemistry" of the neurotic's actions it shows him a new way of defense: not to accept every accusation of the superego but to *fight back*. It also teaches the neurotic the *unproductiveness of his habitual defense of psychic masochism*.

True, the neurotic outsmarts the torturer by changing his torture into inner pleasure. But this pleasure is unconscious; and *every ounce of unconscious pleasure must be paid for with tons of conscious misery.*

Whatever "lesser crime" the neurotic admits to, he always covers up with that disguise the *crime of crimes,* psychic masochism. The justified question arises why the inner law should put psychic masochism in the category of Public Enemy No. 1.

The answer is obvious the moment one clarifies in one's own thinking the fact that the Big Boss in the unconscious is the inner conscience, the superego. If that torture institution is exclusively bent on torture, obviously every neutralization of torture by the belabored ego is unacceptable and "infuriating" to the torturer. Imagine a dictator "wised up" that the torture meted out in one of his concentration camps is made ineffective by a *particular* victim who actually enjoys being tortured. Without fear of torture a dictator cannot operate.

Psychic masochism, then, is neutralization of the superego's power, but a neutralization and pleasure achieved and perceived *only unconsciously.* Consciously the neurotic suffers, and his constitutionally guaranteed pursuit of happiness is made impossible.

How does Freudian psychoanalysis work? It uses transference and resistance, provided automatically by the patient, to elucidate the defeat he sustained in infancy by faulty elaboration of biological and environmental factors. The patient uses the chance figure of the physician as a sort of movie screen on which he projects his bygone conflicts—unknowingly and unwittingly. By contrasting the projected fantasy with the harmless reality some kind of *emotional* understanding is achieved. Before this can happen, before the easily accomplished but sceptical intellectual understanding can be transformed by the patient into effective emotional experience, the long process of "working through" is necessary, meaning the elucidation of what has already been established through the use of ever new material. Analysis uses dream interpretations, free associations, and the connecting of seemingly actual experiences with the repressed infantile past.

Admittedly there exist differences of opinion in analytic circles

What Does Psychoanalytic Therapy Accomplish?

about what constitutes the patient's "deepest layer." Analysis started with the surface of the "psychic apparatus" and found repressed libidinous wishes, concentrated in what became known as the Oedipus complex. Later, libido turned out to be only one participant, and aggression was accepted as full partner with it in the unconscious. Next, deeper neuroses were encountered and the precursors of the Oedipus discovered by Freud—the pre-oedipal phase.

In my opinion the basic human problem is psychic masochism. It constitutes the "life blood" of neurosis and is the *basic* neurosis. *All later libidinous and aggressive deposits are only defensive camouflages, hiding the fundamental problem.* Moreover, the aggression visible in neurosis is only pseudoaggression, and the structure of the neurotic symptom does not constitute a simple defense but is actually a defense against a defense.

Analysis—provided it takes the masochistic vicissitudes into consideration—shows the patient in an emotional experience the impracticality and self-damage embedded in his masochistic solution as well as in his endless procession of admissions of the "lesser intrapsychic crime." It also teaches him to discard his constant camouflage of depression, which simply means an unconscious prayer and alibi directed to the superego: "I don't enjoy my masochism; look how depressed I am."

Emotional "showing" and "teaching" are, of course, ineffective if the patient is not provided with *new energy* to make his new way of life stick. *This energy is provided by splitting off the masochistic energy* so abundantly present in the neurotic. Psychic masochism is, as stated in Chapter 1, only misdirected *aggression,* turned against oneself and secondarily libidinized. *By retrieving the original aggression from the hopeless amalgam the ex-neurotic has the power to fight more successfully the war every human being wages on two fronts: the superego and the obstacles of reality.*

I am adducing three clinical examples, representing excerpts from longer analyses. It is obvious that completeness is not attempted and that these excerpts are condensed in time; what appears as one "discussion" actually represents a running "debate" conducted during several or many appointments. Omissions have necessarily been made too in reporting the details of "working through" the resistances and the transference, in dream interpretation, etc. If more than highlights had been reproduced, one analysis would fill an entire volume.

Dr. A., a well-known surgeon, was in his late forties. He had been married for twenty years to a wife of whom he spoke in disparaging terms; summing up her character, he called her a "shrew with a martyr complex." I pointed out the contradiction in his definition, and he acknowledged it, explaining:

"This is a good example of my impatience, even with words. Of course I put it wrong. What I mean is this: She is a shrew, but independently of being one she uses a martyr technique on me. In other words, when she doesn't get what she wants by being shrewish, she switches her method and plays the martyr."

"Has she always been a shrew?"

"Who am I to judge? She did not seem to be one years ago—I thought her a healthy specimen with some managerial traits."

"You mean that in your good days together you called this quality 'managerial traits,' and in your bad days—meaning the present—you call that same quality 'shrewishness'?"

"Why not assume that her peculiarities have increased?"

"With or without your cooperation?"

"Well, the woman bores me, and I admit that I'm not very good company when I come home dead tired after a heavy schedule of operations. We don't sit down while operating, you know."

"Are you more tired in the evening these days than you used to be?"

"I am."

"Why?"

"Couldn't tell you."

"Are you under more tension?"

"I'm more impatient, yes."

"And the acute conflict?"

"Pertains to my marriage. I'm in love with a young chemist and want to marry her. She's convinced me I'd never have the courage to stand up to my wife. She frightened me into consulting you."

"What is your wife's hold on you?"

"She bullies me. When it doesn't work, she tries her martyr routine. I can sometimes stand up against the bullying; never against the other."

"Why?"

"Pity, I guess."

"But you love the other girl?"

"I am sure. She is much more the love-giving type than my wife."

"What would your best friend and worst enemy, respectively, say about you? What kind of person do they think you are?"

"That's putting me on the spot. I don't know. Can we skip this one?"

"No, we cannot."

"It's such a big order. Do you mean professional or personal friends and enemies?"

"Both."

"I just don't know."

"That indicates that you are thinking about a specific, rather unflattering statement. What is it?"

"Your guess is right. Recently a friend noticed how my wife orders me around—in company, mind you—and said, 'If you were that wishy-washy as a surgeon, I wouldn't dare let you operate on me.' He was half-drunk at the time, but his criticism still hit home."

"And your enemies?"

"My professional enemies claim that only modern techniques of blood transfusion prevent me from losing all my patients on the operating table. They claim that my methods are too radical, and other nonsense of that kind. It's the kind of abuse every innovator expects and gets."

"Do you take extraordinary chances?"

"Can we at least skip this one?"

"For the time being, yes. Why are you so jumpy?"

"I'm caught in the middle between two strong-minded, self-willed, troublemaking women. I'm not a strong man, but this would get anybody down."

"You don't consider yourself a strong man?"

"Now you want my own estimation of myself. Well. I'm a harmless guy who wants peace and quiet."

"And why do you attach yourself to strong-willed women who don't want you to have peace and quiet?"

"You are blaming *me?*"

"You picked these two women, didn't you?"

"They just happened to me."

"We shall see."

In a monotonous, rather depressed recital Dr. A. gave a brief résumé of his life history. His mother, he said, was "a darling, but somewhat distant and unapproachable"; his father, intent on his business, had been a "stranger at home." The child, who had no brothers or sisters, was left a good deal to his own devices. He daydreamed of "becoming famous, because then Mother would be proud of me." He had only vague recollections of the means through which he expected to become renowned; the daydreams, he recalled, dealt mainly with the results of fame. He would see himself entering a theater as the audience rose in respect, or nonchalantly accepting some scroll of honor, or listening, on a street car, as people he had never seen before discussed humanity's debt to him for his great discovery.

I asked: "Where did you place the accent—on being honored or on people's gratitude?"

"What makes you ask that?"

"Two things. Your direct statement that in your daydreams you heard strangers expressing their thanks for your great humanitarian feat—that's one reason. Second, you stated in our first interview that your wife's most effective weapon, if every other fails her, is acting the martyr. That means you identify with the victim, and therefore cannot be 'cruel' to her."

"This would never have occurred to me. You mean I cannot hurt people?"

"I did not say that. I suspect that you unconsciously identify yourself with the weak and helpless."

"I hate this sentimental stuff. While I am operating, I think of anatomical, topographical, technical facts."

"Why do you dissociate yourself so strongly from sympathy and empathy?"

What Does Psychoanalytic Therapy Accomplish?

"Oh, you got me all wrong. As a child I had very pronounced sadistic fantasies."

"Name some."

"Strangely enough, they were connected with two beautiful girls, both much older than I was. They were eleven or twelve; I was six or seven. I admired them from a distance and never spoke to them. I used to get excited watching their legs when we were ice-skating."

"Were you shy?"

"Exceedingly. These girls had something to do with my first fantasy of becoming a surgeon. Yes, it comes back now. While I watched them skate, I created the daydream that both girls get appendicitis (I called it 'something wrong in the navel region'). I, as a famous surgeon, am called in. I operate successfully and save their lives. Great gratitude, tears, admiration."

"Well, I would say the chances are that this fantasy is a later elaboration."

Dr. A. became very uneasy. "What do you mean?" he asked.

"Let's not be naive. The main attraction in becoming a physician —for the child—is the medical man's prerogative of seeing people naked. How about that? Were you curious?"

"I still fail to see the connection."

"Don't be prim. You said that in your fantasy you located the operation as being 'in the navel region.' Why wasn't your daydream about operating on the head or the arm? Isn't it more likely that you were arranging to peep at the beautiful girls under culturally admissible conditions?"

"Every child is curious."

"Of course. But we see here, embedded in your recollections, a banal infantile sexual theory..."

At this moment the patient remembered one of the "most humiliating" experiences in his life. At the age of sixteen he had his first sexual encounter with a girl. Approaching her, he fumbled around 'the navel region,' and was interrupted by the more experienced girl with the contemptuous advice: "Lower, stupid boy!"

"That has happened to more people than care to admit it," I commented. "Well, how about admitting that you did some peeping in childhood?"

A. had indeed been "incessantly" curious as a child. He "took everything apart"; his mother had given him the worst beating of his life after he "dissected" a brand-new doll belonging to a girl in his neighborhood. The two beautiful girls he had already mentioned, he now conceded, were fantasy objects of his "curiosity."

"You agree, then, that your surgical fantasy concerning these two girls had some precursors?"

"It seems so."

"The picture is far from complete. First of all, why did the daydream call for operating on the girls? Treating them for grippe would surely have been sufficient—they would have been undressed, in bed. Second, your own infantile fears have not been mentioned—so far."

"Please be more specific."

"Only a blueprint can be given; you will have to fill in the details yourself. Experience teaches that every child has sadistic-masochistic fantasies about the adult sex act. Experience also shows that every child works his way through an extensive series of fears concerned with having damaged himself with self-play. What about all that?"

"Assuming—but not granting—all this is true, isn't it a far cry from my actual conflict at the present moment?"

"The distance is not as great as you ironically declare it to be. If, as I suspect, your fears were extensive, you may have begun by elaborating on them through masochistic identification with the victim. That would be at least a partial explanation of why you have put yourself in that position, twice, with your two women. As a secondary defense, you may have created, during childhood, the fantasy of the powerful 'sadistic' surgeon—this fantasy would put you on top, and make other people your 'victims.' This island of successful defense, your profession, could not affect other sectors of your life. Your domestic setup is masochistic—why did you choose to marry a 'managerial' woman? Why are you now, with your girl friend, duplicating this experience? You have said that she too is 'self-willed' and 'troublemaking.' And here is another interconnection, hardly distant either—why did your infantile surgical fantasy involve a duo of patients? You could have chosen one girl, rather than both. Who is behind this screen memory? Does it represent mother and nurse? Why do you work on pairs—even now, with your two women?"

What Does Psychoanalytic Therapy Accomplish?

The patient took time out for a few ironic comments on these questions and then produced confirming material. There had been a nurse in his life, even more important to him than his "unapproachable" mother. He had dearly loved his nurse even though she frightened him by telling him "gruesome fairy tales." Yes, his fears had been extensive; he remembered having given all his savings to a gardener's assistant as the price of seeing his sex organ. He had wanted, on this occasion, to find out whether everyone has a "sulcus coronarius" (an indentation at the head of the organ). He had been afraid that he had damaged himself through self-indulgence.

"According to your infantile fantasy, then, you were your first self-damaging patient?"

"Well, the case was dismissed without surgery after ascertaining that the phenomenon was normal."

"But for a long time you did torture yourself with your fear of self-damage?"

"It seems so."

"When did the scene with the gardener's assistant take place?"

Reluctantly Dr. A. admitted that there was a "good chance" that it had happened during the autumn preceding the creation of his "surgical fantasy" involving the two beautiful girls.

"If this is so, you can see how a masochistic fantasy is warded off with a defensive, sadistic one."

"You mean that the popular butcher theory about surgeons is all the bunk?"

"Of course. Sadism in *adults* is merely a defense against more deeply repressed masochistic tendencies."

Some appointments later I asked Dr. A.:

"Doesn't it strike you as curious that you protested so strongly when I first mentioned your identification with the victim? You had yourself brought out the fact that in childhood you had pseudosadistic fantasies, but then you attempted to cancel the admission by saying that your mind was occupied only with objective, technical facts during your operations. You went so far that you objected to sympathy and empathy with the suffering patient; you called these feelings 'sentimental stuff.' What conclusions do you draw from these facts?"

"You tell me."

"Your reluctance reminds me of the saying of the French astronomer Camille Flammarion: 'There are men who would even be afraid to commit themselves on the doctrine that castor oil is a laxative.' Why are you so excessively cautious?"

"This whole business of psychic masochism makes me uncomfortable."

"Let's face a few facts. There is good reason for the assumption that the end of childhood found you with what may be called 'an overdose of psychic masochism.' This was the end result of your specific infantile conflict. After many circuitous detours there were two further results. The first of these was a success: you built up a first-class sublimation—surgery. The second was a defeat: you also maintained a first-class tendency to be tortured by a woman. Your professional and your private lives were exact opposites."

"I'm a tired man today. Make it easy for me and just talk about my success."

"As you wish. Your sublimation has a five-layer inner structure, just as all sublimations do, in my opinion. These are the layers, beginning with the deepest:

"Layer I: This is the end result of your infantile conflict: 'I wish to be masochistically mistreated.'

"Layer II: First reproach of the pleasure-forbidding inner conscience: 'You have no right to harbor this wish.'

"Layer III: First defense of your inner lawyer: 'My client is not guilty of masochism, as the indictment claims. True, he is guilty of an infraction, but his crime is the opposite of psychic masochism. He has deep sadistic desires.'

"Layer IV: Second reproach of the inner conscience: 'This trick will get you nowhere. Sadism may be in the inner lawbook a lesser crime than masochism, but it is just as forbidden.'

"Layer V: Second defense presented by the inner lawyer: 'My client amends his plea. He is neither masochistic nor sadistic. He is socially minded and wants to help people in distress. Isn't surgery an honored occupation in our culture?'"

Dr. A. listened in silence and maintained his silence after I finished my explanation. He gave the impression of wanting to ask,

What Does Psychoanalytic Therapy Accomplish? 89

"What's the catch?" He did not ask his question; no "catch" appeared. He began to breathe more easily and in leaving remarked, with an attempt at lightness, "I am slightly layer-sick. Let me think it over."

It would not have been at all surprising if Dr. A. had plunged immediately into the battle royal of resistance when he arrived for his next appointment, saying "You belittled my natural gift; you attempted to explain away something that doesn't require explanation." Instead he played coy, beginning the discussion cautiously:

"I don't want to pull a Flammarion, as you put it; it's just that I like to hear the whole deduction before I start arguing it out. You've analyzed my success—surgery; now tell me about my alleged defeat."

"We'll start by recording that you have made your objection in advance—by using the word 'alleged.' In the 'defeat corner' of your life, you were unable to follow through what you succeeded in doing in your sublimation: you could not counteract the end result of your infantile conflict. This end result, spelled out, is the ugly phrase, psychic masochism. In your sublimation you were able to claim socially mitigating circumstances. The culture approves of surgeons. But the identical psychic masochism you appeared to have exorcised in your profession caught up with you in your private life. You chose to marry an aggressive woman who could provide you with your daily dose of masochism. What defenses, if any, could you draw on? Only one: 'I'm the innocent victim of my wife's shrewishness.' That means that every time the inner tyrant objected to your beloved pleasure-in-displeasure pattern, you increased your domestic provocations, with the unconsciously foreseen result that more 'shrewishness' came to the fore as your wife's rejoinder. Then, seemingly with good conscience, you were able to claim: 'See how unjustly she is treating me!' Of course this presupposes that you naively but conveniently overlooked two facts—you had chosen the 'shrew' of your own free will; you had consistently provoked her into ill humor. As the Latin saying goes: 'Dixi et salvavi animam meam'—I have spoken, may God have mercy on my soul.'"

"You will grant me the right to point out a few holes in your deduction. In my rebuttal I would first state that you completely disregard my honest contention: at the beginning I simply had no idea of my wife's evil disposition—"

"Interruption, please. You mean you had no *conscious* idea."

"I don't see the point."

"Here is your error. Unconsciously we all possess an unfailing apparatus for ferreting out the other person's psychic make-up. As I have occasion to tell almost all my patients sooner or later: There are no innocent victims in the marital graveyard. The answer to your objection is simple. Unconsciously, you *did* know of your wife's 'evil disposition.' You married her because of it, not in spite of it."

"The burden of proof is on you."

"Correct. Provided you are willing to give me material."

"Such as?"

"Observations during your courtship; little pointers which you observed but disregarded."

"She was energetically—sweet."

"That's a new one. Let's skip the sweetness and light and concentrate on whatever it was that makes you use the word 'energetically.' "

"Well. She took everything into her own hands, I mean finding and furnishing the apartment—"

"Let's get down to brass tacks. Were there any scenes, outbursts, reprimands that could have warned you?"

"Of course there were. But they were always well dipped in a gravy of sweetness, and so I didn't pay any attention to them—except that they did amuse me."

"Examples, please."

"I remember one incident. We were about to go to a party. I called for her and found her in a rage. The shoes she had bought specially to wear on that occasion were too tight. She was just about to trample on the culprits—crush them down with her whole weight —when I came in and saved the situation with some surgical stretching. It was really funny."

"Did this tantrum make you suspicious?"

"Suspicious? Not at all. I admired her energy."

"What is, to you, your wife's most annoying trait? Some time ago you quoted a friend who watched Mrs. A. ordering you around

What Does Psychoanalytic Therapy Accomplish? 91

in company and then made a derogatory remark about your being 'wishy-washy.' What does this refer to, and were there any signs of it before you got married?"

"Why is your memory so accurate when you are busy building a case against me?"

"You are such a passionate injustice collector that you cannot acknowledge the presence of objectivity. We have a problem to solve, haven't we? Why censor or disregard any possible evidence?"

"I just feel that you are building a case against me."

"Don't you see that this is just another transference repetition of your favorite role—acting the innocent victim? Moreover, may I remind you of your 'incessant curiosity' (that's a quotation) as a child and the occasion when you 'dissected' a doll? Aren't you at all curious about what your inner puppet master, your unconscious, made you do?"

"Quite a sales talk, but I'm not buying."

"You still haven't answered my question. What was your friend referring to when he called you 'wishy-washy'?"

"My wife has the unfortunate habit of acting the queen as soon as she occupies a chair. A chair seems to her to be the court of ultimate resort. The moment she sits down she starts issuing orders. 'Bring me this, give me that, do this, why don't you do that?' This endless procession of demands and reprimands catches up with me exactly at the worst time of my day—when I've come home dead tired."

"Do you know that your idiosyncrasy about chairs and sitting down is so marked—it seems to have acquired symbolic connotations—that you repeated it with me during our first interview?"

"What's that? Did I misbehave with you, too?"

"How much of the frightened schoolboy must still be alive in you to prompt your use of that word! No, you did not misbehave. You remarked rather acidly, while we were discussing your chronic tiredness, 'We don't sit down during operations, you know.' I took it, then, merely as an expression of envy on the part of a surgeon, who must stand when he is working, for the psychiatrist, who can sit. I see now that the key word 'sitting' means more to you."

"Do you want me to say 'touché'?"

"You'd better tell what led up to your friend's remark."

"Well, he was out of Chesterfields, which are his favorite brand of cigarettes. They used to be mine, too, for three decades. Recently my wife promoted the idea that any husband who is a gentleman will carry his wife's brand. Hers happens to be Lucky Strikes. I didn't want to load myself down with two packs of cigarettes, so I switched to Luckies, even though I dislike them. My friend, knowing our similarity in tastes, asked me for a cigarette, expecting to get a Chesterfield. That was how he found out about my switch. In his indignation he called me 'wishy-washy.' "

"Well, you are quite a compliant husband."

"Anything to avoid reproaches!"

"How does this fit in with your establishment of a triangle? Does the presence of a second woman in your life also contribute to peace and quiet?"

"I was waiting for that. As you know, my girl friend read your book, THE REVOLT OF THE MIDDLE-AGED MAN. It was from that damn book that she got all the ammunition she is using against me. I read it too and I'll admit that I disliked it intensely. I don't like your idea that in their forties or fifties all masochistic husbands have to establish an alibi—'I want love—the very same love that I don't get at home'—and therefore start looking for a young, understanding woman. And then you give the story a twist. You say that since—allegedly—this is but an alibi—"

"May the author correct the critic: the word 'allegedly' is your contribution."

"Correct. You claim that the real thing—masochism—wins out, and most of these men stay with their wives. My girl concluded that this is going to be the case with me. Why did you have to publish this book?"

"My humble apologies. In this 'damn book' is also included a long chapter describing the different varieties of 'understanding women' these men find during their rebellions. All these women have one common denominator: they are neurotics. If they weren't, they would not get involved in hopeless entanglements with these 'middle-agers,' as one patient called them, very pleased to be able to indicate a parallel with teen-agers. All in all, your résumé was far from com-

What Does Psychoanalytic Therapy Accomplish?

plete. You carefully omitted the book's main thesis: Middle-age revolt is an emotional second adolescence. And did your girl friend find herself included in the types of 'understanding women'?"

"Of course not. But when I read that chapter, I realized that underneath the warmth there is still a good deal of the bitch in that girl."

"Which just proves my point: are you, or are you not, addicted to 'bitches'?" [12]

"I have to think about it."

"This seems to be your favorite out."

The deep thinking so gravely promised appeared for some time to have produced no results. During this interim Dr. A. turned his attention to the "errors" in the theory of sublimation:

"Please explain this contradiction," he said. "How can I be such a flop in my private life and such a success in my profession? You tell me that both the flop and the success are elaborations of the same stuff—psychic masochism."

"Why is it so difficult to grasp that a man has failures *and* successes?"

"Why wasn't I a failure, or a success, in both departments?"

"Your counter-resources were obviously limited."

"But why did they stretch only as far as success in my profession, and no farther?"

"This is a phenomenon frequently observed. I suspect it has some connection with the peculiar 'game quality' of neurosis. You can observe a similar phenomenon in perverted masochists. Why, for example, do they accept and even pay for flagellation and never ask for total resection of the sex organ?"

"Analogies come in handy."

"This is more than an analogy. For instance, your description of your professional life as completely free from the taint of psychic masochism is, shall we say, unprecise. We have two proofs to the contrary already on record. Proof one: What do you get out of working like a slave in your profession? A highly unsatisfactory home life. Be honest! Do you enjoy the fruits of your labor? Proof two: If my allegedly accurate memory is serving me as it should, you were evasive when I asked if you take too many chances in your operations. Do I understand this evasion correctly—are you starting to extend the private department 'psychic masochism' into your official, professional life?"

Gloomily Dr. A. admitted that his curiosity and his urge to experiment sometimes "played tricks" on him. He himself was not always aware of this; often it was a scared or puzzled expression on the faces of his operative assistants that "brought him back to reality."

"Is this a comparatively recent development?"

"Yes."

"Looking back at these incidents, what do you accuse yourself of?"

"Of endangering the lives of innocent people."

"And your conclusion?"

"The sadistic streak in me that I've tried so often and so unsuccessfully to impress on you."

"Once more: a consoling, self-created delusion. Just think of the possible consequences. You could lose your license and go to jail. You call that sadistic? True, the technique you would be using to achieve your masochistic aim gives the appearance of being aggressive; it is, of course, pseudoaggressive. By the way, you can see one of the rules of the theory of sublimation at work here—or perhaps you will call it, again, one of the 'errors' of this theory. When a sublimation begins to collapse—and you are on the brink of such a development—the crisis is preceded by violent attacks from the inner conscience. The inner lawyer is not strong enough to prevent these accusations and indictments, but does its best to fulfill its protective function by trying to shift the direction of the attack that is bound to come. The initial attack is directed against layer I (I hope you don't get 'layer-sick' again)—that means, against psychic masochism. What happens instead? You accuse yourself of 'cruelty'—that means layer III, pseudoaggression, or 'sadism,' as you incorrectly call it. Q.E.D. Your inner lawyer has again successfully put through a diversionary movement by accepting guilt for the 'lesser crime.' "

Dr. A. had no comment, and I continued: "You use the same unconscious maneuver, though in a different connection, when your wife acts the martyr. You identify with her. Then, instead of accusing yourself of masochism, you worry about your 'cruelty' to the poor girl. And a few minutes later, without seeing the contradiction, you accuse her of 'bitchiness.' "

For the first time, something like an admission was forthcoming from the distressed man:

"I better get rid of this damned masochism; it seems dangerous!"

"That's like the very young private, under enemy fire for the first time, who exclaims, 'Gee, a guy can get killed here!' "

Some time later, I asked the patient:

"Has it occurred to you that you are sacrificing a good deal to your perpetual grievance against your wife?"

"For example?"

"Contentment, a happy home life, lack of depression, the 'bothersome' girl friend, and so on."

"To quote you: 'Masochism is a big shot.' Mind you, I say that mournfully."

The further fate of Dr. A. is only tangentially of interest here. His deep masochism was diminished and his tottering sublimation strengthened. His wish to get rid of his wife proved to be poorly founded; he discovered that his wife, when not repeatedly stung by his provocations, was "halfway tolerable." An ironic note was injected when his girl friend decided to enter analysis herself and found out, in the process of analyzing her own masochism, that she was not interested in A. at all but in the "hopeless situation" she had built around him. Proudly she declared that she had no wish to marry him. Dr. A. lived through his "disappointment"—he was greatly relieved. Remnants of masochism can sometimes be an advantage.

Mr. B., a man in his middle forties, came to me twenty-nine years ago, referred by an outstanding specialist in internal medicine. Giving me a preview of the prospective patient on the telephone, the specialist explained: "This fellow had an appendix operation which left him with a slight postoperative venous complication in his legs. He has spent all of the past year in bed, refusing to get up; he claims he has symptoms of angina pectoris. He was a criminal lawyer of some reputation, but he gave up his practice entirely. He is spending his time waiting for death. The G.P. who treated him, a friend of his, read my recent paper on *pseudo*-angina and called me in. After making all the necessary tests I decided that the problem is typically psychosomatic. Of course the patient doesn't believe me. You will have a hard time with him; he is thoroughly disagreeable. Please don't blame me. Good luck!"

Mr. B., a stern, imposing figure, appeared for his first appointment leaning on two heavy canes. Martyred indignation was stamped on his face. He was a dying man, he told me, struggling through his last days without any of the usual consolations of his condition. Instead of admitting that his situation was hopeless and acting accordingly, medical men (and relatives) insisted that his "very real" heart symptoms were psychogenic. "This seems to be the newest trick in medicine," he added.

"Do you wish to be treated?" I asked.

"I'm helpless against this conspiracy. I want to make one condition, however. You must tell me what the internist told you about me."

"Don't you think you're asking me to repeat a privileged communication?"

"Probably. But mine is a desperate situation."

"I have no objection to repeating what I was told. I suspect you will be both disappointed and sceptical."

To reduce Mr. B. to absurdity, I told him of an experience in the the career of the famous otologist, Professor Neuman, an incident that the professor had so relished that he recounted it again and again. Called into consultation by a colleague, Neuman examined the patient (a known miser and misanthrope) and then retired with the other physician to discuss the case in private. "The diagnosis is obvious," Neuman began. "I fully agree with your opinion and the therapy you suggest. That's all there is to say, but if we go back now this disagreeable fellow will be suspicious, so let's talk. One topic needs to be discussed: how much shall we charge this stinker?"

In due time the two physicians emerged from their seclusion, and Neuman informed the patient of their reassuring diagnosis. This was not enough for him; he wanted a verbatim report of their discussion. "Do you really want to know?" Neuman asked. "You are not going to like it." "Am I going to die?" the patient cried out. "No, you will live, but I called you a stinker."

What Does Psychoanalytic Therapy Accomplish?

The amusing story was lost on Mr. B.

"Jokes apart," he insisted, "what did the internist say?"

I repeated the telephone conversation, verbatim. B. remained unconvinced.

"I don't believe you."

"Well, what do you think the internist said?"

"That I'm a dying man who has to be humored."

"Let's assume you are correct. Name one reason for me to have become a party to this supposed conspiracy. If you were a dying man, you might possibly die in my office. If this did happen, would malicious people believe you died of heart trouble? On the contrary. They would claim that psychoanalysis—or I myself—killed that well-known criminal lawyer, Mr. B. I'm still a young physician, you know. Is it logical for me to take chances that could ruin me professionally?"

"You may have a point," Mr. B. said judiciously, but he remained unconvinced.

My first few appointments with the patient were devoted to giving him an introduction to analysis in the form of a series of explanations. During these hours B. kept his eyes fixed on my face; his expression, though not clearly definable, was one of peculiar watchfulness.

"I may be mistaken," I said at last, "but I have the impression that you are waiting for something. For what?"

During the First World War, B. explained, he had held a high position on the staff of the Marshal Provost's office and had distinguished himself by his ability to "squeeze out confessions."

"That's interesting. But how do I fit the bill?"

"I want the truth about your conversation with the internist. You'll break down, mark my words."

"I heard you. To make your task of detection easier, I'm going to cooperate with you. Typically analysis is conducted in this manner: the patient occupies the couch, the physician sits *behind* him. We'll dispense with this rule. You will sit in the chair opposite me, just as you are sitting now. You will thus have no reason to claim that I'm afraid of looking you in the eye. Isn't this satisfactory? And isn't the criminal cooperating?"

Slightly deflated but not at all shaken, B. went right on suspecting that there was a catch somewhere.

B.'s story of his past history was brief, though hardly to the point. He had some grievances against his stern father, who was president of a district court. The father had automatically assumed that his son would follow in his footsteps by choosing jurisprudence as his life work. The boy had feared his father, loved his mother. "That's all," the patient concluded.

"That's not even page one of a novel of a few thousand pages," I countered.

"Look here, I came to you to *get* information, not to give it."

"I understood you came to be cured of your neurosis."

"Do you insist on play-acting?"

"Here we go again. We'd better analyze what's behind this persistent suspicion that I am keeping something from you. Are you a peeper?"

"Your idea of humor isn't mine."

"No humor—facts. Didn't you say that you are especially good at ferreting out other people's secrets? Aren't you up in arms as soon as you even suspect that someone is keeping some fact from you? Reduce these tendencies to an infantile common denominator, and the result is clear—voyeurism."

For the first time I heard this somber man laugh.

"Is this deduction a new way of humoring me, method 'X' of putting up a so-called therapeutic smoke screen?"

"Whether or not my stab at a diagnosis has hit any part of the truth cannot be decided now. We start with this point: your considered opinion is diametrically opposed to my statements. O.K. Let's pretend that I'm kidding you. Be a good fellow and pretend with me. How's that?"

"At least a new note."

"Come on, give."

"Well, you're right, I'm very inquisitive. I always do look for facts behind appearances. That's probably why I always wanted to study medicine. Of course, my father put his foot down and forbade it. I became a lawyer instead, hated it, and still hate it."

"But your father has been dead now for many years, you said."

What Does Psychoanalytic Therapy Accomplish?

"I had to make a living. Believe it or not, I took a job as legal consultant for a large corporation so that I wouldn't have to go into practice and so that I would have time to attend medical lectures. I went to medical school for a year and a half—I can show you my certificates. Then, while I was studying for my anatomy exam, I realized I was trying to do a full-time job on half time, and I had to give it up."

"Are you sure that's the only reason?"

B. gave me a suspicious look and slowly added: "Well, I had a horror of dissecting bodies."

"That's better."

"Why did you ask?"

"Because I supported myself throughout all my years of medical study, and I know that it's quite possible to hold a job and study at the same time—if you arrange your hours and get along on very little sleep."

"That's the second thing about you that impresses me. The first, as if you didn't know, is your tenacity in covering up for your colleague."

"No comment. Better explain about your aversion to blood and dissection in general."

"I decided that at bottom I'm a sadist, and I ward off my sadism with pity."

"Do you know that you've just presented—though imprecisely— a psychiatric precept? Careful! You might become part of the conspiracy yourself."

B. made a derogatory gesture and asked, "Why don't you confirm my opinion?"

"You are wrong. I suspect that your real trouble is the exact opposite of sadism—it is masochism."

"Do you want to emasculate me, too?"

"I want—and this is as sinister as the rest of my designs—to help you to make your acquaintance with your own self."

"Thanks for nothing. I am on good terms with myself."

"I doubt that."

"Give me one reason!"

"What about your attacks? How can you be a 'sadist' if a dozen times daily you are overwhelmed by self-produced fears?"

"When and where?"

"In your pseudo heart attacks. What would you call sadism directed at oneself—activity or passivity?"

"I'm willing to play along, if the nonsense doesn't go too far. How dare you drag in my sick heart?"

"Isn't it interesting that you should be so violent in your resistance to the diagnosis of your symptom? Your diagnosis—a 'real' illness—spells death; my diagnosis—psychogenesis—spells life. Has that occurred to you?"

"I wish I could believe you!"

"Wait and see. Let's assume, just for argument's sake, that you turn your agression inward, against yourself. There are two possibilities. The first is the one you have seen—the possibility that you feel guilty because of some aggressive deed or fantasy, and inhibit the aggression. But the fact that this occurred to you at all strongly suggests that the interpretation is merely a camouflage; if it were the genuine answer the process would remain repressed."

"What's the second possibility?"

"That at bottom you are exceedingly masochistic and deny it. You admit that you are guilty of a lesser crime, consisting of what you erroneously term sadism."

"What's my error in using the word 'sadism'?"

"Sadism is that part of neurotic aggression which becomes connected with sex. If you torture a prisoner and this gives you an erection, you are being sadistic. Other aggressive acts are just *aggression*, provided the aggression isn't a cover-up for masochism. If it is, we speak—as in your case—of pseudoaggression."

"Let's get some order into your indictment. You claim that I overwhelm myself with fear for the purpose of enjoying my fear masochistically?"

"Correct."

"That's simply idiotic."

"What's your yardstick? Logic? If your test is logic, of course that explanation is idiotic. But if you use, for a change, the yardstick of the unconscious—repressed fantasies, guilt, double defenses—it isn't idiotic at all."

"You just don't make sense. I acknowledge the difficulty of your position: you have to keep my mind occupied. But what made you choose this hyper-nonsense?"

"Aren't you being contradictory? At first you claimed my job was to humor you. Now you claim that I'm deliberately irritating you."

"Perhaps you just aren't experienced enough in your profession."

"That's possible. But it's just as possible that I'm on the right track. We'd better explore that possibility too."

During the next few appointments Mr. B. tried to convince me that "basically" he was an aggressive fellow. He gave me "proofs": He had once forgotten an important date connected with an income-tax matter, and this lapse had nearly subjected his employers to a fine which could have amounted to millions. He had been aggressive towards his wife, and he recited the details.

I objected. "Isn't it interesting," I asked, "that you go all out to prove your aggression, and the examples you cite merely show your masochism? If the tax matter had not been arranged, your employers would have paid—and you would have been fired. And your confessions to your wife, were they never turned against you?"

"You should have been a lawyer, not a doctor."

"I take that, coming from a lawyer, as a compliment. Seriously, don't you find it curious that you should be trying to prove your aggression just when you have been 'accused,' as you wrongly put it, of masochistic passivity?"

As Mr. B. rose to leave, I asked him:

"How long are you going on with the nonsense of carrying those heavy canes, or half-crutches?"

"Would you suggest that I lean on your interpretation instead?"

"Exactly."

"I'm a sick man."

"This you are, but emotionally."

B.'s dreams were full of passivity: persons unknown, of unknown sex, perpetually persecuted, victimized, assaulted, and overwhelmed him.

"Does this also prove activity?" I asked him.

"Don't push me into a corner!"

"So I am one of your persecutors, too? Remember what I told you about repeating infantile experiences, using the irrelevant figure of the physician as the new protagonist. This 'transference' is becoming quite evident."

B's reply was an abusive phrase, followed by an apology: "Sorry, but you are needling me."

"How?"

"By stressing my supposed passivity, which I find unacceptable."

"Unacceptable to your conscious ego? Of course. Did you expect consciousness and unconsciousness to coincide?"

This conversation took place in the third month of treatment. During the next few weeks, two tendencies emerged. B. felt physically better, discarded his canes, and began to think about reopening his office. At the same time his doubts and resistances increased. In a series of skillful oral briefs he reformulated his objections: It was senseless for him to return to his profession; there was "no future" in it. What he really wanted was to go on with his beloved medical studies. Unhappily he did not have the money; that path was closed to him. Moreover, my diagnosis of masochistic passivity was "all wet"; his real trouble was (a new accusation) hidden homosexuality.

My answer was not consoling. "What you call your homosexuality is only a tendency to attach yourself to people who are in the habit of kicking you around. There is not the slightest basis for the suspicion of homosexuality. Your heterosexuality is a fact and was never contested. Of course your having fished up this red herring and dragged it into our discussion should make you suspicious. Is masochistic passivity so intolerable that you prefer to be a homosexual?"

B. laughed, and homosexuality was temporarily shelved.

I continued: "The other problem is more serious. Yes, being a lawyer is not easy. Still, it is the reasonable thing for you to do. Take this into consideration too: You are in your forties; it wouldn't be simple to study medicine. It is also possible that a fleeting identification with me is involved in this wish."

"My love for medicine is older than our acquaintanceship."

"That's true. Analysis can remove the obstacles to this sublimation which you attempt to find in medicine. Whether or not you should pursue this ambition is another question, and this decision is entirely up to you."

Some time later I asked: "By the way, are you conscious of the fact that you were not able to go on with your study of medicine not just because of the reasons you originally gave me but because of your masochistic grievance against your father? He insisted, you told me, that you become a lawyer."

"You seriously believe that I preferred a grievance?"

"I do. Not a simple grievance but a grievance plus. This 'plus' pertains to psychic masochism *and* the 'innocent victim' defense."

"Strange."

The analysis progressed; by the time B. had completed fourteen months of treatment he had regained a good deal of his physical activity and resumed the practice of his profession. In a short précis like this it is impossible to reproduce the thousand ups and downs of resistance, the arguments and rebuttals that characterize every analysis. B. progressed—sometimes slowly, sometimes with amazing rapidity.

Interestingly, he chose to use incidents dealing with his own clients (criminals) as material in his effort to convince himself of the reality of masochism. In his professional memories he found ample evidence of "libidinized self-damage." He used the same material for what he called his "resurrection": the occasion on which he lectured to an audience of lawyers on the psychology of criminosis. I was present at this lecture and I could well understand his colleagues' surprise. B. had done an excellent job of public relations in previous years when he assiduously spread the news of his fatal illness, and these people had taken it for granted that his next public appearance would be at his own funeral service. Instead of gathering to listen to a eulogy they witnessed the triumphant reappearance of the living B.

In the end phases of B.'s analysis he repeatedly marveled at the fact that his "harmless" mother could unconsciously have been the malefactor in his case. The apparent contradiction was resolved when I reminded him of the time element: in the crucial nursery stage his father (who subsequently became so important) had no status; his existence was hardly recognized. Somewhat later the fears that had originally been centered on the figure of the mother had been shifted to the father—a switch that was made easier by the father's imposing personality. The shift also explained B.'s periodic conviction of his own homosexuality; during the oedipal phase he had also developed a strong feminine identification. This is typical, always transitory, always inconsequential in its effect upon the normal child. It was this phase that he mistook for homosexuality, a problem arising from completely different causative factors. Once this confusion in his thinking was clarified, B. recollected many occasions on which he had provoked his mother.

At this time too I drew B.'s attention to his determined use of the provocative, pseudoaggressive technique of psychic masochism in the initial stages of his analysis—in the transference.

Eighteen months after our first appointment B. left analysis, a changed man. He had resumed his practice, "forgotten" his heart troubles, and could justifiably call himself "adjusted."

I saw him, socially, at infrequent intervals during the next six years. They were successful years for him; his election as one of the dignitaries of the local Bar Association bolstered his ego considerably. Noted lawyer or not, the old wish to become a physician was still alive in him, and now that the inner obstacles had been removed he managed to return to his studies and acquire an M.D. at the age of fifty-two.

Then came nine years during which B. and I lost contact, mainly because of the Second World War and consequent changes of domicile. When our correspondence was resumed, I discovered that he had become a famous, almost renowned doctor. Despite adverse conditions he felt well and worked hard. He died only a few years ago, at the age of sixty-seven.

There is an element of particular interest in B.'s case: He was one of the few patients on record who checked (though indirectly) with his analyst during fully a quarter of a century. He had come into treatment one of the "living dead," a man who had given himself up, who had become a professional zero, after having been dissatisfied with his work all his life, and was waiting for death. His real interest, medicine (which was of course a defense), was fenced off from him by inner inhibitions. I saw how, after these inhibitions were analytically removed and his other problems solved by treatment, he was able to re-enter life and actually fulfill his childhood ambition. This does not often happen to people who are approaching the last quarter of their lives.

Mr. C. was twenty-four and contentedly waiting to inherit a fortune of fifty million dollars when he first came to my office.[13]

"According to your book HOMOSEXUALITY: DISEASE OR WAY OF LIFE?, I am a homosexual," he said. "But I don't consider myself one."

"If that's the only trouble why not throw the book away? Who cares about other people's definitions?"

"It isn't so simple. You have half convinced me that I am a homosexual."

"But you must have had your suspicions before reading that damaging book?"

"Sometimes I have, when I was bothered by homosexual fantasies. But I never try to uncover the facts behind my doubts. Let's put it this way: intellectually I know that I'm a homosexual, but emotionally I refuse to acknowledge it."

"Very convenient."

"I know I'm being irrational."

"What did the book clarify for you?"

"That homosexuality is homosexuality, whether it's executed in reality or fantasy."

"And before you read the book, how did you manage to convince yourself of the contrary?"

"I suppose you'd call my reasoning a rationalization. I explained it this way: I had never had actual bodily contact with a homosexual. Then I detest the typical and pronounced homosexual. And I believed that I had not yet outgrown my puberal fantasies."

"What type do you prefer in fantasy?"

"A boy between nine and twelve, with a beautiful body, on a beach, naked or in tight trunks. He has to have his hair in a crew cut. He also has to have beautiful feet. With high arches."

"Does the fantasy stop at this point?"

"No. Mutual play with the organs follows."

"And why do you want to change?"

"One can fool oneself for only a limited time. I detest homosexuality. I dread the consequences. Besides, our family is a dynasty in its way, and I have to marry."

"Does your family know anything about your real inclinations?"

"Of course not. My parents would die of shame. Especially my father—who is something of a tyrant."

"There is no reason for them to know. If your inner rejection of homosexuality is as strong as your intellectual objection, this may all be no more than a disagreeable recollection in a few months."

"But my fantasies—with and without masturbation—are, I could say, compelling!"

"That's totally immaterial. The only important question is whether you *unconsciously* want to change."

"I cannot testify to that."

"You were not asked to. Only a trial treatment of a few weeks can answer that question. By the way, have you ever had sexual contact with girls?"

"The way you mean it, no."

We arranged for appointments, to begin in a few months. Reality factors made the delay necessary; the young man was scheduled for a long business trip (he was being groomed to succeed his father as head of the "dynastic" firm), and I did not have appointments available at the moment.

As he was leaving Mr. C. made an unexpected remark: "Please don't tell my father why I'm really here."

"But why should I see your father in the first place? I told you that there would be only one justification for approaching your father with a merciful white lie: if you could not finance your treatment. You told me then that your father gives you more money than you need. We agreed that your family should be spared all depressing information. Why come back to a settled point and talk as if we had not even mentioned it?"

"I just assumed that you would like to get some information about my childhood from my father."

"How could I see your father without your consent? No, that's not a likely explanation. Isn't it more probable that you are casting me in the role of the enemy who plots against you behind your back? And that you want—unconsciously and masochistically—all the trouble you can squeeze out of the situation?"

The young man had nothing to say, but his face showed how he took his first analytic interpretation: with surprise, embarrassment, and sheepishness.

When he came into treatment some months later he received—as all my patients do—a brief explanation of the ABC of analysis. He listened quietly, bored a good deal of the time but occasionally piqued into interjecting a question pertaining to himself. Obviously he wanted to "get into the act" as quickly as possible. I asked him:

"Are you always so intolerant of information imparted, or are you taking this introduction as a sermon? Who preaches to you at home?"

The patient laughed. "Both my parents are given to long discourses."

"Do you know the story of the man who sits in a train screwing up his face in disgust every few seconds and at the same time making derogatory movements with his hand? The passenger sitting opposite finally asks, 'What are you doing?' The man answers, 'I'm bored, and so I'm telling myself jokes. But I've heard them all before.'—Do you think I'm giving you this information to amuse myself?"

"I beg your pardon."

"Your good manners, which I grant you, are not under scrutiny. Your defenses are."

"What's defensive about being impatient?"

"You are *outwardly* impatient with me because of my—you think —long-winded introduction. But what makes you think this *inwardly* constitutes just impatience?"

"What else?"

"Didn't you say that both your parents are given to 'long discourses'? Didn't you also call your father a 'tyrant'? Didn't you also suspect me of intending to see your father behind your back? Doesn't your 'impatient' attitude during your first two appointments show that you think I'm wasting your valuable time, meaning robbing you of your hard-earned money, meaning injuring you?"

"What are you driving at?"

"A duality of factors. First, your tendency to maintain the fiction that your elders make trouble for you, do you dirt, or at least annoy you. Since you're lumping me in with the others, or—if you prefer—had from the very beginning unconsciously tagged me as a provider of nuisances or damage, you cannot (and this introduces the second factor) accept anything useful or favorable from me, even if it is only useful information, without getting jittery. Or, as you put it, 'impatient.' The two attitudes are contradictory; you prefer the former."

"Do you mean that to accept useful information presupposes a favorable state of mind?"

"At school didn't you observe that you learned more from the teachers you liked than from those you didn't like?"

"Yes, of course. But I don't dislike you."

"You misunderstand. I spoke of your having, unconsciously, tagged or typed me. How else do you explain your suspicion that I intended to conspire with your father, behind your back, against you?"

"Let's close this discussion with the mutually agreed-upon observation that I suspect the possibility of a malicious motive even when someone is nice to me. Let's add that this suspicion will have to be analyzed later."

"You are learning the analytic escape technique fast. O.K. Let's put your suspicions in the psychic icebox to be examined later. In the meantime, please give me a personality sketch of your parents. Tell me how you see them now, as an adult, and how you used to see them as a child."

Mr. C. suddenly semed to have a bad taste in his mouth. He was not enthusiastic about either parent in any time division, past, present, future. His father, when not on one of his innumerable business trips, had been a shouting and tyrannical presence in the house; his mother had always played the *grande dame*. In childhood he had seen little of his mother; she had left him in the hands of a series of "disagreeable governesses." And she counted for little in his adult life. She was still the *grande dame,* still full of "silly prejudices," and lately a hypochondriac. Hypochondria was beginning to engulf his father as well.

"Tell me more about the disagreeable governesses," I said.

"I remember one in particular. She was a good-looking, high-breasted girl, but sour and unappreciative. Once in my bath—I couldn't have been more than four—I proudly showed her my sex organ. She scolded me severely and made a disgusted face. She was always impatient with me; she didn't like me and made no bones about it."

"So nobody really appreciated you, and you had to love yourself?"

"Strange that you say that. I am, people tell me, good-looking. I never thought so myself."

"What was wrong with your hair and feet?"

"First, tell me, what gives you that idea?"

"I suspect that the boy of your fantasies is a radiant and improved edition of yourself, before puberty. Didn't you specifically stress the haircut and the beautiful, 'high-arched' feet?"

"I never thought of that! You mean I'm Narcissus admiring himself?"

"Exactly. But not simply Narcissus, an improved edition of Narcissus. Now tell me what you didn't like about your hair and feet."

"The deduction floors me . . . Well, I had flat feet and for years I had to wear high shoes that made me conspicuous, certainly, and, I thought, ridiculous. And the hair? It was too wavy and there was too much of it, and I was forced to display it."

"Wouldn't you say that you masochistically gave up, very early, the hope of being loved by others? Isn't the reasoning 'nobody loves me, therefore I must love myself' rather defeatist?"

"Yes, of course—if you are right, and the boy in my fantasies is really an improved edition of myself."

"Can you, offhand, suggest another model?"

"No, I can't. But that doesn't prove anything."

"Correct. Do you still remember, from your school days, what a working hypothesis is? Instead of saying 'x' or 'we don't know,' one substitutes a temporary theory to work on. It can always be discarded as soon as the original tentative assumption is proved wrong or can be supplanted by another assumption that seems more promising."

"I understand your caution, but, having read your book, I suspect that you don't make use of even a working hypothesis without good reason."

"At the present moment the Narcissus theory seems the most promising."

Some days later the patient brought the Narcissus theory up again; it had been preying on his mind.

"You said that I had a defeatist attitude—nobody loves me—that practically amounts to a form of masochistic abdication. Since then I've been thinking about something that happened to me two years ago in Rome. A young boy, absolutely *not* my type, followed me; I was on my way to my hotel. After a few blocks he came up and spoke to me, promising me the usual 'good time.' I said no; the boy actually disgusted me. I went on, and then I turned back and asked him what made him a male prostitute. Then I noticed that there were two suspicious-looking men; they were watching me very closely. I concluded that these two unsavory characters were blackmailers and that the boy was the bait they used for trapping wealthy Americans. I was frightened; I got an immediate picture of a scare headline: WEALTHY AMERICAN ARRESTED! I went back to the hotel, fast. I told you, and this is important, that the boy was absolutely *not* my type; he disgusted me. Still, this scene comes up time and again in my masturbation fantasies. Why?"

"Can you provide the obvious answer yourself?"

"No, I cannot. I have some inkling, but I can't even formulate what I mean."

"But look at the connection in which you brought it up. You spoke first of 'masochistic abdication,' admittedly quoting me. Isn't the clue in the word 'masochistic'? Obviously what attracts you in the scene you evoke so frequently is not the sexual connotation. You said emphatically that the boy rather disgusted you and that he was definitely not your type. Conclusion: under the disguise of a sexual scene you live out a masochistic fantasy. You are attracted to the situation of danger, as represented by the two 'unsavory characters.'"

"I don't know whether this is the reason or not. At least it makes

What Does Psychoanalytic Therapy Accomplish?

a stab at clarifying something I couldn't explain at all. Is this another 'working hypothesis'?"

"No. It's an interpretation. Nothing tentative about it."

"Are you sure?"

"I am."

"How can you prove it?"

"By asking you to give me more material. I am certain that additional memories will produce a good many clear-cut masochistic incidents."

"You mean real happenings, or fantasies?"

"Both."

"I don't believe so."

"Neither of us is in the prediction business. Let's wait."

The confirmation came quickly. A few days later the patient remembered a "crazy incident" that took place when he was thirteen. He found a hypodermic syringe in his mother's room. Fascinated by the instrument, he began to use it—on himself. First he merely simulated injections; then, having found a spot on his side that was comparatively insensitive to the point of the needle, he half filled the syringe with alcohol and pierced his skin. This recollection brought back a still earlier one. At the age of twelve, during a vacation trip to the Orient, a man invited him to "go for a walk." He refused and ran to his mother. His mother informed the hotel employees, who held the man until the police arrived. The police beat him severely before taking him into custody. For weeks the boy relived, again and again, what he imagined the man had felt during his beating.

A third recollection then emerged, haltingly: he had some vague memory of a puberal fantasy in which he was alone with a man on an island; the man would "torture him."

"Now do you believe my interpretation of the incident in Rome?"

"Half and half."

"As soon as you inwardly digest the fact that homosexuality has a masochistic basis, originally projected on woman and later—in frantic flight—shifted to man. you will not be a homosexual any more. If you want to express masochistic torture fantasies, why not do it directly? Why hide behind homosexuality?"

"But I don't want to be a masochist either!"

"Nobody is asking you to be. First we have to separate the deeper masochistic tension from the more superficial homosexual one."

"And where did my masochistic tension come from?"

"It started so early in life that we can only reconstruct it. Even though you were only four at the time, your famous scene with the governess was undoubtedly a later edition of the original, but buried, basis."

"What scene? What are you talking about?"

"Isn't it strange that I should remember your material better than you do? I am alluding to your penis exhibitionism in the bath, before your governess, that 'good-looking, high-breasted, but sour and unappreciative girl.' I hope you recognize your own words. The governess who scolded you severely and made a disgusted face when you proudly showed your organ. Do I remember correctly, or am I confusing you with another patient?"

Blushing and rather embarrassed, the patient admitted: "You remember correctly. I don't see, though, what you want to prove."

"What I want to prove presupposes some knowledge of theory. To explain it I need both your indulgence and your permission to 'waste your valuable time.' Promise not to be too impatient?"

A smile brightened Mr. C.'s serious face, and he motioned me to go ahead.

"You see," I began, "this scene with the governess is only one of many repressed incidents in your childhood. Perhaps it was the culmination and the turning point in what could be called 'exhibitionistic reparation.' That calls for a somewhat long explanation. Everybody hears about the boy's 'penis pride,' but few people know that this is a rather late development, coming after a feeling that to the adult seems fantastic. What comes first is *breast envy*. It doesn't matter whether the infant boy was breast-fed or bottle-fed; in either case he envies the giantess of his nursery because she possesses a mysterious organ—big, long, and capable of producing fluid. Then comes the tragedy of weaning, one of the last tombstones of infantile megalomania. Weaning proves to the boy that he is dependent on someone else; it shows, finally, that he was wrong in his theory that this 'someone' is a part of himself or a slave obedient to his magical power. The small child's way out is *reparation*. He

What Does Psychoanalytic Therapy Accomplish?

discovers that his own body possesses an organ that he reasons can substitute for the envied breast. It is big, long, and it seemingly produces fluid. He does not see all the objective differences between his mother's breast, or the bottle, and his own penis. Anatomical, physiological, histological, functional, chemical differences are of no importance to him. All he cares about is that he has discovered a substitute, and it belongs to him. In fact, he finds that his 'penis-breast' has superior qualities. It produces pleasurable feelings when he manipulates it. Only one detail seems unsatisfactory, its size. Though he knows that the organ is capable of expanding at certain times—even babies have erections—he never seems to be sure that the mysterious expansion will be repeated; his penis exhibitionism proves this. All male children go through a period of penis exhibitionism, shocking their elders by their 'indecency.' Their purpose is not so much direct exhibitionism as some kind of confirmation; they want to prove 'how big' the organ is as compared with the size of the breast.

"Now admittedly this sounds fantastic when simply stated as a deduction. Let me give you two examples of the material from which this deduction has been drawn.

"In one of my earliest publications, in 1932, I described a case of pseudo mental debility in which the following scene was recalled. The boy was thrown out of school in the first grade because he masturbated in the presence of the whole class. He was then sent to a country school, where he boarded in a house run by the head mistress of the school. This probably meant that he received some special consideration. When he was six and a half he watched a gypsy woman nursing her baby. That gave him the idea for a game: he took a long straw and put one end into his penis and the other into his mouth. He then drank his own urine. Forget the disgusting element and think only of the meaning of the game. Obviously it is an attempt at autarchy, a declaration of independence from the mother.

"In my book THE SUPEREGO I described, among other cases, a recollection that came to the fore in the analysis of a French photographer. He was three and a half and at the beach with his mother. He came out of their cabin naked; his mother scolded him and told him to cover himself. He obeyed—by draping a towel around his neck.

"There are two sides to the story of the boy's frantic penis exhibitionism. He exhibits to confirm his contention that he couldn't have been deprived of the breast (in weaning) because he possesses just such a 'breast' on his own body. The other side of the story is the cultural necessity of inhibiting this exhibitionism, a necessity imposed by his mother or her representatives. Both parties involved feel fully justified, although, of course, their justifications have different motives.

"This leads to one of the real tragedies of childhod. The scoldings, the faces showing disgust or even horror, with which the mother reacts to the exhibitions at best interfere with the boy's attempt at compensatory (and illusionary) reparation and sometimes keep him from using the mechanism at all.

"There are a series of possible results. To name only three: One type—a classification of future neurotics—acquires and keeps the 'complex of the small penis.' These people are constantly concerned with the size of their penis, complicating the matter by taking an unusable standard for their yardstick. This standard is the non-erect organ. Since the size of the non-erect penis is no indication of its size in erection, their self-torturing inspections and comparisons are valueless. Besides, the usable length of the vagina in intercourse is two and a half to three inches. The average erect penis is longer than that, which makes everything above three inches a 'luxury.'

"Another type, the normally developing boy, weathers all criticism of his exhibitionism and solves his problem by mentally reversing the roles played by his mother and himself. As a baby he had been passively fed by the 'long organ'; now he sees his 'long organ' as the means through which he can become the active feeder. Later, in intercourse, he will push a 'duplicate' of the 'long organ' into the vagina, which he will unconsciously identify with his own baby mouth. At the same time, he will unconsciously identify sperm with milk. This 'active repetition of a passively endured experience' enables him to rescue his narcissism and re-establish his shaky self-esteem. No wonder the average man calls his wife 'baby'!

"The third solution is that of the homosexual. I have called his solution the pursuit of 'the reduplication of his own defense mechanism.' Although he has found in his own penis a substitute for the disappointing breast—the vanishing breast, if you like—he is so unsure of his trick that he constantly requires to be re-assured that it works. His partner's possession of a penis confirms his belief that 'nothing is lost—yet.' Ironically, the penis he so eagerly seeks in his partner is unconsciously only a substitute for the breast that he so often finds 'disgusting' in real women.

"There is another facet to the boy's penis exhibitionism. He is also using it as a defense against his mother's prohibition of peeping. When his passive wish to peep is thwarted it changes into its opposite, following an unconscious law, and becomes defiant and active exhibitionism. The formula is something like this: 'Who wants to look at your ugly udder anyway? I have a beautiful penis-breast myself!' Don't forget that you specifically mentioned that the governess was 'high-breasted.'

"Now you will ask what all this has to do with you. Only this: in view of its undoubted precursors the scene with the governess acquires additional importance."

For the first time Mr. C. interrupted. "You agree, then, that her objectively rejecting attitude did damage me?"

"I would not say that. I have seen cases in which the boy's penis exhibition was checked in the friendliest way, and severe after-effects developed. I have seen other cases in which the parents interfered brutally and there were no deleterious effects. It all boils down to the child himself, how he accepts the unavoidable. This is what accounts for my suspicion that children who cannot take the constant unavoidable offenses to their megalomania are sure candidates for psychic masochism. Don't forget that the psychic masochist rescues some vestiges of megalomania under self-damaging conditions. By unconsciously provoking the kick he gives himself the unconscious satisfaction of being able to say: 'This fool thinks he's kicking me, but actually I, through my initial provocation, *made* him kick me!"

"And what determines the ability to 'take it'?"

"Probably the biologically conditioned amount of megalomania, which is different for every child."

"A very disquieting conclusion."

"Did you ever hear the French saying, 'the most beautiful Parisienne cannot give more than she has'? That's the present state of my knowledge. Ask me again in a few hundred years."

The topic of compensatory penis exhibitionism occupied us through many subsequent appointments. I pointed out additional facts: The patient had casually mentioned once that certain sandals worn by men and especially by boys at the beach had some sexual attraction for him. What he really meant was that these sandals attracted him by prominently displaying the big toe, which he symbolically saw as a penis equivalent. The flat feet from which he had suffered in childhood came into the attraction also. His flat feet had made the symbolism personally inapplicable since they left him "nothing to brag about." It was not by chance that he had endowed his improved self-portrait—the boy of his fantasies—with "beautiful, high-arched feet."

At this point the patient—still with perfect politeness—revealed the strength of his unconscious resistance by making an openly defiant, rejecting remark. "You have finally achieved a result: I am totally confused."

"Why do you blame me for the complexity of the psychic apparatus? If you just want to be angry, enjoy yourself—but you should know that you are again playing the masochistic injustice-collecting game in the transference (meaning using innocent outsiders for the repetition of infantile conflicts) and assigning to me the part of torturer and to yourself that of innocent victim. If it's not that you want to indulge your anger, perhaps you have stumbled on one of the famous 'contradictions' that every patient discovers in the course of his analysis. Let's see whether what you call your confusion (why not say disbelief and suspicion?) can be straightened out."

"I really have lost the thread; I don't understand. On the one hand you claim that I created my improved Narcissus type in order to be loved and love. On the other hand, as the Roman blackmail episode shows, you claim that I derive my real pleasure from my masochistic enjoyment of danger. Which is which?"

"There is a contradiction between your two types of homosexual fantasies, but it is a contradiction you implanted yourself, and it is spurious. Every homosexual declares that he wants 'love.' Yet he

What Does Psychoanalytic Therapy Accomplish?

conducts his love affairs in such a manner that masochism comes out on top."

"As simple as that?"

"What do you call simple? The fact that the human mind is capable of piling one defense on top of another in what seems to be an endless tower has occupied the attention of thousands of analysts all over the world for the past sixty years. Is this what you call 'simple'?"

"I didn't mean to be offensive."

"You are invited to be as sceptical as you wish—provided you also cast a sceptical eye on your own scepticism. By the way, this is a good opening for attacking your hyper-suspicion. At your suggestion we once put it in the psychic icebox. Let's take it out of the deep freeze."

"Why? So that you can have another argument against me?"

"Do you really believe that the purpose of this analysis is to attack you? Isn't your statement another grab at masochistic enjoyment, this time by way of falsifying facts?"

"O.K. You have the floor."

"My deduction is short and—you will like this—simple. By being hyper-suspicious, by being unable to distinguish between friend and enemy, you constantly put yourself behind the eight ball and make yourself into an innocent victim, unjustly attacked. Don't you see that by imputing to everyone, everywhere, under all circumstances sinister designs you are still fighting your unfinished infantile battle of suspecting all your educators of underhand tricks?"

"Are you suggesting that I ought to be naive? Wealthy people have to be suspicious."

"Yes. But they don't have to isue a blanket indictment against all of humanity. Is naivety the only alternative? Why not discriminate?"

"Why should anyone do anything for me without expecting a return?"

"Human kindness does exist, or, if you prefer, some people are sometimes not interested in damaging others. Neurotic malice exists, too, of course, but it is—neurotic."

"The distinction is slim."

"I don't think so. Take your own attitude as an example. Every time I try to fix your attention on some new facet of your problem—'new' meaning an aspect not yet discussed here—you behave as though an attack had been launched against you personally. Do you think this attitude justified?"

"Do you claim you are contributing to my happiness?"

"Definitely yes, if you take the long-range view."

"I see that I'm in for a new disclosure."

"My condolences to your dying neurosis. Why you should defend that beast is less logical. Well, this is what I want to bring up: Remember the episode of the syringe you found in your mother's room?"

"What about it?"

"Do you remember how you used it?"

"Of course."

"Would you agree that you must have had some masochistic-sadistic fantasies about the sex act at that time?"

"I don't see that."

"Why did you fill the symbolic syringe with a fluid and apply it—in spite of the pain—*passively* against yourself? Why didn't you experiment on, say, a cat or a dog, playing the *active* part yourself?"

"I don't know."

"Both possibilities did exist."

"That's true. I never thought of that."

"What would you conclude from this selectivity?"

"Do you want me to say 'feminine identification'?"

"I want you to think, not to play the parrot with half-digested phrases. No, it wasn't feminine identification at all. That was your mother's syringe you found; therefore you were acting as her representative. Your game meant: 'Mother inflicts pain—and that's sex.' Is it surprising that you should run away from that 'torturing monster'?"

There was no answer.

"And do you remember a fantasy you had in puberty of yourself imprisoned on an island and tortured by some man?"

"Yes."

"There you have another part of the riddle that troubled you to

What Does Psychoanalytic Therapy Accomplish?

the point of 'confusion.' In your flight from the 'monster,' woman, you ran away to man, at first maintaining your masochistic torture fantasies. Then, as defense, you create the romantic Narcissus fantasy."

"Let me think this over."

A few days later Mr. C. said in a matter-of-fact way, "Your theory is that every time I have a homosexual fantasy I really mean a masochistic one."

"Correct."

"Since I have two types of homosexual fantasy, the romantic and the more obviously masochistic, can I pick any one I wish?"

"I doubt that. Which you choose probably depends on the state of your inner fear of the masochistic danger. I would guess that the romantic fantasy is the stronger alibi."

"A perfect alibi?"

"A very imperfect alibi. You still, alibi or not, run away from both dangers, man and woman; you still work on the reparation level; you still cling to the defeatist conclusion, 'nobody loves me.' I have always doubted the theory that the narcissistic type in homosexuality simply expresses high-pitched narcissism. It seems to me that the narcissistic type begins as a terribly beaten-down and masochistic child who, in his despair, secondarily rescues himself by retreating to the only refuge he knows, his narcissism. In other words, narcissism is not the propelling factor but a defensive island of safety to which the child goes when everything else has failed."

"Once more, nothing to be proud of."

"Let's face it: undigested fears and narcissistic reparations are not exactly heroic. By the way, your romantic fantasy of the boy on the beach contains two 'reparation payments' worth mentioning, aside from the elements already discussed. One of these is the crew cut. This is not just a protest against your own curly and superabundant hair, as you assumed. It is also an attempt to repair and overcome the tragic—to the child—fact that he has no genital hair. It is possible, too, that some Samson-Delilah fantasies are involved, in an acceptance of castration executed by a woman. Second, you prefer the boy in your fantasy to be naked on the beach, or wearing very little. In other words, the boy exhibits defiantly; you tried to exhibit and were slapped down. Again an attempt at reparation."

"What is real about it all? What isn't fake?"

"If you call reparative defenses fake, nothing is real."

"What am I so afraid of?"

"Of woman's power to damage—meaning of woman as the executive organ of your own innermost wishes."

"How can you prove that I'm afraid of women?"

"Well, you are not exactly a woman chaser, are you? And what about the cave dreams you have had repeatedly in the last few weeks? They are all uncanny, all full of danger. I told you—although we haven't yet uncovered any recollections to back this up—that most likely castration fantasies are involved: if woman herself is castrated she may revenge herself by castrating man."

These dreams finally gave the patient what he had been looking for since the beginning of analysis: a partial and pseudo justification for his resistance to the analytic process. No recollections of vaginal inspections in childhood emerged, nor was much material on peeping elicited. He harped on these "missing links" incessantly, until I told him:

"According to Freud, recollections and reconstructions have the identical dynamic effect. Of course we prefer recollections, if only because they are less vulnerable to attack by unbelievers in analysis. Why don't you substitute reality for the reconstruction?"

"Meaning?"

"Look for the girl."

"So early in the game?"

"Five and a half months of analysis is not too early."

After some time Mr. C. began an affair with a young girl who professed to love him. He made it clear that marriage was not his intention; she claimed that she was not interested in marriage either. Mr. C. was potent with her, though he declared himself irritated by her "stupidity." After we had worked out his "irritation on principle," which proved to cover fear, he admitted that he was enjoying his sexual experiences and the affair itself. I then reminded him of his bitter question "Do you claim that you are contributing to my

What Does Psychoanalytic Therapy Accomplish? 121

happiness?" His only reply was a laugh. To the patient's great surprise even his homosexual fantasies disappeared.

An old (though probably outdated) military principle in the training of troops was "ask for the impossible, to get the possible." A commander who wanted his training group to march twenty miles a day asked for forty.

Applied to analysis: we aim at the maximum. We know, however, that many neurotics are incapable of achieving more than a halfway livable minimum. The elasticity of the ego in different people is different.

It is a commonplace occurrence in the practice of every experienced analyst that while treating simultaneously three similar cases, and with the same method, he achieves quite different results—varying from excellent to poor. Obviously the technique, time, interpretations were identical. Still the results are dissimilar.

"Elasticity of the ego," for want of a better term, denotes in analytic therapy the ability to renounce the old masochistic technique of accepting inner torture under manifold disguises. Retrieving and salvaging the original aggression that was unhealthily transverted into psychic masochism has its limitations, different in different individuals.

Not infrequently encountered is a *shift of masochistic deposits from conspicuous to inconspicuous places.* If this happens many patients declare themselves "satisfied." Sometimes it is advisable to recommend continuation of treatment; in other cases the patient's statement is an accurate evaluation of how far he is able to go.

On the other hand, one can state with clinical certainty that the changes brought about in favorable cases are truly amazing. Psychoanalytic psychiatry, as originally devised by Freud, remains the deepest and most promising form of psychotherapy for neurotics.

What changes in the psychic apparatus does successful psychoanalysis accomplish?

Its most important contributions to relative contentment consists in diminution of the power of the "department of torture," the superego. Though the "daimonion" is beyond analytic reach, three basic changes are achieved:

1. The ego ideal (the "department of don'ts and great expectations") is tuned down to real possibilities and the actual abilities of the individual. Since that "silent mirror" of infantile hopes megalomaniacally inflated is habitually misused by the daimonion to torture the ego, one of its most effective weapons is taken away from it. The objection that the "realistic" person can by himself make these necessary adjustments is naive; the ego ideal, being unconscious, cannot be reached without analysis of the unconscious.

2. The repressed infantile taboos (the "don'ts"), connected with pre-oedipal and oedipal fantasies of libidinous and pseudoaggressive content, are partially resolved, especially if it has been constantly pointed out that these "repressed desires" (to use the popular misnomer) are not so much real wishes as convenient hitching posts for taking the blame for the "lesser intrapsychic crime," the basic masochistic conflict.

3. The ego is given a new weapon to fight the daimonion: the newly retrieved aggression from the previously masochistic amalgam (see above).

At bottom successful analytic treatment strengthens the unconscious ego by partial de-masochization and at the same time humanizes the unconscious ego ideal. Thus, though we have no direct access to the daimonion part of the superego, nor to the id, we render both relatively harmless by interrupting and making superfluous the inner neurotic barter system in the form of staggering defenses (neurotic symptoms), denials, masochization. The id is left to "stew in its own juice," and the daimonion has lost its involuntary "moral" helper and dupe (the inflated ego ideal). The "inner trade balance" of the personality is markedly improved.

The irony of the situation is that our therapeutic successes and failures are viewed erroneously by the ignorant environment. For instance, I once treated a gambler who, after shedding the gambling sector of his psychic masochism, declared himself cured, in spite of my strong protests. For his extended circle of acquaintances he be-

What Does Psychoanalytic Therapy Accomplish? 123

came a living example of efficacy of analysis. A few years later one of his acquaintances consulted me, giving as his reason for choosing me the fact that his friend had been "so thoroughly cured that not even his unhappy marriage and recent divorce could throw him back to gambling." That the unhappy marriage was the result of the unsolved totality of his masochism was not known to the new patient.

To turn the tables. I treated a wealthy business man because of homosexuality, and he was freed from that scourge. Among the other neurotic troubles he had produced was the fact that he could only operate in a "favorable environment"; he practically bought the benevolence of his close and distant cronies with expensive gifts. After this neurotic deposition was removed he became more discriminating and sparing in his gifts, and I was blamed by his innumerable hangers-on for having changed him into a "stingy bastard."

And so on.

Obviously the analytic standards of "cure" and those of the environment do not coincide, to use an understatement. Even more difficult is the fact that the analyst's and the patient's evaluations seldom coincide.

What can be achieved analytically in schizoid cases?

The answer depends on the quantity of neurotic admixtures. The scale ranges from zero—*no success at all*—to higher percentages, where the improvement that can be registered is mostly *transitory*. The accent is on "transitory," because the old neurotic defenses are recalled as a life-saver against the fear of "malignant masochism."

Among the books on my shelves there is one by an authoress (plagued for years by writer's block) who through treatment with me became capable of writing a highly praised novel, only to revert in later years to her depressive, alcoholic moods and total unproductivity. Disregarding the inner facts—her malignant masochism—she became my vociferous enemy, entirely forgetting the inscription in her book: "For Dr. Bergler, without whose help this book would not have been written. With many thanks and all best wishes."

I had among my many homosexual patients one of great prominence, with two cases of schizophrenia in his immediate family, who became potent, married, produced children, only to revert after a number of years to homosexual fantasies, without transforming those into "reality." He obviously could not live without the pseudoaggression included in homosexuality. Once more "malignant masochism" was victorious.

CHAPTER 4

ARE THE LIMITATIONS OF ANALYTIC THERAPY INHERENT IN THE MATERIAL, THE TECHNIQUE, THE PATIENT, OR THE THERAPIST?

IN the first decade of the century some of Freud's more naive medical adherents and a few naive laymen (part of the less ambivalent group that did not reject analysis on principle) envisioned psychoanalysis as a cure-all for every psychic ill. Freud himself, a lifelong sceptic, never shared this undue enthusiasm; he even warned against "furor therapeuticus," pointing out that *at that time* (the beginning of the century) the study of the unconscious was more important than therapy. This had two rather ironical results. On the one hand there were colleagues (and one finds them even today) who refused to acknowledge that they treated a patient; according to them they merely "studied" him. On the other hand, since the exaggerated hopes of curing every patient did not materialize, a deep therapeutic scepticism swept whole groups of psychoanalysts.

As usual, neither hyperoptimism nor hyperpessimism was justified. Neither took into account that analysis—a very young science—was still in the process of developing. Although the greatest limitation of analysis is its exclusively *medical* applicability to neuroses (there are, of course, "applied" fields), more and more has become known of previously not even suspected material—and complications.

To name but a few neurotic disease entities either considered hopeless or difficult to cure or unknown altogether whose curability I myself could present to a scientific forum: character neuroses based on oral-masochistic regression; severe cases of premature ejaculation; psychogenic aspermia (a disease entity described by me in 1937); frigidity based on oral regression; specific types of promiscuity; writer's block; pseudo humbugs and hucksters; pseudo mental deficiency (described by me in 1932); retirement neurosis (described in 1944 in collaboration with O. Knopf); writer's cramp; male homosexuality and Lesbianism; alcohol addiction; gambling; middle-age revolt; impostor-like attitudes; kleptomania; coprophemia; logorrhea; bulimia; money neurosis; pathological smoking; depersonalization; alysosis (described by me in 1946); postpartum depression; and the whole visual orbit (22 subdivisions; see Chapter 7).

Conservatism in a still developing science is not only dangerous, it is faintly ridiculous. It reminds one of Douglas Jerrold's famous epigram: "A conservative is a man who will not look at the new moon out of respect for that 'ancient institution' the old one." One could add that, besides "respect," conservatism in science also involves a mixture of mental inertia and fear.

For example, if further research provides added proof that my contention is clinically correct, namely that the basic infantile conflict is psychic masochism and all later libidinous-pseudoaggressive symptoms only rescue stations from that conflict, a revamping and rethinking will become necessary—painful as it may be for "conservatives."

The neurotic patient's curability depends on six factors:

1. The analyst's correct understanding of the patient's basic inner masochistic conflict and his technical skill in handling it.

2. The patient's capacity to renounce his self-damaging defenses (superficially visible in his symptoms, signs, personality distortions) when they are explained and effectively worked through in the transference and resistance situations.

3. The analyst's capacity to distinguish the basic conflict from the "trimmings," without falling for the camouflage of "rescue stations" (libidinous-pseudoaggressive hide-outs).

4. Finding and debunking the "pseudomoral connotations" on which the neurotic structure rests (see below pp. 130 ff.).

Limitations of Analytic Therapy

5. Dynamic, not static, thinking on the part of both analyst and patient.

6. Sufficient time for therapy.

Many psychoanalysts, to use an understatement, do not conform to these indispensable conditions. True enough, not all neurotics in treatment are capable of renouncing their "hide-outs," but *they should be given a chance* to face their real problem. That is exactly what frequently does not happen. The analyst concentrates on the superficial layers, mistaking those for the "real thing."

In my recent book PRINCIPLES OF SELF-DAMAGE I enumerated "fourteen technical errors in clinical analysis in our transitional period" (Chapter XI). The subheadings of the chapter were:

1. Inner obstacles to acceptance of the paramount importance of psychic masochism, based on oral regression.

2. Confusion between aggression and pseudoaggression.

3. Inability to think in terms of megalomania, aggression, and libido at the same time.

4. Rigidity in refusing to modify the analytic technique in orally regressed cases.

5. Misconceptions in regard to the contents of oral and anal regression.

6. Unwillingness or inability to accept pre-oedipal structures wholeheartedly.

7. Unwillingness or inability to apply the five-layer structure in neurotic symptoms.

8. Confusion between legitimate silence and its illegitimate counterpart.

9. The faulty theory that parents are to blame for the patient's neurosis.

10. A certain unwillingness or naivety in handling reality factors in analysis.

11. Misunderstanding of or unfamiliarity with the "voyeuristic-exhibitionistic exchange mechanism" (see Chapter 7 of the present volume).

12. Inability to grasp the difference between the internal and external "lawbooks."

13. Inactivity when facing the patient's masochistic misuse of the transference situation.

14. Dogmatism, heresy-hunting, distrust of the new, according to the formula "my learning days are over."

This chapter in PRINCIPLES, comprising nearly fifty printed pages, needs no repetition; I shall discuss here only a few basic difficulties.

Here is an example seen in my office dozens of times. A patient consults me, having spent two, three, four, or more years with a colleague (or a succession of colleagues) because of, let's say, depression, or premature ejaculation, or street fear, or homosexuality, or inability to solve or repair an unhappy marriage, or writer's block, or any other neurotic symptom. When the patient is asked to summarize in a few sentences the basic interpretations given to him by his analyst, a peculiar vagueness is often registered. The answers range from "he (she) told me nothing" to "unsolved attachment to mother (father)" to "guilt because of my hostility" to "we analyzed only details, I never got an over-all picture." Making allowances for the patient's anger and obvious tendency to disparage the analyst (or analysts) who did not help him (and the amazing unreliability of patients), one fact emerges: even the intelligent and not-too-malicious ones cannot give a clear picture. The analyst was invariably silent, and the patient "suffered in having to squeeze out so-called associations." This masochistic misuse of free associations was not explained; the patient's neurotic pseudoaggressions were taken at face value as real aggression; though the oedipal instrumentarium was dutifully applied in the transference and resistance the pre-oedipal layers were mostly not dealt with; secondary defenses were confused with the deepest repressed wishes; masochistic vicissitudes were declared to be guilt because of repressed (real) aggression; and—this is decisive—the basic masochistic personality structure was left untouched. One should add that in cases where the visual instinct was decisively involved—e.g. writer's block, jealousy, street fear, boredom, stage fright, etc.—the complex defensive exchanges between voyeurism and exhibitionism, as explained in Chapter 7 of the present volume, were without exception either not made use of at all or were misunderstood.

The most grotesque example was reported by a reliable patient whose analysis I continued after five years of treatment with an ex-

Limitations of Analytic Therapy

perienced colleague. According to the patient, the analyst opened his mouth three times during a half-decade. The first time, when the patient's parents (obviously for tax reasons) gave him a large sum of money as a "gift," the comment was "Now you want me to do your analytic work too." The second remark was made in connection with the patient's early difficulties in school: he could not concentrate, forgot the material, learned little. The analyst's interpretation: "When you told me this years ago I suspected that you would repeat the same procedure in analysis too." The third utterance came during the last appointment when the patient informed him that he had decided to continue his analysis with me: "Don't you think that you should discuss it?" "I have talked for five years—you can talk now." But the analyst remained silent during the whole appointment; at the end they shook hands, and "that was that."

Amusingly enough, all three comments were based on the analyst's misunderstanding of the patient's psychic masochism. The first misinterpreted his "wish to get" as genuine; the appropriate interpretation, based on his masochistic elaboration leading to the "wish to be refused," would have been: "Your parents' gift makes your position more difficult. How can your parents have been as 'bad' as you describe them if they are so generous?" The second comment was only a narcissistic proof of "good prophecy," but, though banal, the point should have been explained to the patient earlier. The third remark, a lack of comment, misunderstood the patient's feeling offended; he considered giving free associations as being "drained" and being refused.

In short, many of these analyses, though conducted in the forties and fifties of the century, could just as well have been conducted in 1905 or thereabouts. It is not clear whether the analysts' knowledge was static and fixated on that early date or whether they had the benefit of later theoretical knowledge (and hence of all the progress made since that time) but did not apply it dynamically.

I do not maintain, of course, that if these rather anachronistic errors had been avoided in the previous analyses of the patients mentioned above they would all have been cured. Some were apparently unrecognized schizoid personalities, some were incapable of changing. But many, in fact most, could be helped when their psychic masochism was put in the center. I have reported in earlier books such seemingly hopeless but actually curable cases in which I was the second, third, or fourth analyst.

The decisive point, which cannot be stressed often enough, is that the patient has to be given an analytic chance. He is deprived of this chance when his deep masochistic conflict is neglected and his difficulties explained only in terms of superficial layers; he is simply not familiarized with his real unconscious problem. This does not mean that the patient will always use that unique chance, but that's *his* affair.

Ironically enough, I have seen and heard of a few cases who could not take the interpretation of psychic masochism in analysis with me and consulted colleagues disagreeing with me on that score. They were mostly schizoid cases (see Chapter 1), and these analyses, renewed attempts to "appeal to a higher court," ended in failure.

I should like to stress a phenomenon that is widely unknown or unapplied even among colleagues who do analyze psychic masochism as the basis of every neurosis: the *unconscious "pseudomoral connotation."*

This represents an additional difficulty, by no means basic but one that contributes to the tenacity of the neurotic balance. One has to uncover the "private moral code" of the particular unconscious ego and also to debunk the unconscious irony that has enabled the weak child to beat the powerful educator with his own stick. This infantile mockery of reasonable educational precepts by distorting their meaning while preserving the letter of their form proves that the weak ego uses every available pseudoaggressive means of warding off reproaches concerning the basic conflict, psychic masochism.

Clinical observation has convinced me that every secondary defense (layer V) is deliberately built around an actually indoctrinated educational precept, cunningly misinterpreted so that it sanctions the exact opposite of the original command. The precept serves as a shield magically and effectively inscribed with the slogan "You (my parents) said so yourselves!" This unconscious irony directed against the internalized educators (enshrined in the ego-ideal sector of the superego) is carefully manipulated by the unconscious ego. Moral precepts

Limitations of Analytic Therapy

are literally reproduced at the wrong time, in the wrong place, on the wrong or inappropriate occasion, out of context, and with the wrong intention, thus entirely perverting the original meaning. The result is a *reductio ad absurdum*.

In this way the unconscious ego immobilizes the daimonion. By appearing to fulfill the demands of the ego ideal it achieves one of its rare, effective pseudoaggressive retorts and removes the daimonion's standard excuse for torture. The tactic also strengthens immeasurably the unconscious ego's ability to create and maintain the spurious secondary defense.

The ego ideal was originally established for a dual purpose: to relieve the child of the burden of constant narcissistic humiliation in submitting to parental commands and to remove the basic cause of conflict between child and parents. The creation of the ego ideal marks the beginning of a new educational era in which the child voluntarily performs familiar routines and voluntarily assumes new ones, instead of reluctantly and rebelliously accepting parental suggestions. Within this benevolent inner structure both parental and cultural taboos are incorporated. At first the new regime is entirely satisfactory to parent and child; the parent prides himself on success as an educator, the child on a successful method of avoiding external conflicts and on the tricky means he has found of protecting his narcissism.

Under the surface, however, there are complications. The daimonion, ever on the alert for torture material, finds here a rich new source: for the ego ideal is more than a tabulation of parental and cultural dicta; it contains the grandiose ideas evolved by the child in speculating on his future career, and his overoptimistic picture, to the last luckless detail, remains on record to be matched against his adult achievement. Discrepancies cannot be avoided, and therefore guilt cannot be avoided. The inner structure that conferred so many benefits thus becomes a source of torture.

But the daimonion does not register an absolute victory here. The internalized taboos and the illusions of a brilliant future, though they provide abundant material for torture, at the same time impose a limitation. The daimonion cannot decree punishment for an act sanctioned by the internalized educators. The ego makes good use of this limitation; it constructs a defense corresponding to an enshrined precept. Strangely enough, the precepts that make up the ego ideal can be used to silence both the ego and the daimonion, thus providing material for a *two-way immobilization trick*. The daimonion silences the ego by pointing out discrepancies between the ego ideal and actual achievement, and the ego accepts penance. But the ego can disarm the daimonion by building a defense on a precept in the ego ideal. Such a defense becomes an *abage Satanas*.

Two mechanims exemplify the inner rule.

Silencing the ego: The child who aspires to decorate some future Sistine Chapel with his majestic creations and grows up to find himself a designer of wallpaper is easy prey to the daimonion. The record is indelible, the comparison damning. For this blatant discrepancy the ego inwardly accepts punishment. There can be no excuses for this "failure."

Silencing the daimonion: A masochistic person performing a magic gesture—demonstrating by his actions that he allegedly wished to be treated lovingly and kindly in childhood—is presenting the fifth act in an unconscious drama. Masochistic submission, the first act, has already been vetoed by the superego (layer II); the defense of pseudo-aggression, the third act, has also been rejected (layer IV). But the secondary defense, the magic gesture (layer V) embodies a cultural precept included in the ego ideal ("What's wrong with kindness and love?"), and the daimonion cannot object to it.

Unhappily this victory over the daimonion merely provides a breathing spell. After a short time the attack is renewed and the artificial structure of the defense inevitably discovered. This clears the way for a veto; the new access of guilt calls for a new defense.

The pseudomoral connotation becomes a powerful weapon of resistance in analysis. Many masochistic attitudes cannot be analytically resolved without dislodging this pseudomoral prop.

This fact reveals the nonsensical element in the objection that stressing psychic masochism dispenses with all other interpretations and the patient "hears only that he is a psychic masochist." True, it is possible to schematize the interpretation of psychic masochism. But it is not possible to schematize the search for the hidden meaning in the pseudomoral connotation, which is highly individualized and

Limitations of Analytic Therapy

specific for every patient. In any case, stressing the psychic masochistic substructure is not likely to become a pons asinorum.

To adduce some clinical examples:

A young man with a severe masochistic personality neurosis and inability to work, who also suffered from "psychogenic oral aspermia," [14] persisted for a long time in his refusal to take a particular technical examination. "Take the idiotic examination!" his infuriated father would demand. "I am not thoroughly prepared yet," was the son's constant reply. The superficial layers of his examination fear were easily explained. His father had tried to teach him the alphabet at the age of four and, dissatisfied with the child's progress, constantly complained that he was not "thorough" enough in his studies. Two decades later the son executed his by then full-fledged masochistic neurosis (also manifested in his wish to fail the examination) by pseudoaggression: "Well, I'll give you thoroughness—till you're blue in the face!" Blame for the lesser crime (pseudoaggression) is accepted, and the pseudomoral connotation of the secondary defense is obvious: "What's wrong with doing as Father said and being thorough?" Time, place, and occasion are of course different, so that the father's demand is reduced to absurdity. That the student damaged himself more than his father is another story.

In a consultation requested by a gifted colleague (living eight hundred miles from New York) for a patient of his, the following situation was presented. The young man, a physician, was lackadaisical in his work and had no interest in making money in his profession. He worked in a welfare institution and had become suspect to the chief of his department, who wrongly assumed that his lack of interest in the work was because the job paid very little. The conflict with his chief pushed him into analysis. In analysis with the colleague his quite extensive psychic masochism, connected with the mother image, was correctly explained and worked out. The analyst wanted a review of the case and some explanation of why the changes achieved in eight months of treatment were not too impressive, though externally the patient had improved and had accepted preparatory work for a medical specialty. He felt that "basically" the patient still had the same peculiar personality. It turned out that two facts had been overlooked. First, the idea of studying medicine had come from the young man's mother; his father had wanted him to study architecture. The mother's predilection for medicine was based on the fact that one of her relatives had become a renowned physician and had amassed some wealth. By accepting his mother's wish the patient reduced her to absurdity: he acted as though she had really meant medicine per se and not the money to be earned by practicing medicine. When I expressed this suspicion to the solemn patient a knowing smile flashed for a moment over his face; he also admitted that in general he was "quite ironical." I suggested that the pseudomoral connotation should be worked out. The second point was the suspicion that the patient's indifference was some kind of unconscious negative magic gesture: "You, Mother, treat me as a nonentity whose real wishes don't count. I shall not give you the pleasure and satisfaction of interfering with me. You want me to be subservient and without free volition; I am. Look what you did to me." Of course whether behind all this there was not hidden a schizoid personality could not be ascertained in one appointment.

A young French homosexual was given to all types of masochistic practices in the framework of his perversion (e.g., he would seek out "lovers' lanes" and look for discarded condoms and would smell, drink, or both, the contents, if any; in the identification "sperm-milk," that action is also unconsciously denoted: "What can you get from Mother but unappetizing fluid!") but stated with some pride that he never wished or allowed anal penetration. He could not explain that self-imposed taboo. It turned out that a posthumous irony against the enshrined mother image was involved. In childhood his mother had explained the sex act to him as a toilet affair: the man penetrates and then "goes to the bathroom like urination." He had the impression from his mother's facial expression that all contact with women was a dirty "toilet business." Since toilet meant for him anality he abstained from women and anality. Thus by using the pseudomoral connotation ("I don't do what Mother wanted me to abstain from") he got a "moral" justification for homosexuality. Once more, reducing to absurdity.

In the treatment of a prominent middle-aged lawyer, in analysis because of homosexuality [15] it turned out that his proud and snobbish mother had broken up his early engagement to a girl *"beneath his*

Limitations of Analytic Therapy

station." A short time later, in his first year at college, he started a homosexual affair with a young man of *his own "elevated" position*. The pseudomoral connotation here read: "You objected to the social status of the girl—you have to admit that my homosexual friend is on my level." Thus by stressing the social level he unconsciously and ironically smuggled in something even more abhorrent to his mother—homosexuality. The latter was not mentioned in his mother's sermon.

The ability to impart an unconscious ironic twist to the parental precepts embedded in the ego ideal may take on bizarre forms. Often the analyst is handicapped in his search for these hidden and anachronistic depositories of ironic lip-service conformity because he does not suspect the "intelligent" patient of so strong a streak of infantilism.

For example, the psychic masochist pleads orthodoxy for his pseudoaggression (which inevitably bounces back at him with a retaliatory injury or humiliation) by quoting: "Didn't you teach me to fight back when attacked?"

The cynic avails himself of this parental "confirmation": "Everybody secretly agrees with my forbidden views; shouldn't one look truth in the face and see the humorous side of things?"

The hypocrite plays his trump card: "Didn't you teach me not to offend people?"

The neurotic optimist, bargaining for forseeable disappointment with his philosophy of unvarying sweetness and light, cites this support: "Didn't you always tell me that people were nice?"

The proverbial victim of ingratitude, who always chooses his beneficiaries for their unreliability or their neurosis, thus making sure that his favors are not reciprocated or even acknowledged, who is always consciously disappointed and unconsciously satisfied by a kick in the jaw, quotes this appropriate precept: "Act nicely, and the other fellow will be nice too."

The neurotic reconteur, who infuriates his listeners by never moving an inch from his position in the center of the stage, finds this unconscious justification: "Didn't you say 'Don't just sit around like a bump on a log; look alive; get into things?'"

The neurotic gambler unconsciously points out: "I was told time and again, wasn't I, to take chances, to be ambitious?"

And so on, in endless highly individualized variations.

The pseudomoral connotation infiltrates another half-unconscious mechanism, *rationalization,* a mechanism of self-deception in which the unconscious ego supplies the driving power and the conscious ego unwittingly furnishes the shaky "logic" that purports to explain away the unexplainable.

It is a familiar observation that many rationalizations are peculiarly "hypocritical" in ascribing to their promoters moral or intellectual "superiority." The observation overlooks one factor: elements of the pseudomoral connotation are included in rationalization.

Since one cannot be too cautious in guarding against possible misunderstandings, it should be emphasized that the pseudomoral connotation in neurotic symptoms does not by any means represent the totality of the interpretation. It is an *additional*—though indispensable—element in the construction of the symptom. It explains why, when a problem has apparently been clarified in analysis, the symptom stubbornly persists throughout a long "working through" period.

There are other hurdles at which many an analysis falters, if the analyst is not familiar with these obstacles. I shall mention only three:

1. *Misuse of free associations.*

The analyst maintains silence in treatment for the purpose of getting material from and through the patient's free associations. The legitimate use of silence is to be distinguished from silence for silence's sake and from silence due to the analyst's failure to understand a particular resistance situation. The pillars of analytic therapy are analysis of transference and resistance, not the "analytic couch" and the "analytic easy chair." The couch does not make a neurotic an analytic patient, nor does the easy chair make a mute listener an analyst.

Maintaining silence for the sake of silence openly invites the patient to misuse the analytic situation for his masochistic purposes; unconsciously he enjoys masochistic pleasure and consciously he considers the analysis an "ordeal." I have expressed the opinion that the patient's "suffering" in analysis is chiefly the result of a technical error on the part of the analyst. Suffering is not an intrinsic part of the analytic procedure.

Limitations of Analytic Therapy

Three sources of alleged torture in analysis are most often mentioned by patients: the positive transference, which, not being reciprocated, is painful; the deflation of illusions (rationalizations) and the explanation of underlying reasons for them; and "waiting for free associations" that "refuse to come."

In the first, the analysis of the positive transference (which in the vast majority of cases represents the palimpsest of oedipality overlying oral regression, the familiar defensive rescue station of the orally regressed neurotic) should remove the sting in short order. In the second (as also in the negative transference), if the analyst avoids the technical error of taking the patient's anger (pseudoaggression) at face value and thus reinforcing his neurotic defense, the exposure of his motivations and illusions will strengthen the inner forces opposed to neurosis.

It is surprising that the accounts of ex-patients contain little or no mention of the pleasure of inner strengthening while they vividly recall their "suffering" and inflate it into the bargain. Whatever "suffering" may accompany analysis, no patient fails to experience at least a trace of the narcissistic elation that comes from self-understanding. The self-understanding that slowly grows in analysis has two results: narcissistic aggrandizement and the acquisition of a new weapon to use against unconscious attacks. Why do ex-patients forget, or at least fail to mention, these gains?

This point alone betrays the mythical basis of the widely accepted view of analysis as torture. In searching for the genesis of the myth, however, one should always consider the possibility that it is rooted in the patient's faulty interpretation of a correctly recorded fact. Since only affective, and not intellectual, understanding is therapeutically valuable, some patients misconstrue affective understanding as suffering.

As for the third source of alleged torture in analysis, "suffering" while free associations are lacking, every student of analysis knows that the part played by free associations has undergone considerable change in the course of the development of analysis. Originally the technique of using free associations ruled supreme; this first phase ended when Freud discovered that free associations could be misused for resistance. Since that time the primacy of interpreting resistance and transference has prevailed in every Freudian analysis. Free associations are still important, of course; in fact, their real importance to the course of analysis increased with the elimination of faked associations prompted by unconscious resistance. Free associations are used today when their relative "purity" is assured and with the understanding that a nugget of valuable information will be forthcoming only rarely and not as punctuation to every pause.

This does not mean that free associations *must* be required from every patient and at every point in analysis. Orally regressed neurotics are frequently unable to use free association at the beginning of analysis. If in treating these cases the analyst abandons his icy silence and talks, he achieves two purposes. First, he prevents the development of a premature and unprofitable conflict with the patient which he is not yet prepared to handle. Second, he makes it impossible for the masochistic patient to misuse for his own neurotic purposes the unpleasantness and tension of a vain wait for associations. This tendency, when in time it does crop up with the gradual resumption of the classic technique, can be partly controlled by analyzing the patient's resistance plus his masochistic misuse of the situation.

A good deal of "suffering" of this type, therefore, is again reduced to a technical mistake on the part of the analyst, that of failure to recognize the basic structure of the orally regressed neurotic.

2. *Specific technique in orally regressed masochistic cases— meaning the majority of all neurotic patients.*

Orally regressed neurotics ward off their deep masochistic attachment with the defense of pseudoaggression and they carry this defense with them into analysis. When asked, as part of the classic psychoanalytic technique, to give words, thoughts, associations, they refuse. The situation actually invites them to identify the silent analyst with the cruel, cold, refusing mother. This transference is, of course, essential to the progress of the analysis, but it must not be precipitate and all-pervading; it must be controlled.

For this reason I have developed a technique of giving words—as the procedure works out I talk for long periods—in the beginning of analyses of orally regressed patients. In doing so I indirectly invite the patient's unconscious ego to take over a particular inner defense, that of returning kindness for kindness and generosity for generosity. The essential point must never be overlooked: all orally regressed neurotics are stabilized on the rejection level; unconsciously they want refusal and conceal this aim with either a pseudoaggressive defense or the alleged wish to be generously and kindly treated. By playing up to the latter defense the analyst fosters an inner state in the patient that mitigates his otherwise invariable anger, suspicion, and more or less concealed hostility. It amounts, paradoxically, to a temporary strengthening of the patient's "basic fallacy": "I'm not masochistic, I'm an innocent victim of Mother's cruelty. If my mother had been different I would have acted differently too." Later, of course, the analyst has to resolve the "basic fallacy."

The patient with whom the idea first occurred to me was Mr. D., a young man of seemingly low intelligence, from whose analysis also I first understood the clinical picture of pseudo debility. (Published in "The Problem of Pseudo-Debility," *Int. Zeitschr. f. Psychoan.* 18:528, 1932.) He had started analysis with a female colleague, who had treated him in terms of the Oedipus complex and who had interrupted treatment after a few months because of the patient's agitation, especially his pathological jealousy of her baby. According to the patient's mother this "harmless idiot" had become a "dangerous maniac." In our first interview he acted quite rationally, but his further behavior was decidedly peculiar. He began his "associations" by shouting, "Don't understand! Don't understand!" and all attempts at explanation were countered by his shouts of "Don't understand." After three appointments of this inauspicious behavior it occurred to me that the thing to do was to talk to the patient, for days and weeks if necessary, completely disregarding his endless shouts. This I did. It was like telling fairy tales to a child. The patient himself took no part. I gave him hundreds of simplified examples of fear from the analyses of other patients, but I could just as well have talked about the weather. In any case, talking seemed to me the remedy, though I could not explain my reasons. The patient would listen quietly, but if I interrupted my discourse for a moment he would fill the silence with his shouted battle cry "Don't understand!"

Treatment continued on these terms for weeks, until one day I used an example in which the word "resistance" had been misunderstood. This was from the analysis of a test patient with a low I.Q., chosen because of my interest in determining the degree of human "stupidity" in which analysis was still effective. I had told this patient, "You are under the influence of your resistance." The patient replied, "You're quite right, one should have a good resistance," understanding the word only as meaning resistance against infection.

When I told this story the patient on the couch remarked, "What a dope! He should have known what resistance in analysis means." This was the first time he had said anything except "Don't understand." The ice was broken!

In evaluating theoretically what I had done intuitively, I came to the conclusion that Mr. D. had projected upon his first analyst the image of the "bad mother" who refuses and to whom he was masochistically attached. That masochistic tendency was counteracted by inner guilt, so that he had to establish a pseudoaggressive alibi that would testify to the alleged *wish to get*. This explained his demanding, jealous attitude.

When he came to me he expected to be punished for these wishes and defenses. His shouts reduced to absurdity every connection I might make. Moreover, he was demonstrating a thesis to his mother: "You can't get anywhere with me." He was not really afraid of punishment; what he dreaded was the full flowering of his extensive psychic masochism, and preventively he reinforced his pseudoaggressive defense. My "giving" attitude confronted him with a new problem: "Mother does not refuse; on the contrary she gives." He now seized the opportunity to substitute a new defense, "That's exactly what I really want—to get." On the basis of this new defense a temporary modus vivendi had been established.

After that preparatory phase typical clinical analysis could be conducted. The patient's life history, especially his neurotic evaluation of reality, abundantly substantiated these conjectures.

Here is another example of the hopeless conflict an analyst gets himself into if he insists on following the classical technique with orally regressed neurotics. A patient with psychogenic aspermia who entered trial analysis with a colleague in another country was told to stick to the basic rule, with the result that he became agitated, depressed, and "suffered hell." The analyst broke his sphinx-like silence for the first time after twenty appointments to announce that he

Limitations of Analytic Therapy

considered the patient a case for analysis. The patient left in a fury. He could not explain what had made him so angry since he had spoken only about business matters. When, some time later, he started analysis with me, he said, "If you, too, tell me that I have to use the couch and talk, talk, talk, I am leaving immediately." My answer was that neither was necessary in his case; he merely had to listen.

When these patients are required to give free associations, they feel "drained" and refused (see "septet of baby fears" in Chapter 1), and a favorable atmosphere has to be created artificially in order that analysis can take place at all.

The problem of the analyst's immutable silence involves some amazing misunderstandings and even ironical paradoxes.

If one rereads Freud's five famous case histories, GESAMMELTE SCHRIFTEN, VIII., Int. Psychoan. Verlag, Vienna, one realizes how much he actually talked to these patients. Of course the analyst needs the patient's associations as material to work with. But free associations were never considered an end in themselves—after Freud's discovery that so-called associations could be used as resistance. The idea that the patient should figure out his problem himself is based on a mystical quality unjustifiably ascribed to these associations, disregarding the fact that deep masochism, as well as the superficial diagnoses of all libidinous-pseudoaggressive "rescue stations," must be interpreted by the analyst.

I submitted the question of that mystical quality to two distinguished members of Freud's Old Guard, Dr. Federn and Dr. Jekels, a few years before they died. Dr. Federn laughed and said that Freudian psychoanalysis had always been misunderstood and that there was no self-healing in free associations, nor in the analyst's silence. It is possible, he added, that Freud, who was intolerant of intellectual limitations, talked little to analyzands for whom he had little respect. For instance, he referred the patient of the "door incident"—this man habitually left the door open between Freud's waiting room and appointment room and was told by Freud that his act had this contemptuous meaning: "Why pretend; no other patient will consult you."—to Federn for continuation of analysis with the remark "I could not stand his stupidity."

Dr. Jekels, informed of Dr. Federn's statement, nodded agreement and said, "It was never meant that way. The dogmatism of associations for associations' sake or silence for the sake of silence is nonsense." When I asked him whether Freud's difficulty in speaking during the last seventeen years of his life (he had cancer of the palate and wore a complicated prosthetic device) might not have been misunderstood by some of his later medical analyzands as analytic technique, Jekels looked surprised, began to laugh, and said, "Quite possible." After a second burst of laughter he added, "Malicious, witty, clever, but, as I said, quite possible, even probable."

In conclusion I said to Jekels, "Ironically, one could add that many colleagues who deny the central importance of psychic masochism indirectly acknowledge it by giving the patient the possibility of masochistic misuse of the analytic situation. Unfortunately that indirect acknowledgement is therapeutically ineffective." Again Jekels laughed. "They make their living that way—masochism triumphant in disguise."

On another occasion, a few months before his death at eighty-seven, I asked Jekels, with whom I had had the honor of collaborating in previous years, how generations of analytic investigators could have overlooked the central importance of psychic masochism based on oral regression. His answer was succinct: *"The fourth narcissistic hurt."* Jekels alluded to Freud's famous statement that humanity had suffered three narcissistic mortifications: Copernicus' proof that the earth is not the center of the universe, Darwin's demonstration that man is not the unique crown of creation, and Freud's revelation that he is not even master in his own house.

3. *Handling of "regret depressions" because of missed masochistic opportunities.*

The irrevocability of the cathexis constitutes one of the most amazing facts in the psychology of psychic masochism. Once the cathexis has been "mobilized" for use, it cannot be recalled or put in storage. This explains why masochists frequently experience depression when the inwardly expected defeat fails to materialize, as sometimes can happen, even with a person who specializes in unconsciously constructed defeats. With the worst will in the world there is no way of avoiding a victory thrust on one by an external phenomenon that

Limitations of Analytic Therapy

cannot be influenced. Such upsets plunge the psychic masochist into a *"regret depression"* and leave him with the problem of disposing of masochistic "energy" already on hand and ready for use. Allegedly elated by his victory but in inner reality disappointed by it, the masochist may discharge the cathexis by hastening into his next "mistake."

This masochistic anticlimax is invariably predictable. With severe neurotics it is not enough to prevent masochistic acts. It is also necessary to make them familiar with depressions following the avoidance of these very acts. Otherwise, "unexplainable" relapses are to be recorded. The price of the inner defense of psychic masochism is conscious unhappiness, and even when the defense is rendered superfluous by a favorable event payment is exacted for the preparatory period.

Assuming the psychoanalyst acts according to the rule of putting psychic masochism in the center and makes the distinction between basic masochistic conflict and secondary, variegated rescue symptoms of libidinous-pseudoaggressive nature, can he be sure of achieving full therapeutic success?

The answer is no. He is not operating in a vacuum but is dealing with living human beings whose mental elasticity is different in each specific case. Various degrees of success can be distinguished:

a. *Excellent Therapeutic Result.* In this group are ex-neurotics who gave up great portions of their psychic masochism, converted sizable amounts of this scourge into productive energy (activity), created new interests and sublimations, straightened out their sex life. Their "neurotic trade balance," as suggested in the Foreword, is so favorable that it surpasses that of the average person. Having learned how to handle the inner enemy and become wise to his tricks, they seldom fall back on discarded neurotic mechanisms; if they attempt to, they understand and laugh and so can cope with the situation at short notice. My twenty-one previously published books and 271 papers abound with many examples of this type.

b. *Middle-of-the-Road Improvement.* Every successful or half-successful analysis ends with a compromise, the question being how much of his beloved psychic masochism the patient is capable of renouncing. In most cases the most conspicuous superficial neurotic symptoms are removed, and the patient learns, more or less sucessfully, to fight his basic problem—the remnants of his masochism.

It is interesting to observe the *change of emphasis* that takes place in every analysis, an emphasis produced by the patient alone. At first he believes that the specific symptom that pushed him into treatment is the crux of the matter and the one source of his subjective unhappiness. After being familiarized with the difference between the basic masochistic conflict and the camouflaging libidinous-pseudo-aggressive "rescue symptoms," his appetite for health increases and so does his program; he wants a "hundred-percent cure." In later stages of analysis he switches the emphasis again and starts to prove to the sceptical analyst that "so much has already been accomplished" and the "remnants are minimal."

At this point the roads part again. Not all patients stick it out to the happy end; many leave analysis contented with having rescued sizable remnants of psychic masochism.

It would be erroneous to assume that this choice is a voluntary one. Quite the contrary. The elasticity of the ego decides, and the analyst does well to take the limitations of the material he works with into consideration.

c. *Half-Losers.* Many neurotics are willing to give up only parts of their neurosis. To exemplify a typical occurrence in street fear (agoraphobia): The most amazing feature in this neurotic disease is the resignation with which many of those afflicted with this symptom entity accept their fate, avoid treatment, and—do nothing. This is paralleled by the high percentage of "runners-away" from analysis after a short time. Those who remain in treatment belong in two categories:

(1) Those who give up the symptom altogether—a small minority. In 1935 I published a lengthy case history of such a patient;[16] the favorable experience has been repeated a few times.

(2) Those who "compromise." These patients give up some of the too ridiculous features and retain some less conspicuous ones. For example, a woman living in Brooklyn and incapable of coming to Manhattan changed her place of residence to Manhattan. Previously she could not take a bath (she used "fractional washing"), since

Limitations of Analytic Therapy 145

she could not fully undress, having to be always prepared to run to the physician in case she should have a heart attack. She gave up this precaution, but still, when asked to a party, ascertained the status of elevators, the story in which the host lived, etc.; above the sixth floor she felt "uncomfortable." On the other hand, she became quite at home shopping on Fifth Avenue.

A business man who had been confined to his bedroom compromised extensively but was still handicapped to some degree. Whereas previously walking even around the block was a total impossibility, he discarded that fear, retaining only a distaste for "too long walks." But he never took a vacation, he never traveled, though with his car he was relatively mobile.

d. *Failures—the "empty bag" type of neurotic.* See the case described on pages 48 ff. and the examples given in PRINCIPLES OF SELF-DAMAGE, pages 274 ff.

e. *Schizoid personalities.* Little needs to be added to the deduction in Chapter 1.

CHAPTER 5

HOW DOES NEUROTIC ESCAPISM IN TREATMENT MANIFEST ITSELF?

NEUROTICS use various techniques of escapism in psychoanalytic treatment. Some of these methods are devious and are by no means known to or detected by all psychotherapists. Here are some of them:
1. Interruption of treatment.
2. Naive transference "improvements."
3. Giving up some of the trimmings while maintaining neurosis.
4. Pseudo successes because of unconscious fear.
5. Flight to "love" with an outsider.
6. Postanalytic misuse of preanalytic symptoms.
7. "Reopening of insoluble problems."
8. Premature resignation.
9. Shifting of psychic masochism to points unrecognizable to the patient.
10. Intellectualization.
11. Pathological lies about the analyst.
12. "Acting out" by misuse of the transference.

1. INTERRUPTION OF TREATMENT

There is nothing unclear about the external action of running away, but the story reads differently when the motives behind it are scrutinized.

Miss E., a young Italian actress, had attached herself to a ne'er-do-well, a psychopath with parasitic, homosexual, and drug-addiction

How Does Neurotic Escapism in Treatment Manifest Itself? 147

tendencies. She came into treatment at the urging of friends, who told her that the man was "just no good" and a danger to her career. The reason she consented to treatment was that she had found syringes and drugs hidden in the draperies in her apartment and was afraid that while she was working on location the man might take in homosexual addicts (his friends) as boarders. She well understood that she could not afford to be "negative headline stuff" in the tabloids. She remained in treatment a few weeks, constantly using the argument that "people can change" in referring to the man of her choice. She also made the point that this undeniably "difficult" man was the only one who could give her sexual enjoyment, though she admitted that there were long "stretches in between" when the gentleman "retired from sex," periods sometimes lasting a full year.

It could be shown in analysis that the man unconsciously presented a caricature of her masochistic trends (her mother complained about her unruly attitude: "She is a monster"); that in him she loved herself narcissistically, always being able to point out to her accusing conscience the "difference"—she was a "good girl." Her overdimensional psychic masochism, moreover, deposited in the mother image, was fully taken care of in this hopeless relationship. As for sexual attraction, it could be established that she was very little interested in sex proper. In childhood she had been a tomboy, rejecting the feminine role. She was an only child, and in puberty she looked on sex as a nuisance and with a feeling of "examination fright," questioning whether she could make the grade. The present relationship absolved her of the problem, and the idea of finding another man filled her with horror.

Because of social pressure the man took some kind of job temporarily, making the greatest difficulties about it and asking the actress to provide him with costly outfits, an expensive car, and so forth, to make a good impression on his employer. The job required extensive traveling, and when she accompanied him on one of these trips he paid practically no attention to her. She concluded, nevertheless, that he was a "changed man." Before she left on another trip on location in another continent I reminded her of her analytic agreement not to make any binding decisions during treatment, pointing out that her friend's constant demands that they have a child (as reassurance for his parasitic tendencies) fell in this category and that marriage and establishment of a family should wait.

When she came back—married, pregnant, and entirely convinced that the man had changed—she did not call up and did not resume treatment. Obviously she had made an unconscious decision that masochistic martyrdom was her lot, whatever her conscious rationalization may have been.

Only a year later, after all the predicted facts were once more confirmed by the man's truly fantastic behavior, she came back into treatment, asking for "removal of her sick attachment." Whether or not she will go through with it is unclear.

Mrs. F., a highly paid business executive, came into treatment under pressure from a friend, to whom she had confided that she was "near a nervous breakdown." She had bitten off more than she could chew. She was married to a good-looking nobody with poor earning capacity, had produced a series of children in short succession, held a responsible job requiring great concentration, and so forth. What really plagued her unconsciously was the half-realization that she simply imitated normality with her pretentious and demanding husband, without achieving it. The whole menage was built around her large salary. She was a proud woman who could not admit defeat, especially defeat in the eyes of her mother, to whom she was masochistically attached. Her wish to "collapse" was counteracted by savage independence, which had driven her to extraordinary achievements. But recently the masochistic substructure had come to the fore more and more. She gave two reasons for leaving treatment after half a dozen appointments: my statement that some psychic conflicts cannot be resolved alone, which offended her "independence," and the fact that there were "so many doors" in my office and waiting room that she got confused. Obviously she could not accept help, identifying the therapist with the mother image, before whom she acted out her "pseudo normality."

Mr. G., a homosexual of fifty, came from a distant part of the country for a trial treatment of four weeks. It was understoood that if he was a favorable case he would have to change his place of residence for the duration of treatment. As he was a man of considerable means his only problem was to find some professional "diversion," and he

How Does Neurotic Escapism in Treatment Manifest Itself? 149

had an elaborate plan ready. He was prognostically a rather dubious case though not a hopeless one. He went home, informing me that he was about to make arrangements. A few weeks later I received a letter saying that he had decided not to go through with his plan, one of the decisive reasons being that he could not leave his beloved—horses.

As can be seen from the foregoing examples, it is by no means the severity or negligibility of the symptoms that decide the question —to stay or not to stay in treatment. All three examples, in fact, concerned very severe neurotics. These *"lost souls"* do not want help. Experience proves that as time goes on severe neurotics deteriorate without treatment. Unfortunately, neurosis is a progressive, not a self-limiting disease.

2. NAIVE TRANSFERENCE "IMPROVEMENTS"

The external trappings are so well known that a few words will suffice. Transference denotes the unconscious repetition of bygone infantile conflicts, executed on an innocent outsider. Since these conflicts always contain positive and negative components, both possibilities of repetition exist.

The negative transference is easier to see through than its positive counterpart. It gives the impression of hopelessness, and some nonanalytic psychotherapists feel uncomfortable when it appears. Today the average analyst is prepared for the negative transference and interprets it. What he frequently does not know is that the patient's aggression is only pseudoaggression, a provocative technique to achieve psychic masochistic pleasure.

What he also frequently does not know is that in some cases the positive transference may be a mirage, produced for the purpose of proving to the patient himself that he wanted love and nothing else. It is, in other words, a camouflage for the masochistic picture. If the analyst does not see through the mirage, painful results are encountered: the patient, apparently improved, declares himself (herself) cured—and his (her) masochism has not even been touched. Later, of course, the "cure" collapses, and the patient repeats the performance with a second, third, and nth analyst.

3. GIVING UP SOME OF THE TRIMMINGS WHILE MAINTAINING NEUROSIS

The greatest obstacle to success in psychotherapy is the patient's unconscious wish to "improve" his neurosis by eliminating his conscious suffering. When it becomes clear that the aim of analysis is to destroy neurosis, in short, that the analyst "means business" and is really fighting neurosis, some patients leave and some look for a convenient way out. The "fight between the couch and the door" is frequently solved by the patient's spurious compromise: he gives up a few trimmings and convinces himself that "everything is O.K." The analyst's explanation of this specific resistance is sometimes accepted, sometimes disregarded.

4. PSEUDO SUCCESSES BECAUSE OF UNCONSCIOUS FEAR

This is a preventive mechanism, based on fear. What happens is that the patient projects his own repressed megalomania on the analyst, after which the analyst ranks as "omniscient." As the patient now sees him, he possesses the uncanny ability to discover *all* the patient's secrets. To avoid that feared danger the patient unconsciously proceeds to sacrifice and renounce less important symptoms for a time, in order to keep the basic neurotic structure intact. Superficially, a cure seems to have been effected. This cure turns out to be pseudo all over; in deeper neuroses it is only transitory. (See also p. 54 f.)

5. FLIGHT INTO "LOVE" WITH AN OUTSIDER

Love has the undeserved reputation of being beyond explanation and of presenting its own justification. The layman, moreover, makes no distinction between real love and its neurotic counterpart, pseudo love. Here is an explanation of the difference.

Real love is an episode in the great battle of the conscience. The inner conscience, as has already been stated, is made up of two opposing forces, the ego ideal and the daimonion. The daimonion's typical technique of intrapsychic torture consists in constantly reminding the intimidated ego that it has failed to measure up to its self-created ego ideal. The achievement does not match the promise,

How Does Neurotic Escapism in Treatment Manifest Itself? 151

and the inevitable discrepancy is paid for with depression, guilt, dissatisfaction.

The ego is hoist with its own petard. It cannot deny the grandiose ambition or the relatively minor achievement. And excuses get nowhere with the daimonion, which insists on payment, in the form of guilt. So far, the ego has been hopelessly outmaneuvered, its own weapon seized and used against it. In desperation, it devises another ingenious tactic. The daimonion, a formalist, always asks for a witness who will attest the ego's promised greatness. The ego will find such a witness, a person who has complete faith that the victim will more than fulfill his childhood ambition, who is convinced that only the malice of the outer world has kept him from getting his chance, who actually thinks of him as the most desirable, admirable, successful human being in the whole world!

This is the unconscious preamble to the emotional hurricane of love. *The lover projects his own ego ideal on the beloved,* and in so doing deprives the daimonion of its instrument of torture. Since the object of love approves of everything done by the lover, there is no longer a visible discrepancy between the ego and the ego ideal, and the feeling of guilt disappears. The ego ideal returns to its original benign state and as long as love lasts cannot be used for the daimonion's anti-libidinous purposes. This projection of the ego ideal explains the ridiculous overevaluation lovers put on one another, when the projection is mutual.

Tender love, viewed genetically, is not just a "romantic" addition to sensual satisfaction; it is a *powerful weapon against inner guilt,* in fact the most powerful weapon available. It is available, however, only to the not-too-neurotic, or so-called healthy, person. The neurotic is incapable of feeling love.

Counterfeit love, the substitute the neurotic finds for tender love, consists in endless repetitions of infantile patterns, in other words, in *transference.* In neurosis real people are misused as objects on which an unconscious infantile conflict can be reeled off.

Tender love and counterfeit love are, in my opinion, pathognomonic for health and neurosis. They are the measure of a person's success or failure in his fight against the chronic inner enemy, the superego.

The key to the normal person's ability to feel love lies in his unconscious attitude toward guilt. He avoids it, using various devices, of which tender love is the most potent. Because he is less of a psychic masochist than the neurotic, his reaction to unconscious guilt and punishment is one of pain undiluted with pleasure, and he can therefore be single-minded in his search for antidotes.

The neurotic, on the other hand, does not want to free himself from guilt. It is bound up with his psychic masochism, secondarily connected with the pre-oedipal and oedipal fantasies he clings to, and it becomes their accepted companion, a sort of duenna, since he will not renounce his fantasies. And in his secret deals with his superego the neurotic uses his guilt as a bargaining point: "See how unhappy I am!" The whole structure of neurosis rests on this bribe.

Counterfeit love may look—externally—like the real product; its psychological *raison d'être* is, however, quite different. It is either transference or a cloak to disguise a deep masochistic attachment.

For example, every masochistic neurotic of either sex, embroiled in a hopeless injustice-collecting conflict, informs us that he (she) wants "love, love, nothing but love." By choosing a partner—unconsciously on purpose—who caters to and provides for masochistic needs, he (she) counteracts his (her) own official aim, in order to get what he (she) really wanted—the proverbial kick in the jaw. In my books DIVORCE WON'T HELP NEUROTICS, CONFLICT IN MARRIAGE, HOMOSEXUALITY, extensive material proving this point is collected.

It is a very typical occurrence that masochistic women in analysis with a male therapist start to repeat in the transference a positive feeling belonging historically to a father-brother-uncle image. In simple hysterical cases this may be genuine enough; in masochistic neurotics it is *not*. When the analyst does not see through the unconscious camouflage and does not analyze the masochistic substructure, he is frequently faced with a painful surprise: after what seemed to be a successful analysis (and after apparent solution of the transference neurosis), the patient falls in love with a person with whom a totally masochistic conflict is repeated.

This can be avoided by analyzing psychic masochism. Recently

I witnessed such a case, treated by a colleague who was proud of disagreeing with me on the subject of masochism. After the new "love" marriage proved disastrous, the patient went into a deep depression, but finally settled for continuation of analysis.

6. POSTANALYTIC MISUSE OF PREANALYTIC SYMPTOMS

Every psychoanalyst is occasionally confronted with the baffling and uncomfortable situation of seeing an ex-patient, some years after the conclusion of a successful analysis, return with a new crop of "old" symptoms. After overcoming his feeling of disappointment the analyst's thoughts converge on one problem: the advisability of continuing the analysis himself or referring the hapless ex-patient to a colleague.

The disappointed analyst postulates the following explanations for the situation: (1) The transference situation has not been solved. (2) Deeper layers, not analyzed, were involved. (3) The analysis tapped the dynamically decisive layers but not thoroughly enough, hence more "working through" is required. (4) The diagnosis was wrong in the first place.

Assuming that all four possibilities can be excluded in a particular case and the analyst did a good and thorough job, the fact that the symptoms recurred must still be faced and explained. Aside from the theoretical problem, there is still the matter of the patient, who has to be helped—if possible.

To adduce a clinical example.

Mrs. H., a woman in her early thirties entered analysis because of street fear. She had had two previous analyses, of three and two years, one with a psychotherapist of a split-off group, the other with an acknowledged analyst. She had originally undertaken analysis because of "general unhappiness and depression." Her agoraphobia had developed during treatment; she could not leave her apartment unless accompanied by one of her sisters.

The focal point of her previous analyses had been a purported but never confirmed event in her infancy. Allegedly, she had been sexually mishandled by her father. Several facts contradicted the tale, and the patient's life did not conform at all to the oedipal conclusions.

Still, two analyses had been built on this theme song, with the accompaniment obligingly supplied by the patient.

Mrs. H. was married to an ineffective nobody who was both stingy and brutal. Her well-to-do older sisters had a naive explanation for his hold on her: "He is drugging the poor child." The patient had her own explanation. She believed she had a mission to "improve" her husband's financial position, but it became clear that he could never be more than an underpaid employee, "half-contented in his rut."

Merely listening to her life history provided enough material for the *pre-oedipal* substructure. Her mother's life (her parents had been divorced long ago) was regulated by superstitious compulsions and obsessions involving the dangers of infection. The most pronounced result was that she never kissed her children; kissing could transmit bacteria. This emotional Siberia was faithfully repeated in the patient's marriage. Her husband treated her as coldly as her mother had but added a more direct attack—he hit her.

The patient had no inkling that pronounced exhibitionism was contained in her symptom of street fear; this had never been explained to her in five years of treatment. Why the symptom had developed during analysis soon became clear: treatment to her was an exhibitionistic fiesta. However, it had a strong voyeuristic basis, secondarily warded off with exhibitionism.

Her "general depression" was a misnomer; what she really meant was constant thought of death or illness in her family or acquaintances. These thoughts had been explained in previous analyses as "repressed death wishes for which the penance of guilt is paid." Actually she identified with the suffering people because of the masochistic allure, and her aggression was really a defense. In short, the typical tragic confusion between pseudoaggression and real aggression was involved.

After a year of treatment, working through the psychic-masochistic basis and the pseudoaggressive defense, plus the voyeuristic-exhibitionistic exchange mechanism (see Chapter 7), Mrs. H. improved to an amazing degree. She lost her street fear, divorced her husband, resisted her family's pressure to "marry a wealthy man,"

How Does Neurotic Escapism in Treatment Manifest Itself? 155

and in general emerged from her bundle of fears to become a charming, witty, rather contented person. She married a young professional man and for two years lived happily with him.

Whenever I listened to her friends' compliments on the outcome of her case I was always conscious that the truly dramatic change did not correspond to the "state of her masochism." I saw her a few times during these two years for "check-ups." Her understanding of her psychic make-up was still satisfactory.

Then, after two years, she observed the gradual recurrence of her old symptom. First a feeling of apprehension before leaving her apartment; then she tried to avoid leaving the apartment at all; most of the time she was absorbed in a fear of impending doom.

I saw the patient a few times and, having experienced similar relapses with other patients, arrived at this conclusion:

The new-old symptoms had no connection at all with the original genetic basis. Previously these symptoms had contained a specific psychological meaning, but the new repetitions did not. The reason for them was not insufficient working through; the "shell" of symptoms only served the purpose of providing a place of deposition for the patient's self-allotted portion of psychic masochism. Their starting point was the unconsciously unsatisfactory state of her marriage: she could not stand so much happiness. At bottom the recurrence represented nostalgia for her miserable (though unconsciously masochistically enjoyed) first marriage.

Two problems are of practical importance in such cases: Should analysis be continued? Can the amount of self-allotted psychic masochism be reduced?

In my opinion treatment should *not* be continued, *provided* the analyst is convinced—and I mean *justifiably* convinced—that the genetic basis was properly reached and the patient's *psychic masochism sufficiently analyzed.* One has to accept the dreary fact that each person subsists on a diet containing a specific amount of libidinized self-torture. Analysis can explain, reduce to the infantile basis, emotionally work through, and considerably diminish, this scourge. It *cannot,* however, force the patient to give up *all* his psychic masochism. There is no point in denying that even in favorable cases a good dose of psychic masochism remains. These remnants must be understood—and *accepted*—by the patient.

I believe that "postanalytic misuse of preanalytic symptoms," as described above, taxes the determination and courage of the therapist to a considerable degree (not to mention his willingness to endure unpleasantness for the sake of conviction). It is much easier to continue treatment or to send the patient to a colleague than to accept censure for "cruelty," "lack of consideration," "coldness and lack of interest." The ignorant environment is especially active in heaping these reproaches on the physician. Still, the only correct move is to explain the situation to the patient and leave him to battle the problem through—*alone*.

The patient can appeal from the refusal to continue treatment; there is always a colleague at hand willing to prove that the "pessimistic" analyst had "overlooked" important points. So it was with this patient. She went into analysis with a female colleague, who spent the next year and a half analyzing her oedipal structure and misunderstanding her masochistic substructure. When the patient ventured allusions to the pleasure-in-displeasure pattern and taking her pseudoaggressions at face value, the analyst would cut her short with a stock reply: "I don't know what you are talking about."

Mrs. H. broke off treatment and shortly afterwards called me up, requesting resumption of the analysis. I refused, but I did consent to a limited number of appointments.

A year later she telephoned again, "in a desperate state," this time because of her ex-husband's remarriage. This produced a masochistic "regret depression," which could be worked out in a few months of treatment, of one appointment weekly.

Since then many years have passed. I saw the patient once or twice yearly for a few appointments. Except for some over-drinking and restriction of movement because of remnants of street fear, the patient feels "happy."

In such cases, if one reaches the conclusion that a *neurosis* is at stake, the patient should not be treated *ad infinitum* after a comparatively lengthy period of analysis. If, however, a *schizoid* personality is operative, other principles should be applied. Some kind of "guidance" is advisable and should be continued for many long

How Does Neurotic Escapism in Treatment Manifest Itself? 157

years. But this supervisory attempt to keep the patient out of trouble (whenever possible) should not be called psychoanalysis.

Interestingly enough, some patients cannot wait for postanalysis to perpetrate "postanalytic misuse"; they resort to this technique in advanced stages of analysis. Although great changes have already taken place in the personality and symptoms have temporarily subsided, the mirage of an unconquerable symptom suddenly presents itself. In these cases further analysis of the symptom leads nowhere; unless the phase passes quickly, the symptom simply becomes a depository of masochism that cannot be resolved. It is of advantage to present to the patient the problem of the *"maximum and minimum program."*

The maximum program, of course, represents a cure: the patient learns to devaluate his depressions as bribes offered to the superego; he learns that his guilt does not pertain to his pseudoaggressive defense but to his deeply rooted psychic masochism; he learns to use analytic interpretations as a means of reducing his masochistic self-flagellation. From this effective understanding he progresses to normal productivity and contentment.

The minimum program consists in finding a way for the patient to live with his unchangeable psychic masochism. It should not be assumed that the minimum program is the automatic result of a failure to achieve the maximum; the minimum aim is also difficult to achieve. It is not easy, for instance, to accept the fact that a damaging inner trait is permanently entrenched and cannot be altered. Nor is it easy to see through the consoling fantasy embedded in the psychic-masochistic pattern and learn to check at least one's most damaging ventures into injustice-collecting. But just as a person who has sustained an irreparable injury on the battlefield can learn to live with his handicap, the psychic masochist (under the minimum program) can learn to live within his psychic limitations.

The advantages are patent, if not sweeping. The automatic increase of the neurosis, inevitable if not treated, can be halted. The patient profits by the narcissistic pleasure attendant upon his new ability to recognize other people's psychic masochism. And last, he is fortified, still, by traces of what he has learned in analysis.

Unlike the runaway patient, who conveniently "forgets" the entire episode, the patient achieving the minimum program still retains his awareness of some of the guiding posts mapped out in analysis.

The analyst invariably finds it difficult to decide when he must "throw in the sponge." But even at the risk of being wrong the decision must sooner or later be made.

7. "REOPENING OF INSOLUBLE PROBLEMS"

This type of escapism is truly paradoxical and is distinguished from other types by the fact that the patient seems to go through a partially successful analysis ending with the apparently mutual understanding that, though many facets of his personality have been changed, *one* specific problem cannot be resolved. Then suddenly, months or years later, the patient tries single-handed to storm the very door that would not open. The result is dismal defeat, with gradual readjustment to the old situation, or—in exceptional cases—some success.

Mr. I., a gifted young man, entered analysis because his professional success did not correspond to his undoubted abilities and because of a deeply masochistic conflict with his wife. The result of his analysis was that he became spectacularly successful in his particular field of endeavor, and his masochistic attachment to his wife lessened. Twice during his treatment he fell in love with another woman, only to cool off shortly; he simply could not leave his wife. The whole "melodrama," as he sarcastically called these episodes, had the unconscious purpose of demonstrating how his wife deprived him—of love. Every interpretation in the instrumentation of masochism was tried; he seemed destined to stay in this "indifferent" marriage. It was pointed out to him that his equilibrium, though based on a "boring" marriage, was better served by continuing it.

A year later he "reopened the closed case" by falling in love with another woman, only to find that he could not divorce his wife. He made a spectacle of himself, cried, was indiscreet, telling innumerable people of his troubles. He became angry with the analyst for not having freed him of this particular difficulty. When told that long and repeated attempts had been made in his analysis to do so, the patient admitted this. The end of the story was continuation of the

How Does Neurotic Escapism in Treatment Manifest Itself? 159

"boring" marriage. Then, after more of this "postanalytic rigamarole," he finally did leave his wife. Obviously he could not abstain from "revenge" on the analyst, who was guilty of lessening his extensive psychic masochism.

Not only is unsolved negative transference involved in these cases, but these neurotics work on a peculiar "time table," to which we have no access.

Another, very similar, case had a less happy ending; the man stayed with his impossible wife on some kind of "resignation basis."

Such cases are disagreeable because enemies of analysis, witnessing the spectacle (and these ex-patients are typically indiscreet) can gleefully point out that such things "should not happen after analysis." They shouldn't, but they do. Analysis is an *attempt* to solve inner conflict, not an insurance company.

8. PREMATURE RESIGNATION

Neurotics using this type give up too early, at a time when the issue has not been decided—yet. Some can be convinced that they are the prey of their masochism, some cannot.

Sometimes the premature resignation is part and parcel of their "Weltanschauung."

Mr. J. was a homosexual who did not want to change.[7] He was in analysis to make the best of an impossible domestic situation. What he had read of masochism in my book on homosexuality had "impressed" and frightened him, and what he hoped analysis would do was to help him outsmart his wife, who had forced him into treatment, by freeing him from the tendency to self-damage. As for the connection between psychic masochism and homosexuality, he frankly stated that he "did not believe one word of it." A streak of megalomania also colored his attitude towards the analysis: he had "put one over on me," he thought, by persuading me to take him on as a patient even though he did not meet the standards set forth for treatment in my book. Otherwise, he was highly suspicious.

The first three appointments were taken up with an exposition of the aims of analysis. Mr. J. listened very carefully, as a lawyer listens to an opposing attorney's argument. I asked him at one point,

"Why are you listening so carefully? Is this the way you register information, or are you gathering material for a rebuttal?"

"Why, doctor, you have a dirty—or at least suspicious mind!"

"You shouldn't be talking about 'a suspicious mind.' No less than three times, in our first appointment, you gave me that famous suspicious-dirty look that meant 'Aha, you've been plotting with my wife!' Three times you accused me of conspiring with her. True or fantasy?"

"I'm still not convinced that you didn't."

"I'm going to tell you something that—I hope—will convince you. We analysts don't lie to our patients in general, and particularly not about family contacts. Suppose I actually had gone behind your back and talked to your wife. What assurance would I have that she would not tell you about it?"

Once the introduction was complete, I asked Mr. J. for a short history of his nursery past.

"Nothing, but nothing in my uneventful childhood pointed in the direction of my future troubles. Father: a shy though friendly, quiet man, a postal inspector in a small upstate New York town. He spent most of his free time in the basement of our mortgaged house playing with his inventions—all very minor. His idea of a great inventor wasn't Edison but the man who got the idea of the square clothespin. None of his experiments ever came to anything."

"Did your mother object?"

"She was pleasant enough. No, she was condescending with a sort of ironic kindness. She was the one who wore the pants; she decided everything."

"I asked you whether she objected to your father's hobby."

"Before I answer I would like to know why you are stressing the point."

"There are no hidden strings attached to the question. Your father was a tinkerer and obviously an amateur. You became a mechanical engineer, a professional. Superficially it seems as though you identified with your father and then outdid him. On the other hand, your mother treated him with ironic condescension. That didn't give you a very imposing ideal to look up to and identify with. I suspect, therefore, that behind this pseudo-identification with your father lies a more deeply repressed aggression of some kind, directed against your mother. If she had objected to your father's hobby—a game that consumed time and money and brought no results—then your identification with your father's only interest would appear in a different light. It would mean rebellion against your mother. Satisfied?"

"Is this the way you construct theories?"

"If that's irony, I don't see the point. Yes, that's the way tentative assumptions are built up in analysis. I know from other cases that homosexuality means unsolved unconscious conflict with the image of the mother; therefore you must have harbored that very conflict. On the other hand, you identified with your stepped-on father. Why should you find it strange for me to be following this trend of thought and trying to link the known material with what is still unknown? Please note that I did not give you an interpretation; all I did was ask for specific information. Please answer the question."

"It seems my fate to confirm your hunches and guesses. O.K. You win. Mother did object, and I mean forcefully. From time to time she would go into hysterics about it: he never spent any time with his family, she would tell him in no uncertain terms, he spent every available cent on tools, raw material, and so on. That isn't all. I did well in high school; I was captain of the football team and in general what they call these days a 'big wheel on campus.' Full of confidence, I told her I wanted to study mechanical engineering. She threw up her hands in desperation and said, 'I hope you don't become like your father!' Now I'll ask your favorite question: Satisfied?"

"In a minor way, yes. Aren't *you* pleased when you've made a correct guess? Now tell me this: Wasn't there talk in high school and college because you didn't have girl friends?"

"Who told you that I didn't?"

"If my memory serves me correctly, in our preliminary interview you told me of your reaction when you met your wife: 'I was so elated that I could be aroused by a woman,' you said. Is it farfetched to assume that this was a new experience for you? Or do you suspect that I am in contact with some of the girls you disappointed in high school?"

"Can't overdo it. Aren't you a suspicious person yourself?"

"Of course—when it makes sense to be. But not because distrust is a principle, as it seems to be with you. What about your constant suspicions here?"

"First prove that you are being open and aboveboard with me."

"I certainly am. Since you are the accuser, it's up to you to present the indictment."

"Look, I'm no dope. The fact is that after I told you that I wasn't sure whether I was interested in changing my homosexuality, you should have sent me away. That statement meant that I didn't come up to the standards you yourself set up for treating homosexuality. You printed them in your book. Instead, you took me as a patient. Could it be the money, I asked myself, but I couldn't be satisfied with that answer after you told me I would have to wait two or three months before you could give me any time. If not money, what was it? I told you that I was impressed with your pet idea of 'unconscious self-damage.' Could that have flattered you enough to make you break your rule? I excluded that possibility too; you must be bored to death talking about psychic masochism. How am I doing?"

"Very well, so far. Let's hear the sinister aim you finally uncovered."

"I came to the conclusion that you were an inveterate experimenter. After all, your whole idea of curing homosexuals, when your esteemed colleagues offered nothing but a shrug of the shoulders, was just an experiment—an experiment that came off successfully, if you are telling the truth. I simply asked myself: What does this son of a gun hope to find in me? First I couldn't figure that one out. I read your book again, this time looking for a single clue—a case like mine. I found it, in an unexpected place. In describing the case of a Lesbian—amusingly enough, your heading reads 'example of an unchangeable case'—who did not want to change, you wrote that characterologically she *did* change. Here was your challenge, your opportunity for experimentation! And this was a long time ago; the date you put on it in the book is 1942. Since then you must have

How Does Neurotic Escapism in Treatment Manifest Itself? 163

been tempted to try it again with your 'vastly improved experience' (your phrase) to help. This makes it clear that you are not playing fair with me. Consequently my suspicions are justified."

"I am going to divide my answer in two parts: your suspicions in general and your specific suspicion of my specific motive in taking you on as a patient. The first part is easy. You mixed up your chronology. You gave me the three dirty-suspicious looks *before* we discussed whether or not I would take you on as a patient. Is this correct?"

"Well, perhaps."

"Therefore the statement that you are pathologically suspicious stands."

"Now let's see how you manage to squirm out of the main indictment."

"You misinterpreted the case history. I considered this Lesbian a therapeutic failure and said so in so many words. Her characterological changes were minor. As these things are done today, such a case would not survive the trial period. . . . And you conveniently forgot another item. I expressly stated that I was accepting you as a patient 'at your risk, without promising you anything, and for a trial treatment.' You are here on probation, for four to six weeks. After that we'll see."

"You haven't said anything about your interest in experimentation," said Mr. J., waving the only flag he had left.

"There is nothing to experiment with in a situation that has already been clarified. It is impossible, therapeutically speaking, to isolate a person's masochism and leave his homosexuality intact. Masochism is the basis of homosexuality. But you have not figured out my real motive. You should have figured it out, but you didn't. That's not a criticism of your intelligence but evidence of your neurotic pessimism."

"I'm curious."

"If one has as many dealings with homosexuals as I do in this office, one acquires something like a finger-tip knowledge of them. This 'feel' tells you intuitively how to judge the individual homosexual's real psychic situation. This extra tentacle, if I may call it that, told me that you were inwardly much more ready to change than you consciously knew and consciously declared."

"Don't kid me!"

"Facts. I took a chance on you to test my intuition, not to experiment. Why didn't that positive possibility occur to you? My answer: you were stopped by your neurotic pessimism."

"I'll be damned!"

"I can prove the point from another angle. Didn't you tell me that your father was always conducting experiments that never came off? Isn't it possible that you inwardly identify experimentation with failure? This makes your theory that I took you as a patient in order to experiment on you into a pessimistic prognosis a priori. You will have to grant that some experiments are successful."

It was a short time after this that Mr. J. produced a piece of evidence that "really threw him." In his words:

"I remembered something—a painful incident—that confirmed what you said and frightened me out of my wits. You caught me on the experimentation business. A few years ago I had a partner, a real screwball, but a man with new ideas. He proposed that we develop a new kind of machine, at our own risk. I turned the idea down cold and insisted that we break up the partnership. I have a horror of anything that isn't practical. It turned out that I was dead wrong. My screwball ex-partner got a backer, started producing his machine, and sold his invention to one of the really big manufacturers for half a million bucks. It occurred to me yesterday that I threw away a quarter of a million dollars because of a souvenir from childhood: 'don't experiment.' Boy, oh boy!"

9. SHIFTING OF PSYCHIC MASOCHISM TO POINTS UNRECOGNIZABLE TO THE PATIENT

Mr. K. started treatment because of severe premature ejaculation. He was in great despair; his wife had left him because he could not satisfy her sexually. During his first phases of analysis he behaved like a schoolboy making fun of the teacher. The interpretation of the oral and anal contributaries to his sexual difficulties were for him a never ending source of sarcasm and scorn, and he criticized me constantly. The fact that the furniture in my office was "modern" was a continual subject for merrymaking. He refused to analyze his senseless disparagement and his constant praise of his own antique furniture, with the excuse that axiomatic statements do not need to be proven. Every attempt to show him that his objections on matters of taste covered something else (e.g., sexual comparisons in the transference repetition) was futile, since there was no necessity to agree about such things. One day, after seven weeks of treatment, the patient informed me that he could no longer afford analysis as he had invested the money reserved for that purpose in remodeling his apartment with modern furniture. "A guy has the constitutional right to change his mind," he said, and, furthermore, he "was cured anyhow"; during the last few days he had acquired a girl friend and had repeatedly had normal intercourse. He left analysis, in spite of my objections, and remained potent. His unresolved psychic masochism found an even more dangerous depository; by hiding political literature for his so-called friends of various political parties in his country, in later years he railroaded himself into the position of being repeatedly arrested and having to serve jail sentences, although he himself was indifferent to politics of any kind.

10. INTELLECTUALIZATION

Every person in analysis uses the escape valve of intellectualization—occasionally. The patients I have in mind do it *typically and permanently*. Frequently they are schizoid personalities beyond repair (see Chapter 1).

11. PATHOLOGICAL LIES ABOUT THE ANALYST [18]

Terence once said: "There is nothing a man would not believe in his own favor." This dictum is applicable to technical situations in clinical analysis in which a patient has been caught lying about the analyst and argues his head off to prove that he was fully justified in his presentation of the "facts."

The technique of these *specific* lies is encountered mostly in *psychopathic personalities* and is typically executed in the following situation: The transference neurosis has taken place, and the analyst has been unconsciously identified with the infantile image with whom the original conflict started. If, luckily, the "real" person involved in the original conflict is still at hand, the latter is fed with lies and distortions purporting to have come from the analyst. If, however, the original is not at hand, substitute figures are chosen. In the two cases, the purpose of the procedure is identical: mobilization of fury against the analyst, and masochistic expectation of retaliation from the analyst.

A young man of twenty-eight entered analysis under peculiar circumstances. He was potent with his wife, whom he did *not* love, and impotent with his girl friend, whom he *did* "love." The official reason for analysis which he presented to his father (who was paying the bills) was of course different: the patient explained that he needed treatment because of his inability to get along with buyers in the business he and his father conducted.

The patient's original infantile conflict—consisting of a deep oral-masochistic elaboration relating to the mother—was subsequently shifted to the father. This was easy enough because this father had been an irascible, inconsistent, half-hypocritical educator, a dictator who shouted everybody down. Officially the patient was submissive towards his father, who continued to hold him down even after he became an adult. He was given a relatively large salary when he entered the business, but his father kept the reins securely in his own hands. There were constant quarrels between them, subdued on the son's part, not so subdued on the father's, which grew out of the young man's feeling that his father had become a mere figurehead in the firm, while he (the son) did most of the work without being elevated to a partnership or at least rewarded with an "adequate" salary.

As is usual in orally regressed masochistic cases, the *wish to get* covered more deeply repressed conflicts centering around the *wish to be refused*. The latter wish corresponded to the solution of the infantile conflict along masochistic lines; the former wish was *not* identical with baby greediness (as it originally was) but represented a subsequently established *defensive* cover designed to counter the superego's accusations pertaining specifically to the "pleasure-in-displeasure pattern."

The patient demurred when this explanation was presented to him. He considered himself a hedonist longing for "real love" and "real money."

The contradiction between conscious and unconscious aims could be demonstrated: both in marriage and in business he was in pursuit of rejection. He had married a cold, detached, sexually frigid girl who was totally unresponsive. Her housekeeping was sloppy; she never served him his favorite dishes; she was uninterested in company and isolated him socially. In business the patient also had to swallow his fury: here, too, he was constantly confronted with an inaccessible person (his father) from whom it was easy to extract a stream of "injustices."

As time went on, stronger inner defenses were needed and erected. To counteract the accusation of the inner conscience pertaining to his masochistic, self-created marital misery, a "kind and loving" girl friend was acquired. To counteract the accusation of conscience, hitting at the masochistic submission he displayed towards his father in business, the defensive wish to get money was instituted.

It soon became obvious that this patient could operate only in a climate of refusal. Where there was no refusal, he provoked until he got what he wanted—the proverbial kick in the jaw. This also explained the paradox of the man's potency with his unloved wife and his impotence with the loved girl friend. Obviously he could not provoke his sexually uninterested wife by being impotent with her —she would have been only too glad to dispense with the whole "messy business." Hence potency retained with her meant a repeated demonstration of how unjustly he was treated: he gave sex, and in return got—nothing. However, the girl friend wanted sex. Here he provoked by being impotent.

The patient described his relationship with the girl as rosy, but this was by no means factually correct. In addition to the suffering guaranteed by his impotence, he cashed in on other masochistic pleasures. He was pathologically jealous, "suffering hell." To make absolutely sure that the girl would be an instrument of torture, he had vaguely promised her that he would divorce his wife; of course he did nothing whatever about this promise. Resentment became increasingly visible in the girl.

Having established his "three torturers" (father, wife, girl friend), he proceeded to play for higher stakes by antagonizing buyers in his business. His father understood this danger and suggested analysis.

The patient accepted the suggestion, but for his own reasons: he wanted potency with his girl friend restored.

With undisguised malice the patient told me: "That old fool has no idea why I went into analysis. He is hyper-moral and would hit the ceiling if he had any idea of my real reasons."

The patient's analysis developed along unusual lines. The unconscious reasons for his impotence with the girl were worked out quickly, and the symptom disappeared. The patient did not see any reason for continuing analysis. I warned him against breaking off, pointing out his completely shaky neurotic balance, his conflicts with everybody, his depressions following each new "injustice." I had the impression that he had quite a different motive for remaining in treatment: his father paid the bills, and it gave the patient pleasure to "waste the old fool's money." He concluded with this comment: "I wouldn't get it anyway; let him pay!"

It was difficult to focus the patient's attention on his real inner problem. With unrelenting irony he countered every attempt to explain that what he called his "real" problem was in his case merely a sham, and that in inner reality he desired neither love nor money. "Nothing can satisfy an 'injustice collector' but—injustices," I told him.

The patient did not develop an interest in analysis until his girl friend became belligerent and definitely demanded "clarification": her motto was "Either divorce your wife and marry me, or we are finished."

All at once he needed the analyst. It was the analyst's business, he told me, to convince his father, a devout Catholic, that it was "old-fashioned" of him to object to his son's marrying a Jewess (his girl friend was Jewish). I answered that he would have to convince me first that he really loved the girl. In my opinion he was planning to divorce his wife and marry the girl for only one reason: he was bargaining for more trouble. I suggested that he postpone all plans.

In spite of my definite "suggestions," and contrary to them, the patient decided to go ahead. This simply meant that he was putty in the hands of the quite energetic girl, who was pressing hard for marital status. The father, informed of these developments by his son, was horrified. In conformity with my suggestion ("no decisions

How Does Neurotic Escapism in Treatment Manifest Itself? 169

during analysis"), although for different reasons, he, too, demanded that his son postpone his plans. The patient finally accepted this demand, although with a stipulated time limit of twelve months.

Immediately the patient started a campaign for more money. The father refused: "Why should I help you support two families? A divorce would mean cutting your income in half. If you want a divorce, change your style of living!"

Needless to say, the "injustice" was bitterly exploited by the patient. He also became indignant with me, since I had pointed out that the demand for more money was ill-timed: I practically foretold his father's answer. He did not give credit to the explanation of his masochistic action, but began to accuse me of being "in cahoots" with his father.

The identification between father and analyst was obvious; the patient denied it vehemently. Transference, he declared, "is the bunk. I am dealing with realities, not nebulous fantasies of an even more nebulous so-called unconscious."

This was the *second* of two incidents that made me question whether anything could be achieved with this patient; nothing is more ominous than complete misunderstanding of transference and resistance on the patient's part. The patient's attitude reinforced the suspicion that had been aroused a few weeks earlier by the first incident: The patient's father had reported his son as saying, during a discussion of his divorce plans, "Nothing has been changed by analysis." *On that identical day* the patient had urgently begged me to "convince his father." Obviously the patient was provoking the analyst; obviously, too, he was undermining the strength of the latter's arguments *vis-a-vis* the father. My position was not too enviable. I could not refute the patent lie; I was bound by medical secrecy not to divulge the patient's great secret: his previous impotence with his girl friend and the analytic removal of that symptom. I simply told the father that there must be some misunderstanding; if the son were present, I went on, I would retire with him for a private consultation of about a minute's duration, to remind him of a specific set of facts. After this, I assured the father, the son would be bound to retract his statement. The father understood that questioning me would lead nowhere; from his facial expression it was evident that doubts about his son's veracity had been actively aroused.

The incident was analyzed, and the patient was shown how senseless and ill-timed his lie had been. I pointed out, too, that the usual moral indignation with which the outer world surrounds the word "lie" does not apply in analysis: *analytically a senseless lie is simply a subdivision of the general masochistic technique.* Specific determinants may, or may not, be added. In his particular case, I suspected that inner irony at the expense of the father was involved. With an ironic smile the patient countered: "I had simply forgotten my impotence."

The patient's anger was continually shifting from father to buyers to myself; the circuit was then repeated. I pointed out that he clearly could not live without a bogeyman.

Then came an event which nearly torpedoed the whole analysis. During one of his quarrels with his father the patient "quoted" me as having said that his father was half-crazy and needed analysis more than his son did. The father indignantly informed me of this, and I simply stated that I had never made such a statement. I promised that the young man would be forced to retract the obvious lie. The patient admitted to me that he had lied: his father had been irritating, and he had wanted to throw "something that really hurt in his face." He also admitted the "exaggeration" to his father and retracted the "quotation," telling his father that my alleged statement had never been made.

The next step was—once more—a "reality situation," according to the naive patient. His "fiancée," as the patient called his girl friend, worked as an assistant bookkeeper in one of the numerous companies affiliated with his father's business. Her office was so close to the patient's office that it was possible for him to spend a good deal of time with her during working hours. The patient's father objected to this practice, claiming that it was detrimental to the business morale of the employees. Rumors, suppressed and only partly suppressed, grew rapidly, and the father laid down an ultimatum: "The girl must leave." This infuriated the patient; every attempt the father made to explain the situation was fruitless.

The problem was, once again, dumped into my lap. I tried to

explain that prevailing standards tabooed "affairs" in offices, and that in this case, the taboo was especially strong, since the patient had been "indiscreet" in handling the "affair" (in other words, had *provoked* once more). Eventually a compromise was reached; the patient undertook to persuade his "fiancée" to look for another job. It became clear, very soon, that neither the patient nor the girl had any serious intention of sticking to the agreement, although their reasons for non-compliance were quite different. The girl did not want to leave because she suspected that changing her position might lead to the patient's throwing her overboard. The patient did not want her to leave because she had become a pawn in the provocative masochistic game he was playing with the "powers that be."

At last the father lost patience and told me that if the girl did not soon resign voluntarily, his son would have to leave the business. I tried to dissuade him from this radical step. I discussed the problem with the patient again and pointed out that it would be to his interest to press the point with the girl. I met with the strongest resistance, and the "realistic" statement that the only position she could get would pay $10 less than her present job. I suggested that for the time being he give the girl the difference: a weekly payment of $10 would be less damaging than being thrown out of the business.

It became clear during this discussion that his boast—"The girl does everything I tell her to"—was pure braggadocio; he was completely under her thumb. I told him so, and the masochistic attachment was discussed.

Parallel with these developments went the patient's running battle for "more money." During an analytic appointment *the patient accused his father of having lied to him:* two years earlier he had been promised more money if and when certain provisions of the Federal wage-stabilization law were rescinded. These laws had since been invalidated, and he still had not been given more money.

On the very same day on which the patient told me that his father had "lied to him," he went to his father and informed him that he had decided to break off his analysis: *he had lost all confidence in me, since I had—lied to him*. This was the alleged lie: the patient knew that one of my other patients was a distant relative of his; some time earlier I had quoted "private information" to the effect that relatives of his (also shareholders) did not want him in the business. The story was a complete fake, of course.

Confronted with this alleged statement (repeated to the father), I completely denied it; hence I "lied in his face."

The first to inform me of his decision was the patient—*by phone*. He gave no reason, simply stating that he had decided to break off analysis. I answered that he could do whatever he wished, and that we would discuss this during his next few appointments, since analysis was a month-to-month arrangement, and he had filed his "letter of resignation" (via telephone) in the middle of the month.

The next telephone call came shortly afterwards. It was from the patient's father; he expressed his satisfaction with my answer, and his hope that the few remaining appointments would "knock some sense" into his difficult son.

In the next appointment, the patient was again confronted with the complex net of masochistic acts he had executed via lies. He was told that he was projecting the father image and reminded that the reproaches having to do with my "lie" pertained to his father, whom he had accused—on that very same day—of having lied about the promised salary increases. I also pointed out that he constantly tried to use analysis as a weapon against his father in connection with his plans to remarry. It was not until I had confirmed the fact that his fiancée had to leave the business that he became unable to use me as a counter-weapon in the conflict. I told him that if his father claimed that one and one equaled two, I could not—to please the patient—agree with his dissenting opinion that the total equaled twenty-seven. Once more the masochistic substructure was clarified.

The patient answered excitedly that I had no right "to make an ass of him" by denying his statements about my "lie."

"You had no right to attack me!" he insisted.

"I did not attack you. I simply had to clarify a lie you had told. This is not attack but self-defense. I have told you repeatedly that you are not to discusss your analysis."

"Maybe I made a mistake in opening my mouth to my father. But that's *beside the point*."

"It is not beside the point; it is the heart of the matter. If you attack me by spreading lies about me, I have the right to put the record straight. But you act the innocent victim; you attack first, and when I defend myself you turn around and ask indignantly, 'Why are you attacking me?' When I tell you that your actions began it all, you answer, 'That's beside the point.' To sum up: You cannot and will not take the real analysis of your 'acting out' and your masochistic personality. This being the case, analysis can do nothing for you. You had better leave, but be clear about the dangers ahead: You are bargaining for real trouble. Analysis is a therapy for neurosis; you, however, are suffering from more than a neurosis."

To adduce two other examples:

A blocked writer, a deeply masochistic woman, reported that between the ages of five and ten she had, as she put it, "sold her looks" to an old man who lived across the street. The payment was fifty cents for each exhibitionistic performance. This action could be reconstructed as her first desperate unconscious attempt to cope with her own voyeuristic conflict, for in these performances it was not she, but the old man (father image) who committed the crime of peeping. The mechanism used in this expiation of guilt was, first, projection; second, exchange of one of the visual tendencies for the other; third, identification with the old man's voyeuristic pleasure. The child exhibited in two ways; in addition to giving the peformances, she confessed them to her horrified sister. She thus preferred to take the blame for the defense mechanism (exhibitionism), for the sake of covering up something more important—peeping. But why did she accept money? At that time the child's father was beating her frequently and brutally. Every beating was administered with a specific ceremony which included undressing and formally asking for punishment. Very early the child suspected that her father's motives were not of an exclusively punitive nature. In taking money from the "man across the street," she was unconsciously directing an ironic message to her father: "You enjoy this; you should pay for your pleasure, just as the old man across the street does." Secondarily, unconscious ideas of self-degradation were included: "This is what Father makes out of me."

As already mentioned, the patient was a writer; in her, therefore, oral and voyeuristic tendencies were intensified (see Chap. 7). Her customary behavior was markedly exhibitionistic. As is usual, she used exhibitionism as a defense against more deeply repressed voyeurism. When she was asked why she had done nothing about her father's cruelty, the patient presented very interesting rationalizations. She claimed that she was "ashamed of her bruises" and of the possibility that the neighbors would consider her father "crazy." What the child really dreaded was the possibility that people would perceive her masochistic pleasure in this paternal torture. It became apparent in the transference that it was not modesty that prevented her from making the exhibitionistically conceived complaints that would expose her father. In the transference she projected the "bad-mother-father" attachment upon the analyst; she misconstrued all developments as situations in which she was being mistreated; without understanding what she was repeating she started to mobilize outsiders against analysis. The reason was obvious: since her feeling of guilt had been augmented by analysis of her masochistic wishes, she did *now* what she had *not* done as a child—she complained about "mistreatment." Even there an ironic twist was discernible: "You ask why I didn't complain; well, I'm complaining now." Thus analysis was "punished" for having disturbed her masochistic pleasure.

When this patient took the step of mobilizing outsiders against the analyst, her complaint was that the analyst was "driving her into suicide." Conveniently left unmentioned was the fact that her history recorded three suicide attempts, the first of which had been made at the age of seven! She left treatment, told her "story" to a number of colleagues, and eventually landed with an "understanding" analyst. The analysis with him, of course, was a failure.

Twice in later years this patient telephoned to me, requesting that I take her case again and continue treatment. According to her she was *still* blocked, frigid, unhappy in the choice of her partners. I declined, although the woman claimed that she *now* partly understood what she had acted out with me, and declared she had a "hunch" that the analysis "would work" *this time*. In other words, she still wanted to squeeze out some repetitive conflicts.

Here is the third example:
Nearly ten years ago for some weeks I treated a man of twenty-

How Does Neurotic Escapism in Treatment Manifest Itself? 175

six who possessed many of the traits of the impostor. His ingratiating behavior had persuaded a man from an old and wealthy family to become his business partner. When treatment began, the patient informed me that he was the owner of a business firm; this was the full extent of the information I had. Very soon, the patient's "peculiar partner" came under scrutiny; the partner's motives were totally incomprehensible. Before the situation came to a climax—the partner had fraudulently obtained money from his wealthy family and seemingly had invested this money with my patient as a "speculation"— enough of my patient's rather fantastic past had come to the fore to stigmatize him as a psychopathic personality. "Business reverses," meaning his partner's arrest, made further analysis impossible.

Years later, in quick succession, *three* young women came to me for consultation; each one bitterly accused me of having "prevented her marriage." The prospective husband in each case was the patient described above. Each interview proceeded along the following lines: I stated that I had not seen the man for years. "But how can that be possible?" the young women asked. "He showed me a bill of yours!" In every case the legitimizing bill had been exhibited in a dim light and at a distance; the date (now nearly a decade past) had been cautiously hidden. In any case, further "business reverses" and the progress of his psychopathy had led the man to specialize in promises of marriage; the profit lay in thus obtaining money to cover "divorce proceedings." The lies he used for extricating himself from tight spots were rather remarkable. On one occasion he used the money (half-extorted, half-lent) for a journey to Alabama; he came back allegedly married, claiming that the father of another girl had forced him, at the point of a gun, to marry his daughter. Moreover, he claimed that I had "advised him on psychological grounds" not to marry the girl, etc.

I clarified the lies and warned the man against further use of my name.

What should the attitude of the analyst be when confronted with these damaging lies?

Obviously medical secrecy does not bar self-defense. To protect himself, the analyst must contradict these lies in *general* terms, since other people are invariably involved. On the basis of my experience I would say that such patients, in these situations of heightened transference, are inaccessible to interpretations.

Especially difficult are situations in which an "acting out" patient circulates untruth, and the analyst cannot divulge the facts which would expose the statement as a lie. An example is the statement made by the first patient described here, in which he declared that nothing had changed during his analysis; the patient had simply omitted the cure of his potency disturbance. Another example is to be found in the second case: the patient's story was that the analyst was "driving her into suicide," when actually her first suicide attempt had been made at the age of seven, and the attempt had subsequently, but long before analysis, been twice repeated.

As soon as one discovers that one of the masochistic techniques of a particular patient consists of repetitive lies, it must be concluded that what is involved is not a simple neurosis. And, unfortunately, analysis is not too effective with psychopaths of the schizoid variety. The simplest procedure would be to ease the patient out by gradually interrupting treatment. Regrettably, the patient more often takes the initiative by provoking violent conflicts.

Such cases are more than a nuisance; they are dangerous. This is especially so because these patients are not bound by normal self-preservation: masochistically they advertise to outsiders most of their conflict with the analyst, in an attempt to mobilize the outsiders against the analyst. The whole problem falls into the category of professional risks which cannot always be avoided.

12. "ACTING OUT" BY MISUSE OF THE TRANSFERENCE

In spite of the extensive literature on acting out, the following clinically important points are frequently overlooked:

    a. What is acted out is a defense, never an original wish.

    b. Acting out is a proof of the deepest masochistic passivity, warded off with a pseudoaggressive gesture; confusion here means unchangeability.

    c. The acting out of a dramatized defense should not be confused with the "unconscious repetition compulsion," a mistake frequently made. The dramatized defense is an inner alibi performed for the

How Does Neurotic Escapism in Treatment Manifest Itself? 177

benefit of the inner conscience, whereas the "unconscious repetition compulsion" is an *active* repetition of an experience that once had to be endured *passively,* with the purpose of narcissistic reparation.

d. Acting out in the form of a "negative magic gesture" is a denial of inner masochistic tendencies by impersonating the "cruel" parent, the recipient of the "cruelty" being cast in the role of the "actor's own mistreated self." It demonstrates, in caricature, how unkind the parent really was. It is often a defense against a previous "positive magic gesture"; hidden behind both disguises is an aggressive reproach and, still further hidden, psychic masochism.

e. Acting out with the analyst as a projection figure to be "fought to death," as was not possible in childhood.

Mr. L. suffered from personality difficulties of a banal masochistic nature, regularly maneuvering himself into situations where he was "mistreated" by a woman. His analysis began with his recital of his childhood troubles with his mother. Whenever he got into a temper with her he would run away from home, usually finding refuge with an aunt. He was always brought home by force and severely punished. His retaliation was *"taking an oath not to talk to my mother;* once I stuck it out for *six days."* This information came at the end of an appointment. When he arrived for his next appointment he gave me a friendly greeting, proceeded to the couch, and then lapsed into utter silence. None of my openings elicited a single word from him. At the end of the appointment he took his leave with a friendly civility, not at all ironical. The next appointment followed this precise pattern.

I began to suspect that his silence had some connection with the infantile "oath" he had mentioned, which was now being repeated in the transference situation. He had "stuck it out," he said, for six days; the question was, how long had he intended to keep his oath of silence? Six weeks, I hoped; but months passed, monthly bills were paid, autumn gave way to winter—and still the patient remained silent. During all this time I interrupted his silence at ten-minute intervals, explaining what he was repeating in the transference neurosis: "Sorry to intrude on your private life, but you are paying me for that." No response. As time progressed, it became more and more clear that the patient would "stick it out" for six months

(I optimistically excluded the possibility of six years) and that this time limit probably corresponded to his original "oath."

Once during this period Mr. L. did open his mouth; at the end of one appointment he said in a completely matter-of-fact tone, "Things are getting more and more complicated." There was not even a response to my laughter; he just looked blankly surprised.

It is difficult to reproduce the tragicomedy of the situation; I though that remark was the funniest I had ever heard.

Exactly at the end of six months Mr. L. broke his silence. He had remained completely blank during his silent appointments; it was "like being in a daze," as he expressed it. My beautiful interpretations of his "oath" and his system of showing his mother how "helpless" she was had been entirely wasted; he had heard nothing. The quantitative factor (and the desire to show his "mother" that he was powerful enough to win the battle of silence) was stronger than his appreciation of reality and my analysis of his resistance.

Last but not least, another group of "escapists" should be mentioned: *neurotics who never enter treatment,* despite knowledge, money, opportunity.

In my opinion the subjective suffering which every neurosis produces is *not* the real reason why a neurotic consults the psychotherapist. Only if the inner balance between inner masochistic wishes [19] and inner punishment for exactly these wishes is disturbed does the neurotic seek help. This assumption explains why not all neurotics who have enough money, knowledge of the existence of psychotherapy, and the necessary time and opportunity, do consult us.

A good example is a case I described in ONE THOUSAND HOMOSEXUALS:

Mr. M. was a successful business man of thirty-eight, a confirmed homosexual who liked his way of life but had recently become impotent in his "exciting favorite sport." He was in danger of losing his "wonderful friend," and he asked anxiously whether his potency disturbance could be cured in psychiatric treatment. When I told him it could not, he accused me of not wanting to cure him, of being a hypocrite and a moralist. I explained to him that his difficulty

How Does Neurotic Escapism in Treatment Manifest Itself? 179

showed that an inner objection to a neurotic trait—homosexuality—had been built up and was being propelled by inner guilt and that a neurosis within the framework of neurosis could not be treated. "The same masochism that pushes you into homosexuality," I told him, "is now preventing you from satisfying your 'wonderful friend.' It's obvious that unconsciously you want to lose him."

It came out in the discussion that his friend was a parasite who was taking advantage of him in business as well as in his personal life. I warned him that the next step would be a lot more expensive: threats, extortion, blackmail, and what not. Crestfallen, Mr. M. asked: "What am I to do?"

"Understand that you yourself, by means of your newly developed potency disturbance, are making sure that your friend will leave you—at least sexually; he may continue to exploit you financially. Without knowing it consciously you are approaching the point of no return in your homosexuality. Sooner or later this inner development will penetrate into consciousness. When it does, come and see me again. Perhaps then you can be cured of your homosexuality."

What this means is that Mr. M. was able to take all the masochistic suffering and to strike a balance. But when his added difficulty—impotence—appeared, the balance became shaky. Still, I never heard from him.

CHAPTER 6

ARE THERE NEUROSES OF THE "GRAND DESIGN" TYPE ?

THERE are, in general, two techniques that enable the psychoanalyst to learn something really new and never before described. In the first he makes an observation that is intuitively [20] understood in its implication and later elaborated on and checked clinically. The second consists in being dumbly fooled by the unconscious of a patient (or succession of patients) and learning post facto from the failure. The first technique is implicitly included in the observations of every analyst with productive intuition and the ability to verify these flashes clinically. The preceding and following chapters of this book abound with examples of this type. In the present chapter I would like to describe a contribution to the second, unheroic, technique.

Some failures in psychiatric-psychoanalytic therapy are due to the fact that certain neurotics harbor—unknowingly and unwittingly—an unconscious "grand design" that fools both the analyst and the patient. This type of very severe masochistic neurotic can be defined in this way: they are *dominated by one, and only one, climactic unconscious fantasy*—mostly reducing the mother image to absurdity by total masochistic submission via pseudo-identification ("you wanted me to be that way," partly a negative magic gesture) and/or by "outdoing" the mother—and they spend their lives creating the prerequisites for this form of acting out. Their whole existence seems like an appurtenance of the "great moment"—the *grand masochistic fiesta*—which, if achieved, is protracted as long as possible. When

Are There Neuroses of the "Grand Design" Type?

these neurotics come into treatment they don't use therapy for changing but for strengthening, bolstering, and speeding up the expected "great moment." This attitude accounts for both the amazing changes (which turn out complete duds) and the unapproachability that cannot be explained.[21]

In other words, patients of this type may achieve short-range "successes" that fool the analyst just as much as the tenacious stubbornness in some other cases surprises him. Both the pseudo success and the total failure are simply subordinated to the misunderstood unconscious aim of the patient's "grand design."

Such a neurosis is difficult to detect in analysis because the "grand design" has *not* been materialized—yet. It is hard to analyze *future possibilities;* only clinical facts are available. The patient may show scores of symptoms, never the "grand design." *The neurosis treated and the "grand design" are never identical.* The only solution would be a prophetic one, a *construction of future possibilities* from the infantile history, provided the analyst is familiar with this peculiar type of neurosis.

CASE 1. Mrs. N., a woman of forty-seven, consulted me first four years before she entered analysis, and not on her own account. Her husband was having an affair with his secretary. His "strange behavior" at home had aroused her suspicion, and he had finally confessed to her. His reason for confessing, however, was a decidedly odd one: he wanted his wife's approval for his affair with his secretary. After she had given him her answer, "over my dead body," he agreed to consult me himself. When he was told that his behavior was a typical example of "middle-age revolt" (his wife had already made him read my book on this subject), with the added twist of confessing and asking for approval, the man took an even more unusual line. "What's wrong with having an affair?" he asked. "Weren't there courtesans in France during the reign of the Bourbons?" When this nonsense had been disposed of, it was made clear to him that he was simply bargaining for masochistic troubles. This did not impress him, and he arranged to take a rather long business trip, accompanied by his wife, as an excuse for bowing out after five appointments.

During the next two and a half years I saw Mr. N. three times, once every six or eight months. His story was always the same: his wife had started a campaign to persuade him to sever his connection with the profitable chemical business in which he was a partner (he was a specialized chemical engineer). Her plan was that they should both study history at a university; they would thus be together, united in a common interest. N. was horrified at the prospect of not working. He always asked the same question, "Should I give up my work and sell my share?" My reply was always the same: "Do you want to?" "Definitely not!" "Then don't." These visits were paid for with checks drawn on a special account in a distant city, with the purpose of keeping them a "deep secret" from Mrs. N. Of course I had my doubts whether so severe a masochist was capable of holding back any incriminating material and was sure that he would do exactly what Mrs. N. wanted him to. I told him so, explaining my impression that she wanted him to get rid of the business instead of the secretary and intended to have him under constant, twenty-four-hour surveillance in the new life devoted to history.

A year later Mrs. N. appeared and wanted to be analyzed. Her husband, of course, had sold his part of the business; and they were both studying history. But—and this worried her—Mr. N. was only paying lip service to the brave new life she had carved out for them. He wanted to go back to work in his field, though he wouldn't admit it. She was firm, however, in her conviction that when one had achieved relative security, work was just "idiotic, unnecessary, a silly prejudice." She summed up her situation: "For twenty-five years I have led the life he wanted. I moved from one place to another, according to his jobs. I produced, brought up, and married off seven children. We are financially independent; let him, for once, do what I want. If he won't, I shall leave him." When I objected that work was an inner necessity above and beyond making a living, that she just wanted to have her husband under continual supervision because of the affair in the office, that she had better analyze the reasons for her unusual demands, Mrs. N. would have none of it and went into long discourses to prove how right she was. This went on for some time, until I told her that she should either begin her analysis or leave.

Are There Neuroses of the "Grand Design" Type? 183

Under this pressure I got some material from her childhood. According to Mrs. N., her parents had an exceptionally good marriage. There was some mystery about their background: it seems that they had both been previously married, somewhere in northern Europe, and both had had children. They fell in love and ran away together to the United States; it was not clarified whether or not they were actually divorced in the old country. Afterwards they lived happily in a city in the West. The father was a musicologist and music teacher and gave lessons at home. Of her childhood "there was little to say." She was a very independent child and repeatedly ran away from school, the first time when she was in kindergarten.

As far as one could reconstruct in a few weeks, Mrs. N. was repeating her parents' marriage. Her father stayed at home; her husband should do the same, in an improved version: Her father worked; her husband did not need to. Her constant threat of leaving her husband corresponded to the old infantile megalomania—she herself had repeatedly run away when things did not go her way. It was also pointed out to her that there must be more to it: What was missing was her masochistic elaboration of her parents' happy marriage. She must have felt excluded, and it seemed that she now wanted to duplicate that fantasy; by destroying a perfectly workable marriage she put herself into the masochistic position of the "poor little girl left out in the cold."

Mrs. N. reacted with a decision to divorce her husband. I objected, pointing out that our "analytical contract" excluded such a decision during analysis. Mrs. N. insisted, and first behind my back, later with my knowledge (though not my approval), instituted divorce proceedings. The whole thing was over in three weeks. Not to disturb the patient, I told her that we agreed to disagree. Whether or not she had done a masochistic thing would be clear later on, depending on how she felt about it after a few years. We parted amicably.

The denouement could only be reconstructed indirectly, from telephone calls and letters from *Mr.* N., who started immediately to "inform" me. He went through something he called a "nervous breakdown" and went to another analyst, who after four weeks was said to have declared him completely "normal." Obviously his severe masochistic personality distortion was not seen or dealt with, if Mr. N.'s report was accurate, of which there was no proof. However, the colleague had two sessions with Mrs. N., "to get information" from her, and it seems she so infuriated him, or left such a peculiar impression, that he told Mr. N. he should be glad to be divorced from this "very sick, man-hating" woman.

In the meantime Mr. N. had again taken up relations with his secretary, discontinued nearly two years before. When he told Mrs. N. about this (just as he had told her the first time, just as he had told her of his "secret" visits to me) she was furious and accused him of "spoiling everything." Obviously it did not even occur to her that, after a divorce she herself had pushed through against her husband's and her analyst's wishes, she had no right to complain. (Mr. N.'s agreement to a fantastic financial settlement on a fifty-fifty basis— in a state where "community property" was unknown—may be mentioned in passing, to show the extent of his masochism.)

At this point I received the following letter from Mr. N.:

Dear Dr. Bergler:
Thank you for the opportunity to talk to you by phone.

I really think Mrs. N. got the divorce to *jar me* to my senses, so I would have an opportunity to prove that I still loved her. Maybe I was too hostile and slow-witted to realize this. In any case, I've had plenty of panicky periods since: I was really scared I was going to crack up—thus the sudden rush to your colleague. When I started to see Ann [the secretary] after a 15 months complete gap (and after the divorce) that settled it for Mrs. N., I think. She felt *that* proved she was right about me in the first place. And in a sense she was correct, as had I been truly in love with her at that time, I would have waited.

I am going to take a job in Africa, and am leaving in a few weeks.

I'm giving this information to you to keep you posted, as it is very possible one of us may be seeing you again sometime.
                                                    Sincerely, etc.

Besides the fantastic masochistic submissiveness, the letter clearly reflects ideas implanted in him by Mrs. N.

In retrospect, it seems that Mrs. N.'s unconscious grand strategy was an outdoing of her mother—in the mysterious first marriage in Europe. Her mother ran away—that was the official version—but Mrs. N. as a child must have concluded that her first husband threw her out. She herself, nearly half a century later, reversed the roles: she threw her husband out, got half his money, and still—he came back. There was probably more to it: Mrs. N.'s unreasonableness in begrudging her ex-husband the right to associate with another woman after divorce perhaps represented the imagined fury of her father's mythical first wife, with whom she masochistically identified.

CASE 2. Mr. O., a Dutch intellectual of high caliber, consulted me. He was having an affair with a "loving and understanding" girl, whom, as he proudly informed me, he had rescued from an "impossible Lesbian affair." He was clever enough to arrange to have her analyzed as a "precaution" before marrying her. For reasons unrelated to the case he had a very high opinion of me and was disappointed that I could not take her on. I referred her to a gifted colleague with the proviso (stipulated by Mr. O.) that if the analysis should not work out I would take over.

A few months later Mr. O. again appeared and complained indignantly about the colleague's analysis, which "simply gives her new arguments for her provocations." She had in the meantime moved into his apartment, and this was the description he gave of his domestic life:

"It seems that all my habits, attitudes, predilections, likes and dislikes are somehow wrong. I have to get rid of all of them and start again from scratch. She has a slogan that nobody can quarrel with—'to live together, work together, share together.' But the way it works out is that I'm being trained to be her servant—and trained the hard way. What I want doesn't count at all. If I object to what she wants she pouts, turns sullen, and then goes on to tears, shouting, and violent scenes. Do you remember Oliver Herford's wisecrack, 'My wife has a whim of iron'? So has this girl.

" 'Working together,' as she interprets it, means that she prevents me from working and expects me to conduct my business as she sees fit. 'Living together' means that I'm not supposed to see people alone even on business; she insists on being present. 'Sharing together' means *my* sharing and accepting her ideas—there's no other side to the picture. I have to walk the dog. I have to do the marketing. She's a terrible cook and a sloppy housekeeper. What's more, the dirty jobs are all left for me—I'm her servant, as I said. I don't pretend to know what she's acting out. As far as I can gather, there are two tendencies: cruelty and not permitting me to enjoy solitude for even a minute. She started out to reform me, and now she has me in a reform school. And after all, I'm not exactly a wayward child!"

Mr. O. was adamant in insisting on our initial agreement (that I would take over if the analysis with my colleague did not work out satisfactorily), and I was forced to begin treatment with the girl. Even before this the colleague had wanted to resign from the "hopeless task."

The future Mrs. O. was a beautiful girl of twenty, very tall and very blond, who told me that intellectually she understood the reasons for her provocative behavior, *afterwards,* when they were explained to her, but never at the time of her tantrums (her story sounded rather hypocritical). It turned out that the colleague had done a good job in explaining her neurotic-masochistic attachment to the mother image, which had led, among other things, to Lesbianism.[22] But it had been impossible to penetrate her really mulish stubbornness and her complete conviction that she was entirely guiltless in the irrational conflicts described by Mr. O. He was the one who needed analysis, not she, was her refrain.

I told her that she had an amazing ability to fool herself about her behavior, explaining that not every case of injustice-collecting could be solved, and suggested a three months' period to work out her problem. If after that time she still persisted in her attitude, we would call it quits.

During the next few weeks an extraordinary change came over the girl. She showed what seemed to be real understanding of her problem, gave up her provocations, and, in short, was changed to a degree that surprised both Mr. O. and me. My explanation was that results prepared in the first analysis became apparent in the second.

Are There Neuroses of the "Grand Design" Type?

Mr. O. married the girl, and after a short time—at an even increased tempo—she reverted to her previous behavior.

What really happened could only be understood later: marriage was the prerequisite for her "grand design" neurosis.

Analysis of Mrs. O. clarified some of her attitudes. She was the child of a broken marriage. Her mother had dominated her childhood; the divorce had taken place when she was four. After the divorce her mother had taken a lover, and the affair had to be kept secret from the man's jealous wife. Periodically there were reconciliations between Mrs. O.'s mother and father, but these invariably "failed to work out."

Mrs. O.'s mother had been a hard taskmaster. Part of the time she was disagreeable and nagging, the rest of the time she was detached and uninterested.

One could gather from Mrs. O.'s behavior in the analysis that she had elaborated masochistically on her infantile conflict. Everything the analyst said or failed to say was perceived as a deep injustice. Before entering analysis she had displayed the same pattern of repetition, constantly accusing Mr. O. of "excluding and humiliating" her. In her opinion he had chosen her because he thought she would not stand in the way of a perpetually bachelor-like existence in which she would be completely disregarded. There was no doubt that she unconsciously hoped her marriage would fail. Her mother's reconciliations with her father had always been short-lived; without knowing it she steered her marriage in the same direction. She was a captain of disaster.

Unaware of her deeply buried real wishes, Mrs. O. proudly and frequently referred to her conscious formula for an ideal marital partnership: "Living, working, and sharing together." Her demands were extravagant, so unrealistic that they were doomed to failure. The simplest way to ensure disappointment is to demand too much. In this way she smuggled her unconscious desire for rejection into her carefully constructed defensive alibi: her formula for happiness in marriage.

Mr. O. was quite correct in accusing his wife of cruelly attempting to make a servant of him. In so doing, Mrs. O. was caricaturing her mother and reducing her husband to the image of herself as a child.

Unconsciously she was actively repeating passively endured experiences. She was, in this, declaring her desire to revenge the wrongs done her by her mother in childhood. But this false show of aggression was merely defensive; underneath the superficial—though still unconscious—need to prove aggression lay the deeply buried, decisive need to enjoy psychic masochism by repeating her mother's marital fiasco.

Her conflict with her husband seemed to reproduce the infantile guilt for aggressive thoughts (taking the father from the mother), but this was merely a smoke screen. Guilt was assumed for this "lesser crime" to conceal its real source—her masochistic attachment to her mother.

First by campaigning for her husband's reform and later by putting him under a reform-school regimen, Mrs. O. provoked him mercilessly. Ironically, her slogan—"living, working, sharing together"—was, as he conceded, irreproachable. In her methods of applying the slogan to daily living, however, she showed that she wanted to be rejected. She reduced the reasonable to a caricature. Evidently the caricature was in some way symbolic and cued to her mother, literally inseparable from the child. By asking for too much she got too little. Her inner aim was to get twenty-four hours of disappointment in return for asking to be loved twenty-four hours a day.

Still another defensive mechanism became visible. To diminish her own infantile guilt, she had to prove that her father had been "really impossible." This too was a smoke screen, for Mrs. O. had not married the image of her father but that of her mother. She had reproduced the masochistic pattern and in defense had to repeat the pseudoaggressive alibi as well. This accounted for her hatred, disparagement, and humiliation of her innocent-guilty husband.

Why do women like Mrs. O. marry at all? Often they feel that marriage is not for them, but this conviction rarely stands in their way. Evidently they need marriage to achieve an exact repetition of the childhood situation. Mrs. O. had to be married before she could repeat the unconscious game of marital reconciliation that her mother and father had played throughout her childhood.

Are There Neuroses of the "Grand Design" Type? 189

CASE 3. Mrs. P. was the wife of a brilliant young South American physician residing in this country, an internist with great respect for analysis. Again because of reasons unrelated to the case he had great confidence in me. The young woman came into treatment because of "writer's block"; otherwise everything was "O.K." with her in her own estimation. But her husband complained about constant procrastination in fulfilling household duties, a certain coldness and detachment towards him, disorder in their apartment, and so forth. She made light of these complaints.

In analysis this charming woman used a special form of resistance that I have never seen before or since: all anger in the transference repetition was ironically mimicked as a joke (like an accomplished *diseuse* she would say, "If I were a naive person I would tell you that you're unjust to me"). At the same time her understanding of her original conflict with the mother image (her mother was a psychotic woman, repeatedly in state hospitals) was excellent, after the following recollection came to light: At the age of four she had bought a little bottle of perfume for her mother's birthday, a sample the man in the drugstore gave her for a few cents—she had saved the pennies for months. She put the miniature bottle in front of her mother's door while she was taking a nap. When her mother came out of her room and found the bottle, she said, "It smells like cheap perfume." The child never admitted it was her present.

The analysis of Mrs. P.'s writing block proceeded satisfactorily, according to the principles outlined in Chapter 7 and elaborated in my book THE WRITER AND PSYCHOANALYSIS. After some months she started to write again, produced a few good short stories, and began a very ambitious novel. She also had a child and shortly afterwards became pregnant again. She considered herself cured, and I saw no reason why her treatment should be continued, especially since her husband had decided to enter analysis.

The next five years revealed that all this remarkable improvement was only a mirage. Instead of writing, the lady became a child-bearing machine, producing in rapid succession, and against her husband's wishes, four children—the identical number of children in her family in childhood. After they bought a house in the suburbs she was a slave to house and children. Her technique was simple and effective:

she could not find a maid and she successfully sabotaged all attempts to remedy the situation. She bitterly reproached her husband for the miserable life she led and reacted with intolerant fury when he tried to show her that she herself masochistically created the very troubles she complained of. In short, she became a martyr. Her husband claimed that the closets in the house were in indescribable disorder, that their sex life had deteriorated, that she embarrassed him in company with her "silly talking jags, in which she acted the half-idiot."

It seems that Mrs. P. simply misused analysis as a "certificate of health," and in possession of the imaginary document (constantly held up to her poor husband [23]) she played the role she was forced to play as a child: from the age of eight, every time her psychotic mother was committed to an institution, the burden of the household fell on her. The unspoken reproach against her mother was: "Look what you did to me!" Once more the spurious improvement in analysis was only a stepping-stone to living out the "grand design."

CASES 4 AND 5. There are two other cases in my files corresponding in principle to the preceding examples; unfortunately they concern people and circumstances that could be recognized and so cannot be divulged.

In general, I can say that without knowledge at least of the existence of the "grand design" type of neurosis the thought of such fantastic potential repetitions does not even enter into the analyst's deliberation.

The practical consequences are of clinical importance. Suspecting at least helps the analyst's peace of mind; whether the patients (sometimes schizoid) can be helped is another, rather dubious, question. The analyst's knowledge can, however, sometimes protect the marriage partner. Here is an example:

CASE 6. Mr. Q. was a man of many conflicts. Both he and Mrs. Q. played the typical injustice-collecting game of psychic masochists in their marriage. Both felt misunderstood and slighted. Mr. Q., my patient, described his wife as a kill-joy who poured cold water on any interest he might have. He felt uncomfortable in her presence;

Are There Neuroses of the "Grand Design" Type?

once he characterized her as a "criticizing governess." To complicate matters Mr. Q. had homosexual tendencies, confessed to his wife several years before, and it was this difficulty that led him to consult me. Even after the resolution of his homosexual inclinations in analysis there remained the question of how to deal with the difficult personality of Mrs. Q. Finally she was persuaded to enter analysis with a female colleague I recommended. The snatches of "reports" Mr. Q. received were such that he became highly suspicious whether her part in their neurotic partnership had been explained to her (or whether she understood it). These reports, which he described in horror as "à la *Ladies Home Journal*," combined with Mrs. Q.'s unwavering conviction that she herself had no conflicts and had entered analysis only to help him, made him request an interview with his wife's analyst, if his wife would consent. Mrs. Q. refused but, oddly enough, had no objection to my having a conference with her analyst. The final straw that broke the camel's back (or Mr. Q.'s patience) was a dream his wife had and recounted to him. The dream, which followed a conflict about "free evenings," was simple: Mr. Q. was condemned to die in the electric chair. Quite reasonably Mr. Q. asked whether she considered the dream a simple expression of fury or the ego's pseudoaggressive retort to an accusation of masochism made by the superego ("Why did you allow yourself to get into such a situation in marriage?") Mrs. Q. looked blank and seemed not to be informed of the difference.

My discussion with Mrs. Q.'s analyst had this result: Of course she was given thorough explanations of her psychic masochism; of course she seemed to understand what it was all about; of course her resistance was strong and she could only gradually accept the fact that her conflict centered round her mother image. In contradiction to this information was the fact that Mrs. Q. played dumb in discussing her analysis with Mr. Q.

At this point two things became clear.

First, why Mrs. Q. refused Mr. Q. permission to see her analyst but consented (even half suggested) that *I* see the analyst. It seems that all three—Mr. Q., her analyst, and I—were being used as "messenger boys" to inform the mother image (in the transference repetition the female analyst) that Mrs. Q.'s "acceptance" of analytic explanation was only lip service, totally ineffective and totally ironical—unconsciously.

Second, it became obvious that Mrs. Q. had an unconscious "grand design" scheme. She wanted to be declared analytically hopeless and was working (without consciously knowing it) towards a divorce. This would force her to live with her mother—and to be entirely and masochistically under her thumb. This she achieved; Mr. Q. divorced her a few weeks after he understood the situation. Mrs. Q., as was to be expected, immediately gave up her analysis.

The great difficulty in even spotting the neurosis of "grand design" is its *occult nature—the material is latent and has not been lived out—yet.*

Preventive analysis of conflicts not yet materialized and lying in the future is impossible, as Freud pointed out in "Analysis, Terminable and Interminable." He was speaking of conflicts understood by the analyst. The cases I have in mind are more complex—the analyst cannot fathom the not yet visible conflict.

The only conclusion one can draw is that one cannot be careful enough and should never underestimate latent masochistic possibilities if even the slightest hint is given. Admittedly an exasperating problem.

In retrospect: In CASE 3 the hint was perhaps the wish for an immediate second pregnancy. The reason given was that one child is unhappy alone, and Mrs. P. wanted to have time for writing later. In CASE 2 the sudden change before marriage was—perhaps—suspect. In all the other cases there were no hints, even in retrospect.—One hopeful note: Mrs. P. reentered analysis after five years; at the present time she is in treatment. The feeling I have is that—perhaps—something can be achieved, because explanation of her "grand design" made a shock-like impression. Who knows?

CHAPTER 7

HOW DOES THE VISUAL DRIVE, THE LEAST EXPLORED CHAPTER IN PSYCHOPATHOLOGY, CONTRIBUTE TO THERAPEUTIC FAILURES?

UP TO the present time *looking* and *showing off* and the neurotic symptoms and healthy sublimations connected with them have been *the* stepchildren of psychiatric-psychoanalytic investigations. Neglect of them has been so general that there is not even a vocabulary for dealing with them. The *visual drive* has no English name—only the related opprobrious epithet Peeping Tom (of Lady-Godiva fame)—and neither the French derivative *voyeurism* nor the British scientific neologism *scopophilia* is understandable to the nonspecialized physician, much less to the intelligent layman. There is the same lack of terminology for the tendencies connected with showing off. Exhibitionism has many disparate connotations, and its mental department is equally unfamiliar and equally nameless.

The term *"visual neuroses"* is more appropriate for the purpose of subsuming both tendencies—voyeurism and exhibitionism—when they miscarry. Freud elucidated one part of the connection between them in stating that both are "partial drives" and that an interflow of *unconscious* identifications takes place: The exhibitionist, while he is exhibiting, identifies himself with the one who watches him; while peeping the peeper also identifies himself with the one who exhibits. In this assumption peeping and exhibiting are put on an equal basis. My investigations, conducted over a period of more than thirty years, have convinced me that *this parity is spurious; only voyeurism is an original drive; exhibitionism is a later defense.*

Not only is exhibitionism only a defense; it is a very specific one. It contains *"confessional elements,"* the admission that one has actually *passively* seen (or imagined seeing, or wished to see) what one now—*in active repetition*—exhibitionistically repeats, frequently in exaggerated caricature and on one's own substitutive organs ("repetition in reverse," see p. 205).

These "confessional elements" in exhibitionism are highly paradoxical. On the one hand, they serve as *guilt-diminishers*—simply by implying that imitation is involved; therefore other people (the imitated, active ones) have the responsibility. On the other hand, the mere fact that there is an admission of having seen sometimes makes the transition to exhibitionistic self-assertion impossible (or difficult) in some children; *shyness* results.

Shyness may be masochistically unproductive or, by increasing autarchic imagination, productive. (The second solution is that of shy people among creative individuals in all fields; if the first solution ensues, these people, in spite of effort, are frequently sterile.)

The upshot is whether the ego can convince the superego, which is averse to the guilt-diminishing excuse of imitation and puts more emphasis on the forbidden early peeping.

It should be noted that the "confessional elements" in exhibitionism are *both an inner defense and an invitation to punishment.* The relative strength of the two components determines the outcome.

Moreover at the infantile crossroads where peeping is exchanged for exhibitionism there is also (under unfavorable inner circumstances, meaning weak ego, strong superego) a *meeting point with infiltrating psychic masochism.* The unavoidable transition can be accomplished normally—with *spite* and aggression. Or it can be accomplished masochistically and halfheartedly; in this neurotic solution *looking becomes a proof of having been denied sight,* masochistically exploited.

Every neurosis connected with the visual drive and its defensive derivatives is based on the masochistic elaboration of the infantile peeping conflict.

When seeing (the breast, the mother's body) is unavoidably thwarted, two elaborations (each with several subdivisions) become possible:

1. EXHIBITIONISTIC DEFENSE.
a. *Normal solution:* spiteful refusal to look, leading to defensive exhibitionism ("Who wants to look at your ugly udder? I want to display myself!").

b. *Half-neurotic, hence typical, solution:* peeping is partially maintained (in combination with the exhibitionistic defense given above) but elaborated according to the masochistic "allure of the forbidden," hence half expecting punishment. Thus the average man is a surreptitious peeper at innuendos of the female body (see the author's book, FASHION AND THE UNCONSCIOUS).

c. *Masochistic grievance,* leading to half-attempts at reparation in the exhibitionistic defense while seeming to maintain the voyeuristic "wish"; this "wish," however, is not identical with the original peeping but is masochistically imbued. The clearest example is later perversion voyeurism in man, in which, under the disguise of wanting to see the woman, unconscious masochistic enjoyment of woman's injustice in refusing to be looked at is paramount (see Section III no. 21).

2. IMAGINATION AS FLIGHT FROM THE DILEMMA OF VOYEURISTIC DEPENDENCE. *Imagination* "opens shop" in the sphere of voyeurism, excluding the refusing object. This is an attempt at *visual autarchy.* The following solutions, therefore, are encountered:

a. *Subjectively creative fantasies,* e.g. daydreams.

b. *Objectively creative fantasies,* e.g. those leading to literary and artistic work or creative work in any field. These sublimations are of various types (see Section III).

c. *Imagination of disaster*—perpetuation of masochistic rejection. Nothing productive about that.

It is superfluous to mention that these "solutions" overlap and can be encountered in the *same* person, though in different quantities, in different sectors of the personality, and at different times.

The *genetic-historic picture* in the visual drive—voyeurism as basis, exhibitionism as defense—should not be confused with the *clinical picture,* observable in the adult, where a peculiar *"exchange mechanism"* is put into operation: *secondarily* voyeurism can be used unconsciously as a defense against exhibitionism, and vice versa.

The complexity of the problem becomes apparent when one hears the rationalizations of people caught peeping: "I didn't do anything —I was just looking"; "I wasn't peeping, he (she) made me look, by exhibiting!"

It seems that infantile peepers have a special code: only overt and *active* performance is reprehensible, whereas the *passive* "taking in" of a visual impression to them appears harmless. Moreover, infantile adults mix up the internal and external lawbooks; thus (according to epistolary information from a friendly assistant editor of a psychiatric journal) a young man caught peeping defended himself in this manner. "I wasn't peeping at the girl undressing in her room; I just wanted to see whether she was already asleep—I wanted to steal her car."

The activity-passivity problem goes even further. It would lead too far afield to discuss the whole theoretical gamut of what constitutes activity and passivity. That activity is *not* identical with masculinity, nor passivity with femininty, is analytically acknowledged. In 1933 I suggested (in collaboration with L. Eidelberg) in "The Breast Complex in the Male" (*Int. Zeitschr. f. Psychoan,* Vienna, 19:547-583, 1933) using the oral stage as a paradigm in which *activity denotes giving, passivity denotes receiving* (the mother *gives,* the child *takes*). This was applied in that study to voyeurism and exhibitionism, voyeurism as the "taking in of impressions" being classified as passive and exhibitionism, the "giving of sight," as active. I still subscribe to this theory, which includes the oscillations between activity and passivity (nobody is only active or passive; only specific partial actions are alluded to; moreover, one can be very "active" in pursuing a passive aim, e.g. sucking; movements of the female in intercourse, etc.).

The peculiar immunity of the passive "taking in," personally self-bestowed, probably has its inner reason in unconsciously equating ocular intake with food intake (see Section I below): didn't the mother actively feed the child, the child being the passive recipient, and isn't the active one "responsible"?

The activity-passivity series in visual problems, later connected with guilt, explains actions in adult neurotics that are otherwise baffling. For example, a patient, a well-known physician, was a truly fantastic peeper and at the same time completely inhibited in his imagination. He could not "think," read, imagine a face, had no foresight in the simplest things. Why the contradiction? In looking at woman's anatomy *she* "took the responsibility" by displaying it; he was helpless when he had to perform actively even in sublimated peeping—no guilt-relieving excuse was at hand.

Why are some neurotics "more papal than the Pope," *more severe in visual affairs than their educators actually were?*

For instance, in the case of a blocked writer of forty-six, the recollection emerged that at the age of seven, having been called by his mother, he entered a room in which she was dressing before a mirror. Her breasts were half-exposed and he immediately withdrew, although his mother said, "Come in, I want to talk to you." "But you aren't dressed," countered the boy.

A blocked song-writer of twenty-six remembered specifically that his parents were rather indifferent to his running around half-clad and that he never had reprimands connected with peeping. Still, even talking about peeping in analysis was hard for him; otherwise his sexual inhibitions were nil. (He had difficulty in taking a book from the shelves in my waiting room, though there were obviously no secrets.)

I suspect that the reproach another patient, a famous theatrical director, threw at his parents ("they never taught me anything, not even how to wipe my ass") was *only a masochistic elaboration of a peeping conflict.* He became a peeper, listening to other people's intercourse in hotel rooms.

These and similar cases show that no direct repetition of parental reprimands is involved. On the contrary, parental dicta on peeping are *magnified and made more severe to maintain the fiction that parents were "mean" and sight-depriving.* One can also suspect that the *emphasis on privacy is a magic gesture;* the child's privacy is constantly invaded by the parents, although they themselves retire at night "to their privacy."

It is because voyeurism is a subdivision of orality (E. Simmel) that the impact of "oral withdrawal" (weaning) is so strong.

Here the connection with "direct peeping" comes in. For example, the blocked writer mentioned above, though a lifelong homosexual, paradoxically liked to look at breasts. (Most homosexuals "hate" the breast.) They excited him though, put to the test, his penis shrank ("expanded in the other direction," he added ironically). The situation must be similar to that of the perverted voyeur—"woman is mean and sight-refusing."

The visual orbit covers a very wide field. In its *neurotic* elaborations these symptoms and signs are observable:

1. Shyness.
2. Blushing (erythrophobia).
3. Fear of confined places.
4. Street fear (agoraphobia).
5. Fear of heights (acrophobia).
6. Fear of examinations.
7. Jealousy, pathological curiosity, and logorrhea.
8. "Writer's block" (painter's, sculptor's, composer's "block").
9. "Block" in scientific, photographic, journalistic endeavors.
10. Depersonalization.
11. Stage fright.
12. Boredom (alysosis).
13. "Negative exhibitionism."
14. "Thinking block."
15. Lack of imagination in perceiving external phenomena and lack of "business acumen."
16. Temper tantrums.
17. General inhibition in reproducing verbally or graphically what has been seen or heard.
18. Coprophemia (active and passive utterance of obscene words).
19. The "demonstration character" of neurotic and psychosomatic manifestations.
20. "Sham shame" and the fear of "being found out."
21. Perversion voyeurism.
22. Perversion exhibitionism.

None of these disease entities can be analytically resolved without applying the specific principles governing the visual drive. Since these are partly unknown to our colleagues, partly unapplied, most analysts have trouble with visual neuroses, which thus make their contribution to therapeutic failures.

Sometimes one also gets the impression that a contributing factor to the nearly universal analytic uncertainty (to use an understatement)

The Visual Drive

in dealing with visual neuroses is not knowing to what level of development the visual instinct should be assigned.

I. THE "FORBIDDEN BREAST"—THE CENTER OF INFANTILE ATTRACTION AND PERMANENT CONFLICT

"In the beginning was the word," claimed the poet Goethe of poetry and science. An interesting assumption for an adult artist in words but certainly not exact for the infant, baby, small child. Long before the child could actively utter one word with his mouth, or do one deed, he used a "substitute mouth" for passively "taking in" visual "food"—impressions through the eye.

The only worthwhile early contribution to Freud's pioneer work on the two "partial drives," voyeurism and exhibitionism, (contained in a few sentences of THREE CONTRIBUTIONS TO THE THEORY OF SEX, 1905) was Ernest Simmel's conjecture in 1922 [24] that voyeurism was a subdivision of the *oral* drive, that impressions were "taken in" just as the child takes in food. Many expressions current in all languages make this analogy: "to devour with one's eyes," "greedy eyes," "devouring a book."

Later investigations confirmed Simmel's assumption, though the course of further discoveries in this field was rather circuitous and puzzling. In investigating cases of depersonalization,[25] I found (in collaboration with L. Eidelberg) that these seemingly incurable neurotics were curable by centering attention on the fact that their repressed buttocks exhibitionism was warded off with a *double* defense: the exhibitionism was first transformed into *pleasurable* voyeuristic self-observation and then changed into consciously *unpleasantly* perceived self-observation according to the formula "I must observe myself because I am sick." [26] These transformations were performed under pressure from the accusing inner conscience (superego). Why exactly buttocks exhibitionism should be so predominant in the neurotic disease entity "depersonalization" could not be clarified at that time.

What was most surprising about these data of 1935 was a practical and theoretical consideration. In practice the curability of a, till then, hopeless neurotic disease entity [27] was established and clinically proved. Theoretically, a whole rattlesnake brood of questions opened up: Can voyeurism be used as a defense against exhibitionism? Are there two different kinds of voyeurism—"unpleasant" and "pleasant"? Why was buttocks (anal) exhibitionism singled out in depersonalization? How many layers of defense are involved? How could the prevailing view of the three-layer structure of the neurotic symptom (unconscious wish—superego veto—unconscious defense) be reconciled with the above experience pointing in the direction of a *five-layer* structure (unconscious wish—first superego veto—first unconscious defense—second superego veto—second unconscious defense)?

All these questions remained unanswered, although my further studies produced more and more material showing that *voyeurism can be warded off with exhibitionism and exhibitionism with voyeurism.* In blushing (erythrophobia), for instance, the two blushing cheeks unconsciously represent the breast, and the very obvious exhibitionism is superficial, hiding a more deeply repressed voyeuristic substructure.[28] The same holds true for street fear.[29] However, exactly the opposite is clinically visible in depersonalization and fear of heights [30]—here exhibitionism is warded off with voyeurism.

In another disease entity, boredom (alysosis),[31] voyeurism is totally repressed, and no apparent substitute appears, except for faint exhibitionistic innuendos designed to demonstrate the extent of the individual's ennui. It is well known that people with vivid imaginations never really get bored. The alysotic unconsciously acts the "good boy" by emptying all mental compartments of incriminating material that is voyeuristic in scope.

By utilizing my experiences the above-mentioned disease entities became therapeutically accessible, but without clarifying the theoretical question marks concerning the over-all picture of "visual neuroses" in general.

What finally convinced me of the typicality of the *"voyeuristic-exhibitionistic exchange mechanism"* was my studies on writers.[32] Before the writer can write he must have a plot, produced by "imagination," which is genetically rarefied peeping. The French writer Joubert very aptly called imagination "the eyes of the soul"; the poet Heine, more than a hundred and ten years ago, when asked what he had been doing lately, answered, "I have been giving

The Visual Drive

audience to my fantasies." Later the writer writes down and elaborates on the plot, thus exhibiting before the reader. If there is a disturbance in the form of writer's block, two distinct difficulties arise, depending on what section of the visual orbit is involved: some blocked writers are devoid of ideas (voyeuristic disturbance), some have a superabundance of ideas but cannot elaborate and write them down (exhibitionistic disturbance).

This, of course, is not the whole story of "writer's block" but only the part affected by the visual component (see Section III, no. 8 below).

After the "voyeuristic-exhibitionistic exchange mechanism" (or vice versa) was established, the question of its genesis arose. Oddly enough, the starting point—depersonalization—furnished the answer. In 1950 I published a study entitled "Further Studies on Depersonalization," [33] in which, on the basis of clinical material, I concluded that the *buttocks* exhibitionism (anal exhibitionism) of the depersonalized is in inner reality *breast* exhibitionism, an unconsciously fantasied display produced for two purposes: to negate the lack of breasts *and* to invite being beaten. Thus the question that could not be answered in 1935 finally did find an answer: in cases in which *beating fantasies are combined with extensive visual tendencies, depersonalization is used as a typical defense mechanism.*

The *spolia opima,* the highest prize in the internal tug of war of all the visual neuroses is the *breast.*[34] Looking at the breast, even for children who are breast-fed, becomes taboo after weaning, hence after six, eight, or ten months of life. Experience has proved that on the visual "front" it makes *no difference whether the child is breast-fed or bottle-fed.* Every child gets tactile impressions of his mother's breast when carried in her arms, hugged, or kissed. It is not even necessary to assume deep archaic or biologically transmitted intuitive knowledge; the child wants everything he doesn't possess. And these two bulging organs are noticeable even in clothes, sometimes even exaggerated in size by the fashion of the day.

In the "battle for the breast" every child is the loser. Neither can he get to see the breast after some time, nor does he possess the organ himself. Gazing at it is strongly prohibited and inhibited, and for good. The boy performs an amazing tour de force: he finds on his own body a substitutive organ—the penis. True enough, anatomically, histologically, physiologically, functionally, the two organs are dissimilar—but all this is unknown to the baby. He sees the oblong shape, the pendulousness, and the "fluid-producing" capacity. Besides, beggars and babies in urgent need of "narcissistic reparation" cannot be choosers. Thus the forbidden sight of the breast is eradicated by a declaration of the male baby's independence: "I have just such a thing myself (penis)! Who wants to look at the ugly udder anyway!" *Thus voyeurism changes into defensive exhibitionism—for the first time.*

Everything is "perfect," with one exception: there is doubt concerning the size of the organ. And so begins a search for confirmation that can only be executed via demonstration. The result is the penis exhibitionism of the boy that startles adults so much. As the child grows older his elders are no longer amused; angry rejection, disgusted facial expressions, and punishment follow.

The result is the beginning of one of the great tragedies, so abundant in the nursery: parents must, out of cultural necessity, implant in the child the accepted standards of decency. On the other hand, the child sees in their educational dicta only one thing: *The masters of the nursery reject his reparative attempt by not letting him show them that he possesses this wonderful breast-penis himself!*

Thus, in the nursery—the place that may well hold the world record for misunderstanding by all concerned—arises the great doubt about the size of the penis that haunts millions of men. *The yardstick is never the real organ but the unconscious comparison with the giant breast.* The *"complex of the small penis"* (correctly named but incorrectly explained by S. Ferenczi) has its origin in that very spot. Ironically, since the real problem is unconscious, the comparisons actually made are senseless; the size of the non-erect organ is compared with that of other boys and even adults, surreptitiously peeked at. No conclusions can be drawn from the non-erect organ about the erect state. Besides, only much later will the poor comparison-maker find out (if at all, and too late) that the usable length of the vagina is no more than two and a half to three inches. Since even "small" penises are longer, everything above that length is—luxury.

The Visual Drive

Besides this more or less typical solution there exists the *masochistic solution* of early voyeurism, previously elaborated on (see p. 195).

What about the girl? [35] Not being in possession of the "substitutive breast"—the penis—the little girl cannot solve her voyeuristic difficulty in the same way as the boy. This anatomical difference gives rise to the only psychological divergence in the development of boy and girl in the oral, pre-oedipal phase. Both have been confronted with the giantess of the nursery. Both develop the "septet of baby fears." Both live on the basis of infantile "autarchic" misconceptions; both are plagued by the great troublemakers—infantile megalomania, aggression, libido, unconscious conscience, reality. In coping with the deprivation of the breast their courses part.

What psychological use does the girl make of the physical difference? At first, in the usual infantile manner of cavalierly ignoring painful facts, no cognizance is taken of it. Of course, at the baby stage no possibility of comparisons exists—except that both breast and bottle, compared with the child's own size, is "overdimensional"; and so the experience of the "enormous" fluid-carrying "organ" (the bottle-fed child identifies the bottle with the person who gives it) is established.

As for the first sensations in the genital region, they center round the clitoris. These feelings are initiated by stimuli reaching the child in two ways: through the mother's cleaning procedures and through the child's own "organ expeditions" and discovery. The baby also discovers that clitoris and nipple have a very similar consistency. And the differentiation of production of fluid? The orifice of the female urethra is located directly below the clitoris; one doesn't expect the baby to distinguish the fact that two organs are involved. Even many adults are amazingly ignorant of the anatomy of the female genitalia.

The infant girl thus establishes the same identification of nipple (breast, bottle) with clitoris, her "female penis," as the boy does with an organ better suited for it. Although a consoling one, the initial identification, however—and this distinction is later of great importance—can make use only of the nipple, *not* the whole breast (bottle).

Then comes the inescapable tragedy of weaning. Whereas the boy can use his whole "long" penis to repair and negate the loss of the "long," now withheld organ, along the lines of "repetition in reverse" (see below), the girl has much less "length" at her disposal. Nevertheless, the "reparation" is installed. There are, however, two obstacles to its success.

The first, which occurs even in families where the girl is completely isolated from boys and allegedly never has an opportunity to glance at her father's organ, is simply seeing the contours of her mother's breasts through clothes (sometimes even magnifying in their effect). Here the "injustice" of being deprived is demonstrated ad oculos. This not only strengthens the fantasy of the mother's cruelty but diminishes the value of the defense: "I haven't lost anything; I have a similar organ on my own body." The second obstacle is that, sooner or later, the little girl sees the boy's penis. Her reaction is "penis envy," as stated by Freud, leading to the vain hope that the clitoris will grow to the size of the penis. However, here too the maternal breast is the original yardstick.

The reason for "penis envy" can be understood only from the "breast complex." "Mother did not give me that thing," is the girl's bitter conclusion. The resentments and fears attached to that conclusion differ; they range from the accusation that her mother "cut it off" to "mother maliciously refused." In any case, fury and fright are reinforced, and so is the "septet of baby fears," now concentrated at its last component, "castration fear," after the principle "What next?" [36]

One might ask what all this bitterness is about anyway, since later on the girl will have two advantages over the boy: her ability to bear children and fully developed breasts. The question is academic, as these compensations come too late. The psyche, it must be remembered, is formed between the ages of one and three.

Thus the grandiose "reparation" of the trauma of weaning is attempted by the girl as by the boy, but in her case it works out rather poorly because of the "poor" material available for the process of "repair." All this strengthens the typical "psychic-masochistic solution." As we have defined the human tragedy as an overdose of psychic masochism, the female of the species seems to be worse off than the future "he-man."

Actually the opposite is true. Women are the stronger, men the weaker sex. Three reasons account for this strange fact. First is biology; there is a higher mortality for the male from the prenatal period throughout the whole of life. Second, the woman's early bitter disappointments, although masochistically elaborated, can be built into her biological function; childbirth and rearing of children consume an enormous amount of productively used masochism. Third, her "passivity" is not under social pressure, like that of the man, and so cannot be used as material for reproaches by inner conscience.

To what degree the breast, or breast equivalent, is *the* yardstick for the small child is visible in the psychological superstructure of intercourse. Again one could say that a biological function does not have to be "explained." Quite true. But what does have to be explained is the superstructure built upon the biological function.

The first experience of the child is that of having an object, breast or bottle, pushed into his mouth. At this point the first cornerstone for the equation activity-passivity is laid down: the pushing mother is *active* (giving), the object of the pushing is the baby, *passive* (receiving). "Psychological" observers are frequently confused by the fact that the baby may suck quite forcefully; as stated previously, one can be quite active in pursuing passive goals.

What happens later in man's intercourse? A complete reversal of roles according to a "repetition in reverse": [37] the active-giving man pushes his oblong, "liquid-producing" (actually liquid-carrying) sex organ into the passive-recipient vagina. Here mouth and vagina, breast and penis, milk and sperm, are unconsciously identified. No wonder the average man calls his wife "baby"—she half represents the baby part of him, while he half represents the giving mother.

Those who doubt this deduction may observe the neurotic reactions when these "repetitions in reverse" (from passivity to activity) do not take place. If the male child identifies unconsciously not with the *giving* mother but with the allegedly *refusing* mother, stinginess in sex (and in money, words, affection) results. (This is, of course, already a pseudoaggressive defense, covering masochistic elaboration.)

The sexual disturbances of this type of neurotic are either premature ejaculation or psychogenic aspermia. For elaboration, see my book COUNTERFEIT-SEX.

Another important residue from the lost "battle of the breast" is visible in *various hopeless attempts to achieve autarchy*. We have already met one example, the narcissistic reparation of the boy in identifying his penis with the unachievable breast. But these normal children do not go all the way—they don't refuse food and don't live on "self-produced urine." Some become poor eaters, some constantly "prove" unconsciously that though their mother feeds them the food is spoiled ("weak stomach," hypochondriacal complaints). All the different elaborations of the "septet of baby fears" (first stated in THE BASIC NEUROSIS) are encountered. These fears were summarized in Chapter 1 of the present volume.

That not all children react gracefully to the "disappointing" breast (disappointing chiefly in not belonging to the child, since, according to Freud's suspicion, the child perceives the breast as part of himself) is visible in some peculiar games:

A patient remembered that, at the age of seven, watching a Gypsy woman suckling her baby excited him. He arranged a "game" in which he put a long straw blade into his penis and taking the other end in his mouth, drank his own urine. Here penis and breast, milk and self-produced urine are clearly identified.

The high point of these refusals to accept dependence is seen in one of the variations of the Narcissus myth. The youth so much admires his image reflected in the brook that he "forgets" to eat— and dies of starvation.

What happens if a baby *girl* does not accept with good grace her dependence on the breast? Various types of frigidity on the oral level of regression result (for elaboration, see COUNTERFEIT-SEX).

After clarifying for myself the complexities of the "voyeuristic-exhibitionistic exchange mechanism," two questions resulting from the 1935 study on depersonalization remained:
1. How is it possible to explain the confusion manifesting itself in oscillations between voyeurism and exhibitionism used reciprocally

The Visual Drive

as defenses? How could voyeurism be used as a defense against exhibitionism in some disease entities, while in others exhibitionism is used as a defense against voyeurism?

2. How can the riddle of the three-layer or five-layer structure in neurotic manifestations be solved?

The second question has already been discussed in Chapter 2 (pp. 61 ff.).

The first question could be solved by *differentiating* the *genetic* from the *clinical picture* in the framework of visual components.

The *genetic* picture comprises voyeurism as the basis (a subdivision of the oral drive) that is changed into the exhibitionistic defense—after the external inhibition of peeping and, even more important, after the establishment of narcissistic restitutions (penis exhibitionism and reassurance).

The *clinical* picture, built up after the genetic one has been established, comprises mutual exchangeability of the two components, voyeurism and exhibitionism, as defenses.

It is of great importance to be clear about the *specific unconscious features in the defense "exhibitionism"*:

1. It represents a "repetition in reverse," an *active* repetition of a *passively* endured voyeuristic experience.

2. The term "experience" is used with reservations. This does *not* mean a photographic reproduction. It incorporates the infant's misconceptions and misinterpretations, imaginings, fantasies, wishful thinking, and so forth, including especially his caricaturing exaggerations and reductions to absurdity.

3. The defense "exhibitionism" contains a *"confessional element";* in "reproducing" the "experience" an admission is made that one has seen the copied or caricatured the "forbidden" original.

4. The *fight between the confessional-admitting element* in exhibitionism and the *guilt-relieving shift of responsibility* ("I just copy the original") leads to pitched battles in elaboration. Living out the confessional element in disguised form is more "normal" than inhibiting it, which results in "pathological shyness."

5. In the clinical picture both exhibitionism and voyeurism can be connected with *psychic-masochistic elements*.

6. All attempts to correlate visual elements *clinically* with *specific genetic levels* of development (oral, anal, phallic) are *useless;* the defense lends itself to *all* levels. However, genetically both *partes constituentes* belong to the oral level.

7. Exhibitionism is never an original drive, *always a secondary defense.*

8. *Not distinguishing between the genetic and the clinically observable* elements of the visual components results in hopeless confusion.

9. As long as the superego can point out that a person's peeping is *imbued with infantile elements* normal elaboration in the form of *sublimation is not possible.*

10. The problem of *passivity versus activity* in the framework of the visual drive is of paramount importance (see p. 196).

11. Voyeurism and exhibitionism are used in the "battle for privacy" (see p. 197).

The case in which I encountered the greatest difficulty in deciphering complexities in the visual sphere—and the one in which I first learned about the "confessional element" in the voyeuristic-exhibitionistic "set-up"—was that of Mr. R., a brilliant scientist of forty, a man of original ideas, in analysis because of a banal masochistic conflict in his marriage. This shy man once mentioned in passing that in high school, or its equivalent in the country of his origin, drawing was considered an important subject and that whereas in every other subject he was a candidate for *summa cum laude, in* drawing he was a "complete anti-talent." He added, ironically:

"Even today I cannot draw a thing—excuse me—except a cube."

"What about a circle?" I asked, without knowing why I thought of that particular question.

"You would be surprised at the caricature of a circle I would produce. One thing is clear: anti-talents are not directly transmitted. My two boys are excellent in drawing, and one of them has a distinct talent for painting."

It was difficult to fix the patient's attention on his childhood "drawing block," since the problem had no practical importance for him. However, when he mentioned another "amusing anti-talent"

The Visual Drive

of his, inability to imagine a person's face when the person was absent, it could be proved to him that analyzing his visual block could be of practical importance. Who could foretell whether his scientific imagination might not ultimately be involved?

"I became conscious of my inability to draw between the ages of ten and fourteen, and these drawing classes were a nightmare for me. When a vase or a branch was given as a model I was paralyzed. Condescending schoolmates helped me; otherwise I would have failed and lost time. Afterwards I went to another school where drawing was no longer required."

"And the inability to imagine faces? Does this apply to your next of kin too?"

"Yes. To anybody. Sometimes the veil is lifted and I see the familiar face, somewhere on the upper outer quadrant of my eye, but only for a second. Then it disappears. On the other hand, I have an excellent memory for faces—if I see them before me, or on the screen. I seldom forget a face."

"And why is a circle 'impossible' and a cube 'possible,' though a cube is more complicated?"

"I have no answer to that.'

Sometime later Mr. R. remembered that he had been frequently teased as a child because of his stocky build and was often described as "square."

"Fortunately," he added with some irony, "the modern connotation of 'square,' the beat generation's term for a contemptible Philistine, did not exist then. Perhaps you have there, in that joke, my predilection for drawing cubes."

"What seems a joke to you is actually important. If the square represents you, why the more complicated cube, making the square multidimensional? And what was the purpose of asserting yourself, and your complexity, before yourself?"

Several days later the patient spontaneously returned to the subject.

"When you were discussing my drawing difficulties, why did you ask whether I could draw a circle?"

"The question was asked without thinking it through. I suspect that at that moment I unconsciously understood your conflict about drawing better than I did consciously."

"Meaning?"

"Obviously I was referring to your peeping experiences centering round the breast."

"That's foolish!"

"Perhaps. I have respect for these 'unexpected, involuntary visitors,' as Thomas Paine called such thoughts in THE AGE OF REASON. His advice was to 'treat them with civility.' That's exactly what I'm doing."

"Intuition, eh?"

"Unconscious understanding, preceding the conscious. Sometimes these are false leads, sometimes pearls."

Then the patient remembered the wet nurse his six-years-younger sister had had (wet nurses were usual in his country of origin). Though "poor at faces" he at once saw "that mean peasant face" in his mind's eye and remembered often sneaking into the half-dark nursery and watching with excitement her "enormous breast" being taken out of her blouse to feed the baby. The nurse objected to his presence and complained to his mother, who gave him a severe reprimand.

"What do you mean by 'watching with excitement'?"

"Red face, beating heart, unexplainable general emotion."

"You will agree that there is 'circle' material in you. Obviously wet nurse number two must have been a screen memory for earlier experiences. Did you have a wet nurse too?"

"Yes. Of course I don't remember her. But my mother told me some peculiar stories about her wanting to prolong her stay, as she was being given special food. That peasant woman, it appears, had gotten the idea that as long as there was 'something wrong' with the baby she would not be discharged. She seems to have stuck hairpins high up into my anus, with the result that I was constantly bleeding —probably only staining. Finally a specialist in the distant capital city of the province, where they took me, pronounced judgment— and suspicion. The nurse was discharged and the bleeding stopped."

"Well, you had some realistic 'mean' encounters with nurse number one. No wonder you called your sister's nurse 'mean-faced.' Was she really?"

After searching his memory the man had to admit that she had a longish, "cowlike" face, placid, rather expressionless.

"Since you cannot possibly remember your own nurse you probably projected feelings of fear and bad intent upon nurse number two. The question arises: what excited you in watching your baby sister being suckled, the breast or the masochistic fantasy?"

"What do you mean by 'fantasy'? According to my dead mother—and she had no reason to lie—the torture inflicted by my nurse was real enough."

"Quite probable. But later it was masochistically elaborated and fixed—by *you*. Reality is only the raw material. What the child does with it is his, and exclusively his, business. For instance, you could have acquired a distaste for 'torturing' wet nurses and avoided the sight of them when 'in action.' Who asked you to sneak into your sister's room? You were not exactly invited."

"That's true."

"By the way, when did your mother tell you the wet-nurse story?"

"After I was grown up."

"Can you *now* connect these experiences and their elaboration with your inability to draw?"

"No. I cannot."

"I know from analyses of writers that peeping is defensively changed into exhibitionism. First the writer has to have a plot (*inner peeping* at a scene played for himself in the internal theater), which he later elaborates on paper—for the reader; hence he *exhibits* before him. If we assume that this defense is typical, according to the inner lawbook peeping seems to be a felony (didn't the nurse complain to your mother?), sublimated exhibiting an accepted and unpunishable half-misdemeanor. All this presupposes 'sublimation,' hence transformation of something instinctual, infantile, and tabooed into something socially accepted. But—and the but is decisive—sublimation also presupposes that the ego can convince the superego —inner conscience to you—that it is doing something *adult* in his act. When the superego objects and can prove that the alleged adult is only a little child in adult's clothes, still holding on to his original 'dirty' peeping or exhibiting, the sublimation cannot be established and a neurotic symptom or inhibition, for instance 'writer's block,' results."

"But in my case no sublimation appeared."

"Precisely. Take the vase you were given to draw and couldn't. Assuming your conscience said to you, 'You dirty peeper and dirty little enjoyer of torture!' what could you have answered?"

"You mean that in drawing the vase *I would have had to admit that I peeped?*"

"That's it! There seems to be a *confessional element* in exhibitionism. The defense of exhibitionism also seems to be a guilt-reliever: 'I'm just imitating, sometimes in a caricature, what the *other* person did; therefore I am not guilty!' "

"But why didn't I use this guilt-reliever, as you call it?"

"Because to do that you would first have had to confess to peeping to enjoying the masochistic experience of being pierced by breast —or hairpin."

"If I understand you correctly, the change of a peeping experience into an exhibitionistic act of any kind is more normal?"

"Yes. It uses *active* repetition of a *passive* experience, a form of 'repetition in reverse.' You never got that far."

"And the cube?"

"Represents your defense: 'I did not peep, I only *look at myself.*' Didn't you say that they called *you* 'square'?"

"Fantastic!"

"Quite true. But look at the further results of your peeping inhibition. You don't even allow yourself to see faces in your mind's eye! And your choice of profession is also involved."

"How is that? I have inventive ideas!"

"Yes, but with the proviso that you observe the material you work with first. Shift of responsibility. 'The material did it, not I.' "

"If that's true, every scientist uses that subterfuge!"

"Also true. These sublimations could be called 'sublimations with half-renunciation.'[38] What differentiates the scientist, the journalist, the photographer from the creative artist, for example the writer, is this shift of responsibility. This is best shown in criticisms of these people. The most telling argument against the creative writer is *'He*

The Visual Drive

has no imagination.' And the corresponding strongest reproach to the scientist reads *'He does not stick to facts!'* "

In the framework of normal and neurotic elaborations of the visual components there are numerous subdivisions. The next section will deal with twenty-two clinical pictures in the neurotic orbit. At this point I should like to mention a few quasi-normal, half-neurotic, and neurotic elaborations.

Re: normal.

We have already met two of these. First the boy's penis exhibitionism, contradicted by the educational process; if in his *"mechanism of stubborn reparation"* the boy weathers this defeat without falling into the trap of the "complex of the small penis" (see p. 202) and later, as an adult, reverses the roles in coitus, he is at the beginning of the homestretch leading to normal sex. The other quasi-normal mechanism is *"sublimation with renunciation."* The example of the scientist Mr. R. (described in the preceding pages) is paradigmatic. Under the condition that the guilt for peeping is shifted from one's own imagination to the "objective material" worked on, imagination (peeping) is allowed. The photographer and the journalist, to name only two other professions, work on the same principle. (See Section III, no. 9.)

In creative writers and creative artists in general another, still quasi-normal, defense is encountered: *"sublimation on probation."* In no other sublimation is the element of the "temporary" so stressed as in that of creative people constantly haunted by the fear of "drying up." That fear will be dealt with in Section III.

Re: Half-neurotic cases.

"Incognito exhibitionism" is a term I suggested for people who are entirely *unable* to accept even normal display or—if necessary —the limelight unless they are under pressure from specific inner camouflaging conditions. The genetic basis of incognito exhibitionism is common to four completely dissimilar phenomenological types:

(a) function (any direct display of oneself) fully impaired;

(b) function not quite impaired but performed only under penalty of the severest fear;

(c) function seemingly unimpaired but performed under "peculiar" inner prerequisites, manifested in bizarre external conditions;

(d) function not only unimpaired but apparently exaggerated, containing, however, specific restrictions on other parts of the ego, e.g. inability to do anything but work in a highly restricted field.

a. *Self-display fully inhibited.* Behind this difficulty is the child's failure to accept narcissistic restitution, or to accept it fully. The shift from voyeurism to exhibitionism is made, but inner guilt becomes attached to the exhibitionistic defense and it can be used only in substitution. A case of this type, a photographer who was unable to attend public functions or make an informal speech about his work, is described in Section III (no. 9, Block in Scientific, Photographic, Journalistic Endeavors).

b. *Self-display partially inhibited and performed with extreme fear.* The mechanisms here are the same as in type "a," but with a slight lessening of tension, that is, the function can be performed but is paid for with extensive production of fear.

Fear, in my opinion, pertains exclusively to psychic masochism. Two subterfuges are used. Inner fear of conscience is shifted outside; the fear-sufferer seems to be afraid of an external danger. Second, the guilt, actually belonging to psychic masochism, is fastened to pseudoaggression, which takes the form of overstepping educational commands. This shift to the outside and the trick of "taking the blame for the lesser crime" of pseudoaggression constitute the maximum assistance the unconscious ego can provide in the fight against the inner conscience.

Sometimes a peculiar compromise is reached inwardly. Self-display is performed, but instead of emotions, coldness and detachment appear on the surface. The performer "freezes up," and his "act" is lifeless.

I once analyzed a man of this type (described in THE BATTLE OF THE CONSCIENCE), a politician, amusingly enough, whose friends objected to the coldness of his speeches and suggested that he use more "oomph" and more gestures. As a practicing lawyer in his pre-political days he had used one particular gesture: spreading apart the second and third fingers of his raised right hand, the space between pointing at the imaginary enemy. In analysis it became clear that in this gesture he identified with a mathematics teacher he had had as a child. The teacher's reputation had been rather shady; he had been tried for fraud and acquitted because of insufficient evidence —a mercy verdict. The second finger of the teacher's right hand had been amputated as the result of an accident. The patient was able to recall the occasion on which, to his amazement, he had for the first time made use of his gesture: when he had feared, though innocent, that he was going to be accused of embezzling a client's funds. The gesture, therefore, signified both half-admission *and* defense—for the teacher had been acquitted. There was a further complication since the gesture had an inner connotation of masturbation: "Look, I'm using my hands for gestures, not for masturbation." Though defensive in scope, the gesture also included a good deal of self-indictment and self-punishment (the empty space between the fingers also signified castration), and it consequently became too compromising for use. Bereft of his gesture, the man became even more a prey to his fears.

Patients of this type are never free from the inner fear that conscience will see through and unmask their disguise of defensive exhibitionism. This fear is shifted to the spectator or the audience. Superficially these patients seem to be suffering from castration fear; underneath lies the whole pandemonium of the orally based "breast complex" with its "septet of baby fears."

c. *Self-display made possible by adherence to specific "impossible conditions."* Paradigmatic for this type was the patient in whom I first observed "incognito coitus." This man would request the girl to recount to him *during coitus* the detailed story of her sexual performance with another man, described in "popular terms"—meaning obscene language. He thus performed the sex act incognito; and on the occasions when he attempted to do so without this crutch, "in person," so to speak, he would fail completely.

Only one phase of this symptom is of interest here. The patient was rather shy and could exhibit only when he slipped into someone else's "skin" (he could not even undress in the girl's presence). Via oedipal identification (both positive and negative) he seemingly repeated a sex act that he had observed his parents performing; even at puberty this scene had been the conscious content of his masturbatory fantasy. Why was all this retained in his conscious memory and not repressed? The explanation was that the memory served as a defense against more deeply repressed oral-masochistic components, visible in the injustice-collecting pattern of his personality in general. They were visible also in his attitude towards his sperm, which he would scrutinize closely after every ejaculation; originally he had believed that masturbation caused bleeding. More deeply repressed was the fantasy that he had "fed" the girl with his heart's blood, so that she was bleeding him to death. When he attempted intercourse without the "incognito" he suffered from impotence or, at times from "psychogenic aspermia."

This peculiar prerequisite for sex pointed to strong voyeuristic components; defensive exhibitionism was poorly developed (see type a), and the patient also had moralistic notions about exhibitionism. One of the reasons, for example, for his constant quarrels with his fiancée was his accusations that *she* exhibited by giving people chance but generous glimpses of various parts of her body. He could exhibit, therefore, only via feminine identification.

d. *Hyperexhibitionism as a defense.* The paradigm for this type is the actor, or professional "exhibitionist," whose case is discussed in Section III (no. 11, Stage Fright).

Another mechanism of borderline solution of the problem is the *"seeing only a little"* technique in some writers, the preponderance of details.

An example is the French writer Stendhal. The real power of Stendhal's novels is hidden in an unending stream of the subtlest psychological details, described with unsurpassed candor, according to his motto *"Il n'y a d'originalité et de vérité que dans les détails."*

The rather fanntastic fact is to be recorded that Stendhal has to his credit five psychological achievements, each with implications that only modern psychoanalytic psychiatry can make understood. Stendhal discovered his individual Oedipus (see his autobiography, LA VIE DE HENRI BRULARD, written in 1835) sixty years before Freud clinically proved the universality of the complex. In DE L'AMOUR Stendhal created a unique narcissistic theory of love. He is one of the precursors of the technique of "free association." He was a pioneer in the technique of indicating general significance through details

The Visual Drive

in fiction. And finally he was the first novelist to put the accent squarely on psychological details, treating the pure melodrama of his narratives with irony and contempt. The question arises: what made him do all this, and more important, what unconscious forces gave him the magic power of psychological vision?

The simplest way out of a psychological mystery is recourse to biological facts. In the case of a writer the pat reply, acceptable to naive people despite its redundancy reads "talent of the genius." The "genius" in turn is credited to unknown biological conditions. The sterility of the answer is obvious. Its inaccuracy is less obvious, but dodging the question with biology can be admissible only after the psychological approach has proved insufficient. I believe that Stendhal's psychological achievements can be explained psychologically.

"What does the writer express in his work?" is a question that has been asked again and again. The preanalytic answer was either that the poet is only the vessel of higher powers (Plato's "Poets utter great and wise things which they do not themselves understand"), or one who modifies *conscious* experience by poetic embellishment. Early psychoanalytic theories contradicted these assumptions, pointing out that the writer gives expression to his *unconscious* fantasies. This was a long step forward. Nevertheless, clinical experience has proved that the step was not long enough. For more than twenty years I have been promoting the theory that the writer's work expresses only the *secondary unconscious defenses* against his unconscious fantasies (see THE WRITER AND PSYCHOANALYSIS). Assuming, for the sake of argument, the correctness of the formulation, the next question presents itself: How are we to explain the variety of conflicts described by different writers?

If, as contended, the basis is always psychic masochism and the defense is always pseudoaggression, why is not all writing uniform? The argument is spurious; every neurotic unconsciously attempts to climb from the deepest layers to the more superficial ones. Since in this attempt there are varying and different "rescue stations" (corresponding to the various levels of regression) the secondary defenses are different too. It is not the variety of the basic conflicts but the variety of defenses—individually conditioned although also unconscious—that provides the kaleidoscope of literary subjects. As Mark Twain said, "It is difference of opinion that makes horse races." The psychoanalyst might add, "It is the difference in individual defense mechanisms that makes variety in literature."

The second set of inner alibis unconsciously created by the writer pertains, strangely enough, to a visual conflict. The writer's imagination had its humble beginnings in the nursery, as infantile peeping. Since this voyeurism is severely rejected by the inner conscience, because of its link with the sanctified rulers of the infantile world, a defense is put into operation which transforms the little peeper into a big show-off. The formula reads, "I am not a Peeping Tom, I am an exhibitionist." By writing down his imaginings the writer exhibits before the reader.

This formulation of the writer's unconscious "battle of the conscience" explains the frequently astounding *unconscious* knowledge encountered in writers. Psychological truth which under other conditions would remain repressed comes to the surface under pressure of inner guilt. It is exactly the *unconsciously forced admission of the "lesser crime" that makes for psychological insight.* That insight is produced because it corresponds to the *specific* writer's required *specific* defense. That singular psychic situation—though completely subjective—can further objective knowledge. This applies to Stendhal's psychological achievements.[39]

Stendhal is truly analytical in his minute, slow-motion descriptions, in his recognition of the psychic importance of details. In HENRI BRULARD he says, "Instead of telling a story, I dwell upon minor events which must be noted with precision because of their microscopic form."

A detail, if significant, is not only a microcosmos; it also contains a quantitative factor, the element of littleness. This littleness can also mean the smallest dose of unconscious self-knowledge still admissible, a subterfuge in the battle of the conscience. The redeeming feature and excuse of the defense, presented to the cruel conscience, denotes also: "Don't pay attention, let it pass, only a detail is at stake."

The suspicion that something of this kind was involved in Stendhal's superabundance of details is borne out when one scrutinizes the

The Visual Drive

nature of his detail observations. As far as unconscious mechanisms are concerned, his famous details pertain to three sets of facts: observations on *psychic masochism* (without recognizing it as such), *voyeurism,* and *narcissism.* Interestingly enough, the generalization of his observations in this triad was drawn by Stendhal only for defensive narcissism, in his theory of love. This may be interpreted to mean that isolated spots of observation in matters of psychic masochism and voyeurism may have had the purpose of the inner defensive prayer directed to conscience: "Don't pay attention."

Added to this defense is the playful-aphoristic technique of his detail observations, which always pertain to *someone else.* Never does Stendhal apply his observations of psychic masochism to himself; the farthest he goes personally is the admission that he is "hypersensitive." Finally, a preponderance of details indicates an inhibition in the sphere of voyeurism. By concentrating on details, this inner defense is furnished: "I look (observe) only a little."

Stendhal's *intuitive* knowledge of psychic masochism was amazing. Fabrice del Dongo is happy only when in prison and facing death. Julien Sorel, according to M. de Frilair, commits "some sort of suicide" during his defense—("I have premeditated the act of killing," says the defendant); he does all he can to assure his own conviction (for instance, he continuously provokes the jury); he remains calm when death is imminent and humorously observes that, odd as it may seem, the verb *guillotine* cannot be conjugated in all tenses. Masochistic enjoyment of the pleasure of fear pervades LA CHARTREUSE: Fabrice, when in great danger, talks about a "nice fear," and when he faces death, "there is, thanks to a *bizarre circumstance about which he did not ponder,* in the depth of his heart a heavenly joy." Most of Stendhal's heroes enjoy love only when they are in danger or about to die. Stendhal turns love itself into the climax of pleasurable self-torture, and in DE L'AMOUR he establishes the principle. "Love is a precious flower, but one must have the courage to pluck it at the edge of an abyss." And of Lamiel Stendhal says: "Even in the wildest of pleasures her glowing fantasy strives for immeasurably more, and above all for peril, for delight without peril is no delight to her."

Another subdivision of Stendhal's detail mania pertains to voyeurism. In his autobiography Stendhal mentions the direct connection with his mother: "One evening when I happened to be put to sleep on a mattress on the floor of her [his mother's] room, she jumped gaily and lightly like a hind across my mattress to reach her bed more quickly." It is likely that the boy gratified his voyeuristic desires and held his mother responsible; he did not intend to look, but her exhibition gave him the opportunity to look. In other words, he shifted the responsibility.

In LE ROUGE ET LE NOIR, having come furtively to his beloved, Mme. Renan, after braving danger, Julien Sorel insists on turning on the lamp, over her objections. "Do you want me to have no memory of how you look?" he asks her. "Is the glow of love in your sweet eyes to disappear, unseen by me? Am I not to see the whiteness of this beautiful hand?"

In LA CHARTREUSE DE PARME Fabrice del Dongo's happiness in love consists in boring a hole in the wooden boards lining the window of his cell, in order to see the governor's daughter, Clelia Conti, with whom he has fallen in love at first sight. But Fabrice wants to be seen by Clelia too, Stendhal emphasizes. Set free, Fabrice repeats the scene by moving into the house opposite Clelia's. Clelia herself vows never to look at Fabrice and "receives him only in the dark"; thus they beget a child. Undoubtedly Clelia's voyeuristic conflicts represent projections of Stendhal's infantile voyeuristic prohibitions.

In HENRI BRULARD Stendhal mentions his voyeuristic desires several times. He reports that his uncle Romain (a provincial Don Juan) "had fun with me and permitted me to be with him when, at nine o'clock in the evening, before supper, he would take off his good clothes and change into his dressing gown. That was a delightful moment for me." And in another passage: "Later, around 1805 in Marseilles, in the Huveaune, under high and shady trees, I had the sweet pleasure of seeing my mistress, who was extremely well built, bathe by the summer cottage of Madame Roy." In a letter to Mathilde Dembrowska (Volterra, June 7, 1819) he mentions his "terrible longing" to see her, who so completely governed and confused him. In this connection should also be mentioned Stendhal's enthusiasm for Ariosto's idea in the ORLANDO FURIOSO of a ring that made its wearer invisible (Diary, September 8, 1811).

The Visual Drive

Stendhal's voyeurism was later shifted to psychological observations. What Nietzsche called Stendhal's *voluptas psychologica* has this humble substratum. Still, in his individual "battle of the conscience" Stendhal achieved only a partial victory; he could observe details but not the whole of an interconnection. His relative sterility of plot-making and his constant plagiarism belong here.

Re: Fully Neurotic Solutions

As an example of how everything can be neurotically misused I am adducing the above-mentioned "mechanism of stubborn reparation":

A young homosexual, previously described in Chapter 2, was attracted to young boys, especially on the beach and wearing scant penis covering. As was to be expected, he unconsciously identified narcissistically with these boys. In so doing he stubbornly denied an early "shock": at the age of three or four, while his governess was giving him a bath, he proudly exhibited his erect penis and met with a contemptuous and angry response. Years later, in projected self-admiration, he seemed to say, "It is possible to do exactly that and be admired."

His tendency of "stubborn reparation" went so far that it accounted for an otherwise inexplicable incident. In a stage of analysis when he had already accepted woman sexually, he was in bed in a darkened room with a girl who, after permitting one lustless (for her, that is) intercourse, was unwilling to give in a second time as he requested. He got disgusted, lost his erection, and switched on the light to dress. The moment the light was on, his erection came back, though the girl's attitude had not changed.

II. EXHIBITIONISM IN THE SERVICE OF THE "PSEUDO-MORAL CONNOTATION" OF NEUROTIC MANIFESTATIONS

It has been my experience that the mere spotting, explaining, working through in the transference and resistance situations of the *contents* of neurotic manifestations, including the basic psychic masochism, does *not* fully solve the specific neuroticism. Something is *missing* in the interpretation: *destruction of the unconscious prop that maintains the neuroticism,* the "pseudomoral connotation." This was elaborated on in Chapter 4. Every neurotic who enters analysis is not only an analysand but also an "ironisand," regardless of whether or not he can consciously boast of a sense of humor.[40]

Exhibitionism lends itself to the expression of the ironical "pseudomoral connotation." Once more, exhibitionism is *genetically* the defense against voyeurism; before the child can ironically reduce parental attitudes to absurdity, it must have observed them. *Clinically* there seems to be a reservoir of exhibitionism and voyeurism at the disposal of the unconscious ego, used independently of the historical source.

Even here one has to distinguish between two types: conflicts entirely unconnected with visual elements, in which exhibitionism is just the means of expressing the conflict externally, whatever its origin (type I); and those in which visual elements actually were at the source of the conflict (type II).

Any neurotic conflict in general will illustrate type I (elaboration in Section III, no. 19).

Here is an example of type II:

A well-known journalist, in his forties, was offered the opportunity of conducting a lucrative television program. He refused—with horror. He said that his inability to exhibit went so far that he never looked at the byline in his syndicated newspaper column; if anyone mentioned his column favorably he was "deeply embarrassed." Analysis of his inhibition produced a curious phenomenon: among other bitter complaints against his mother was that of having forced him as a boy to "wear unbecoming clothes made of unbecoming material." Without realizing it he accused her of pushing him into "negative exhibitionism" (see Section III, no. 13). To ward off that masochistic danger he mobilized the inner defense of refraining from exhibitionism altogether. To this was added a pseudomoral connotation that consisted in holding up his mother's dicta against "ostentatious display." The upshot was the inner alibi "I don't want to be masochistic via exhibitionism since I hate it and abstain from it entirely." This was the end effect, preceded by a phase of wearing "under protest" the "unbecoming clothes" as pseudoaggressive proof of how mean his mother really was. The more psychic masochism was smuggled in, the stronger the defense became. It was also ironical

The Visual Drive 223

that the patient was given to temper tantrums—thus exhibiting negatively, though strongly inhibited at harmless social and professional occasions.

III. TWENTY-TWO TYPES OF NEUROTIC ELABORATION OF THE VISUAL DRIVE IN SPECIFIC DISEASE ENTITIES

1. SHYNESS

Every psychoanalyst confronted professionally with a "shy" person registers in his thoughts two preliminaries: "There is something wrong with his castration fears *and* his exhibitionism." The only difference is that some put these thoughts in this order, some put exhibitionism first and castration anxiety second. Otherwise there is unanimity.

Both thoughts are correct and—therapeutically of little or no help. Both preliminary diagnoses overlook one fact. If a prospector drilling for oil chooses a location where there actually is oil ten thousand feet down but stops at one thousand feet, the fault is not exactly with the spot chosen but with the prospector.

Certainly there is something wrong with the exhibitionism and the castration fears of the shy person. The real basis of his difficulty, however, is not his oedipal fixations and his phallic exhibitionism but his "septet of baby fears" and the *prehistory* of the "voyeuristic-exhibitionistic exchange mechanism."

In Section I of this chapter the genesis of voyeurism in boys was defined as being connected with the mother's breast, later tabooed. This disappointment is worked out via the mechanism of "stubborn reparation"; the boy discovers a substitute breast (or so he thinks) in his penis. This leads to penis exhibitionism, also forbidden and tabooed, for reasons of cultural decency, something entirely incomprehensible to the child. From his "point of view" that "mean" mother simply did not want to acknowledge that he too had a wonderful breast, thus endangering his whole "narcissistic restitution."

Here the roads part:
  a. Some—later normal—children survive the shock, unconsciously

maintain the fantasy, and use it later in the coitus situation (see p. 205).

b. Others acquire the "complex of the small penis."

c. Others later become homosexuals and spend their lives running after the "reduplication of their own defense mechanism," as stated in Chapter 2.

d. Still others, though maintaining heterosexuality, have a difficulty lying elsewhere: they *cannot use the defensive penis exhibitionism because of the "confessional character" of exhibitionism in general;* exhibiting means the acknowledgment of having seen the original, now displayed in a substitute. These are *"shy people."* They are also inveterate "injustice collectors," meaning severe psychic masochists; one should not be deceived by their external demeanor, which seems to ask forgiveness for their very existence.

Of course these deeply masochistic people went through the more superficial stages too. Since all deeper mechanisms are, in the course of development, expressed in the "language" of the more superficial layers, every beginner can detect the superficial layers in everybody. Only the experienced analyst can distinguish between an oedipal *blind,* covering deeper repressions, and a *true* oedipal conflict actually responsible for the specific neurotic difficulty (see Chapter 1).

Without understanding of the oral-masochistic regression, the psychic apparatus is not decipherable. In my opinion, psychic masochism is *the basic neurosis* (see THE BASIC NEUROSIS).

What about the little neurotic girl and her edition of the later "shy woman?"

Not all the shyness is, as generally assumed, the result of the fear of exposing her "castrated" genitals. This is the superficial layer. The deeper layers have a connection with oral-masochistic accusations against the mother, blamed for having "cheated" the girl of her breast equivalent, the breast-penis. True, the small clitoris, originally endowed with hopes and growth possibilities, did not grow, and nobody likes to be confronted with the graveyard of his unmaterialized hopes. How imbued with repressed infantile fantasies this whole area is can be demonstrated by the fact that the penis-lack is compensated for with the achievement of the originally desired: the adult girl *has* breasts. It doesn't help; the infantile yardstick is applied and a "too late" dictated.

The whole problem of modesty and shyness contains a grotesque paradox:

Man's unconscious fears and woman's punishment for being the innocent target are both inexhaustible. Fantastic rules governing conduct during the menstrual period are common to aborigines in all parts of the world; evidence of similar rules and of the superstitions that are their aftermath can be found in the classics of Western civilization. The adjurations in Leviticus 15 were literally interpreted by the Jews, and women "put apart seven days" until Rabbi Akiba's reinterpretation of the chapter in the second century of the modern era. Akiba ended the Jewish woman's ritual isolation, as well as the penalty of "uncleanness" that adhered to any Jew who touched a woman during her period. In Pliny we are told that wine turns to vinegar if touched by a woman who is menstruating, crops are blighted and seedlings killed by her touch, fruit loosened from trees, mirrors clouded, razors dulled, metal rusted, bees killed or driven from their hives, and so on. Similar superstitions are recorded from other sources.

Among aborigines the first appearance of menstruation is especially subject to taboos. In their practical effects these elaborate restrictions transform the adolescent girls into biological lepers, in some cases *for years*. The girls are segregated, and the taboo often requires that they neither touch the ground nor see the sun. One needs hardly more than a trace of imagination to get a graphic picture of the torture imposed on women by man's fear.

The details of these taboos vary from tribe to tribe. The rules range from the very stringent and elaborate to the simple; isolation from men is invariable, but in some tribes seclusion in the menstrual hut, especially at the time of the first period, is made the occasion for social gatherings of the young girls of the tribe. The unchanging theme in all cases is the fact that menstrual blood is "dangerous," and in one way or another imperils the village. As a logical extension of this theme, food taboos are imposed; some of these continue for as long as a year after the initial menstrual period. Frazer, in THE GOLDEN BOUGH, mentions the belief of the Dieri of Central

Australia, who are convinced that all the fish in their river would die if a menstruous woman ate one and the river dry up if she bathed in it. The Arunta, a near-by tribe, eat large quantities of a certain bulb; they forbid menstruating women to gather these bulbs on the theory that the crop would fail if the rule were broken.

There is a curious twist in some of these customs that can be explained only by the assumption that the magical and malevolent power accompanying menstruation is an active force and not a passive contagion. Man's deeply rooted fear that injury will come to him through woman, especially during her menstrual period, is illustrated in Frazer's account of the Kolosh Indians of Alaska. In this tribe it is believed that a menstruating woman who so much as looks at a hunter, fisher, or gambler will destroy his luck. It is also believed that a woman can turn objects to stone at this time, merely by looking at them. The classical as well as the still persisting European parallels to these beliefs—the legends of Medusa and the Basilisk, and the evil eye—come immediately to mind.

A revealing sidelight on the purposes of the menstrual taboo is reported by Margaret Mead in an account of the Manus of New Guinea. Their taboos differ from the usual ones in that they mark what is ostensibly the only menstrual period the girl will have until she is married. The fact that all women menstruate regularly after puberty is kept a complete secret from the males of the tribe. One can conclude that the purpose is to lessen their fear of approaching marriageable girls.

A detailed investigation of the unconscious reasons for these more than fantastic nightmares of suspicion and punishment for being a woman would lead too far afield. It is sufficient to state that man's fear of the bleeding and "castrated" female genital is beyond question and is clinically confirmed in every analysis.

The fear of the genitally "castrated" woman not only revives man's phallic anxieties but the *earliest infantile "septet of baby fears" as well*. In addition to the supercilious, he-man attitude, man has three ways of warding off these Hydra-like fears.

First, he flees the sight of horror—he forces woman to cover the "wound" and the body.

Second, he declares woman "cruel." He-man's deprecatory judgment, "She is *only* a weak woman," is typical, if not universal, but at the same time every man (I said *every* man) harbors the opposite view as well, which is the fantasy that woman is by nature cruel and after man's scalp. Shakespeare's statement in TWELFTH NIGHT, "Lady, you are the cruell'st she alive," expresses a tenet that man keeps in perpetual readiness in a hidden corner and brings to life and illuminates when the "necessity" arises—which is every time a *real* woman fails to correspond to his infantile fantasies of a pretty doll. There is no reason to conceal the fact that women (especially when infuriated with the illogical amalgam of baby and he-man) have a good-sized aggression at their disposal. It is only man's silly fantasy, which tells him so authoritatively "what women are like," that causes his terrified "surprise."

If further proof of the above statement is wanted, it may be found in Chapter 1, where the "septet of baby fears" is listed, detailing all the evil intentions attributed by the immature ego to the giantess of the nursery. Or, if proofs drawn from folklore are more convincing take the old (older than Grimm) tale of Hansel and Gretel, where the cruel step*mother* convinces the father that the children should be left to die of *starvation,* where the cruel *witch* lures the children into her gingerbread cottage and fattens them up to provide her a delicious *cannibalistic feast.*

When we consider how these unconscious fantasies influence man's sex life we can see some of the reasons for impotence produced by castration fear and also some of the reasons why woman is more alluring to him dressed than nude.

Man's fear of women is not a modern invention; most likely it is as old as the relation of the sexes. To mention only one example, the evil powers attributed to witches (hence women!) with respect to man's potency. MALLEUS MALEFICARUM (The Witch Hammer), the official lawbook governing ecclesiastical diagnosis and the punishment of witches, written in 1486 by the inquisitors Heinrich Kramer and James Sprenger and authorized by Innocent VIII, has a long discourse on the subject, under Question IX, "Whether Witches Can Create an Illusion by Trickery about the Male Genitals so that they Seem to be Wholly Absent from Bodies."

Man's third method of warding off his fear of woman is through sugar-coating it, by finding *unconscious* "pleasure in punishment and fear," by *psychic masochism*.

If one were to ask how *neurotic* man typically combines all these defenses, the answer would be: he marries a shrew, acts the he-man with her, is slapped down, complains about her cruelty, and unconsciously enjoys his masochistic suffering, heightened by his poor potency.

Numerous theories have been put forward in the attempt to explain the origin of sexual modesty. To name a few:

1. *The religious explanation,* proclaimed by St. Augustine (DE CIVITATE DEI), states why solitude is sought even for conjugal intercourse: "Because that which is by nature fitting is so done as to be accompanied with a shame-begetting penalty of sin." St. Augustine also declares that sex and lust were originally distinct from each other and that the taint of lust in sex was the result of punishment.

Religious beliefs are *not* an object of scientific scrutiny. Religion is the most personal affair of man's life, and works on a psychic level entirely different from that of science. There is no contradiction between the two approaches, as is visible in the fact that some scientists are devoutly religious. (For elaboration, see THE BATTLE OF THE CONSCIENCE, p. 1, and THE BASIC NEUROSIS, p. 104.)

2. *The theory of protection,* promoted by Stendhal, among others. As Stendhal put it in DE L'AMOUR, this is the argument: "People have noticed that birds of prey hide themselves to drink; the reason being that, obliged to plunge their heads into the water, they are at that moment defenseless." Westermarck correctly objected that sleep is even more dangerous.

3. *The theory of guarding against disturbance by rival*s also fails to explain why sex is so discreet a matter. Ward, in his DYNAMIC SOCIOLOGY, argued that "where there are several cocks, they seek to separate their chosen mates from the rest in order to enjoy complete immunity." To which Westermarck, in THE HISTORY OF HUMAN MARRIAGE, ironically objected, "The cock avoids the presence of other cocks, but not the presence of other hens besides its mate. So also the fear of rivals might have inclined men to avoid intercourse in the presence of other men, not in the presence of women. But how, then, could such fear have been the originating cause of sexual mod-

The Visual Drive

esty, considering that men exhibit this feeling chiefly towards *women*, and that it is even more marked in women than in men, or at least in young virgins compared with young men of the same age."

The "cock" argument is also senseless because psychological facts from the animal kingdom, when applied *directly* to human beings, are always misleading. We have recently witnessed the one-sidedness that results from the use of this biological fallacy in the Kinsey Report.

4. *The "domestication theory"* of modesty seems to have been prompted by a study of the habits of the elephant and the camel, which retire to the depths of the jungle or the desert before copulating. Confronted with the obvious contradiction offered by domestic animals' lack of reticence, the proponent of this theory, L. Tillier, argued that domestication teaches animals that they may feel safe without taking the precaution of secreting themselves during intercourse. This sophism only washes out the argument, since it is unclear why homo sapiens should be less domesticated than his dog.

5. *The "disgust theory"* of the genesis of modesty has found many adherents, although nobody has ever been able to explain why urinary and anal functions are disgusting. At one and the same time sexual acts are declared disgusting because of anatomic proximity to the anal and urethral orifices (*"inter urinas at faeces homo nascitur"*), and anality and urethrality are adduced as argument to prove why sex proper is "dirty" and "beastly." The inherent contradiction is invisible to the proponents, or ignored by them.

The contradiction reaches rather grotesque proportions when one observes the concern and concentration with which the mistresses of the nursery (mother, nurse) judge the amount, color, consistency, frequency, etc. of the baby's bowel movements. It is only at a later period that anal and urethral functions become taboo, to be mentioned not at all or with circumlocution. It seems that adults are permitted to have a rational approach to excretory matters only during the first few months of their children's lives. During the fifties and sixties again, when enlargement (benign or malignant) of the prostate in man, cancer of the rectum in both sexes, or at least digestive troubles may appear, some kind of rational aspect is reintroduced with medical blessings. In between there are only taboos.

On the other hand, scatological jokes and allusions are, statistically, no less frequent than those pertaining to sex proper. The official taboo seems to be counteracted by a strong inner "attraction."

It may be, as some aesthetes claim, that humanity tends to progress in the direction of purification from "animal functions." In putting this claim forward the aesthetes have failed to clarify either reason or purpose. They have not explained why so strong a weapon as shame has to be mobilized as penalty, nor have they suggested any substitutes for the mechanisms of excretion and elimination. And finally, they have never informed their adherents why they consider a new car beautiful and the motor pipes and exhaust—"dirty."

6. *The "evil-spirit" theory* bases its assumptions on primitive peoples' numerous fears of magic influences affecting the male genitals. The most pronounced example is probably that of the natives in Tanna (New Hebrides), where, as Summerville reports, "the closest secrecy is adopted with regard to the penis, not at all from a sense of decency but to avoid the Narak (the bewitching force), even the sight of that of another man being considered dangerous." Therefore the natives use rather fantastic protective measures; they wrap the organ in many yards of calico, "winding and folding them until a preposterous bundle eighteen inches or two feet long and two inches or more in diameter is formed."

Tannaits have never been analyzed; experience with Western neurotics leads to my suspicion that the evil spirit is probably the bad, castrating mother (later father) of their early babyhood, conveniently shifted outside. The fears of these people are frequently thinly veiled (leading to segregation of the sexes and even to taboos on men and women eating together). Sometimes they are directly connected with women.

7. *The "woman as property"* theory injects economic factors into the psychological discussion and is almost invariably linked by its proponents with the argument of masculine jealousy. Jealousy is a complicated phenomenon, which may explain why the layman prefers taking it for granted to inquiring about its psychology or trying to dissect his own reactions. The husband in the *New Yorker* cartoon who flies in a rage at the sight of his wife sitting undressed before the television set, watching (and presumably watched by) the man

The Visual Drive

on the screen, is more than a merely ridiculous figure; he also has a psychology of his own, which is not included in the joke. Without a discussion of the psychology of jealousy (see Section III, no. 7) it is impossible to point out why the "woman as property" theory is entirely inadequate as an explanation of the genesis of modesty.

8. *The "olfactory" theory* suggested by Lombroso and Ferrerro stresses the decomposition of the vaginal secretions and the consequent reaction of disgust on the part of men. Other theorists go so far as to claim that the artificial waistline in clothing, which separates the upper from the lower part of the feminine body, has the same precautionary origin. No one, as far as I know, has tried to reconcile this theory with the fact that extremely tight waists were in vogue during the notoriously odor-impervious eighteenth century, nor with the fact that in the finicky twentieth century there were periods of repeated revivals of sack-like dresses without any waistline whatever. Obviously no purely hygienic measure can be so inconsistent as fashion nor produce so deeply rooted an emotion as modesty or shame.

9. The most reasonable theory promoted by earlier anthropologists in explanation of the genesis of modesty is the *"anti-incest" hypothesis*. This theory still has some validity, even though the real depth of the problem did not become clear until after Freud's psychoanalytical investigations and Roheim's anthropological field-work. There is no doubt that shame is also the second line of defense where originally there was wish and prohibition. Every child goes through a period of incestuous wishes, not because of the attraction of common blood but only because the parents are "just around" and sexually inaccessible.

These and similar theories hardly begin to explain the genesis of modesty and cast no light whatever on who "created" that strange though familiar feeling. Most of the theories disregard unconscious mechanisms altogether. In all of them there is exclusive concentration on rational factors—an inevitable dead end when the problem to be solved is one of irrational feelings.

An example is the "theory of protection," alluding to reality dangers. He-man is indeed in need of protection and consequently wants privacy in sex, but *because he is mortally afraid that his sex technique, the size of his organ, his general clumsiness, his partial or real impotence, will be ridiculed.* Nearly thirty years ago Ferenczi described "the complex of the small penis," the fantasy, common to many neurotic men, that their sex organs are too small. This uncomfortable feeling, in my opinion, is one of the contributory factors in man-made "modesty."

Man's fear of being exposed as possessor of an inadequate organ in adult sex makes secrecy and the absence of witnesses imperative. As a result children are given the impression that adult sex is "uncanny" and "mysterious." Repeat this experience over the course of many generations, and one of the pillars of sexual modesty is firmly established.

Clinically we are well acquainted with the havoc played among neurotics by the fantasy "sex is forbidden." This prerequisite was linked by Freud with the unsolved infantile connotation of sex. In this conception the *aggressive* defiance of oedipal prohibitions not only contribute to the enjoyment of sex but actually becomes an indispensable requirement.

Through the study of a long series of cases in which this peculiar partnership of sex and the forbidden was evident, I have become convinced that the aggressive layer conceals a more deeply repressed, pre-oedipal structure. For these neurotics do not simply "enjoy" sex within the atmosphere of taboos they create for themselves. The "enjoyment" is accompanied by deep anxieties, fear of being caught, found out, punished, involved in a "scandal" leading to loss of social standing. Often the element of fear becomes so intense that it assumes the quality of the *uncanny*.

In my opinion,[41] the feeling of uncanniness is a specific form of psychic masochism, in which is embodied in capsule form the whole history of infantile megalomania, including its eventful and painful end.

In 1919 Freud described the uncanny as a special variety of the fearful, and distinguished two types of uncanny feelings: one produced when some impression brings repressed infantile complexes to the surface again; the other when the primitive beliefs we thought we had overcome seem once more to be confirmed. In practical experience, Freud declares, the two types cannot always be distin-

The Visual Drive

guished from each other, since primitive convictions are most intimately connected with infantile complexes and are in fact derived from them.

In dissecting the feeling of uncanniness each stage of psychic development leading to psychic masochism can, in my opinion, be clearly discerned: megalomania, fury, the subduing of megalomania through one or another branch of the septet of danger (later subsumed under the "septet of baby fears"), the turning of aggression against oneself, and finally the libidinization of fear. Perhaps the most powerful of all the fears that beset the human being is the feeling of uncanniness. To a large extent this accounts for the tendency to capitalize on its "game" quality and enjoy uncanniness in the theater, in movies, "thrillers," ghost stories, and, of course, in spiritualism. Thus masochistic pleasure is combined with the comforting reassurance that it is all "just child's play." It is the element of condensation in uncanniness that differentiates it from other types of fear. The entire aftermath of infantile megalomania—the victory *and* the dreariness—is passed in review in an instant. To begin with, the aggressive contents of infantile megalomania are reaffirmed, in a brief repetition of the fantasy of omnipotence that prevailed in infancy. This explains the megalomaniacal, though repressed, pleasure derived from uncanniness.

The recapitulation continues, passing on to a later stage in the history of infantile megalomania, its masochistic end. It should not be forgotten that both the clinical *and* genetic pictures of psychic masochism include remnants of megalomania. The unconscious process which, when complete, is psychic masochism, begins: *"I* create, unconsciously, a situation in which somebody refuses, denies, inhibits *my* wishes." These defeats—self-selected, self-determined, self-perpetuated—contain visible if pale traces of the original megalomaniacal glow.

The feeling of uncanniness is therefore seen to have a double purpose. It reaffirms the aggressive component in the first of all human fantasies, that of absolute power, and at the same time emphasizes the masochistic elaborations which amend and weaken that fantasy later on. The unconscious pleasure derived from the feeling of uncanniness may seem to pertain to the aggressive connotation, but it does not. Since the aggressive and the masochistic elements are superimposed on each other, it is clear that it is the combination, and not one or the other individual element, that makes uncanniness so alluring.

As in all fear phenomena there is overemphasis on the aggressive connotation and willingness to accept blame for aggressiveness as a disguise for the more deeply rooted, more serious offense, that of psychic masochism. Here again there is resort to the familiar ruse in which aggression is used as unconscious defense against the accusation of psychic masochism.

One can compare the situation with that of a dethroned king who consoles himself in his exile with fantasies in which he is still in power and still signing death warrants. Behind that false, megalomaniacal daydream of aggression is hidden the whole history of defeat: his unconsciously self-damaging tactics, his acceptance of his overthrow, his unconscious pleasure in his own "pain and humiliation."

The feeling of uncanniness is actually an asset if judged from another point of view. The lightning stroke of this emotion saves a person from the prolonged discomfort which would otherwise accompany the memory of his first defeat: the realization that his cherished belief in his own omnipotence was a myth. Uncanniness therefore prevents protracted anxiety and much psychic work.

The adult is not capable of the intensity of feeling that characterizes the emotions of the child. I believe that the profound terror which accompanies the feeling of uncanniness is only a reflection of the child's original reaction when he encountered situations that contradicted his fantasy of omnipotence. The most extreme terror experienced in uncanniness multiplied by one thousand is still only an approximation of the child's emotions during the period of the septet of baby fears.

The element of condensation in uncanniness has the effect of partially reviving that infantile terror. The intensity of the shock experience, plus the fact that it is all over in an instant, has the paradoxical effect of cushioning the blow. In this sense uncanniness is a "fear to end a fear." It can be only momentarily successful in this aim, however, because of the connection with "pleasure in fear."

The Visual Drive

Like all other fears, that embodied in uncanniness also serves as a warning signal. The human being's unlimited capacity for suffering explains the tendency to run the whole gamut of terror in uncanniness. Terror is conquered by the device of "pleasure in pain," and then the signal, warning of even greater damage, cuts the masochistic pleasure short, at the same time ending the uncanny feeling.

In analyzing neurotics whose prerequisite for sex is the "condition of uncanniness," I have observed that their fears are more closely connected with the septet of baby fears than with simple castration anxiety. Only on the surface is the aggressive component dominant. Actually this surface component is a defensive layer concealing the more deeply repressed masochistic temptation. It therefore represents pseudoaggression.

It is of course granted that, even in our presumably outspoken culture, every child links sex with the forbidden. The child sees sex as a great mystery, discussed hesitantly in fumbling terms or not discussed at all. This does not explain why one individual is capable of adjusting his inner views to the requirements of objective reality and another individual cannot. In my opinion the individual who is more deeply involved in the tangles of masochism cannot make the requisite inner adaptation because of the allure of uncanniness.

The neurotic connotation of sex can become the source of an imposing series of difficulties. Most important is its effect in devaluating marital sex; the result is that the husband is impotent with his wife, the wife frigid with her husband, since the essential atmosphere of the "forbidden" is lacking. The consequences may be divorce,[42] in which case the identical process of depreciation will ruin the second, third, or nth marriage. More frequently a solution is sought in sexual escapades, which become increasingly risky. The social consequences can be damaging indeed—not to mention the financial ones.

In attenuated form the fantasy of the forbidden, with all its masochistic connotations, is one of the primary reasons for man's attraction to women's clothes. They help to restore for the child in the grown-up man one of his infantile and repressed connotations in sex. Moreover, clothes make it possible for man to "progress" from the frightened pre-schoolboy who peeps at the forbidden to the *would-*

be-superior pre-schoolboy. The latter, now dressed up as an adult, is no longer aware that the former is still within him. The would-be-superior "adult" is still the frightened pre-schoolboy, which accounts for the typical he-man attitude of aggressive peeping and undressing in thought. If, as some men complain, they pay through the nose for their wives' extravagance in dressing, they have only themselves to blame. They should adjust their bookkeeping systems and charge these bills up to a special account called "My Unconscious Alibis."

Women's clothes, beside unconsciously activating the infantile "situation of the forbidden," also act as a catalyst for another subdivision of infantile fantasy. The "long, long thoughts" of youth, as Longfellow called them, have the quality of being endlessly protracted, the quality of durability and endurance. The characteristic insistence of children on hearing the same story, told in exactly the same way, again and again, is a case in point. This consistent and *protracted* pleasure that children derive from their erotic, aggressive, and narcissistic fantasies is not experienced by adults, whose pleasure is of the short, *orgastic* type, as far as the direct sexual-erotic component goes. The sexy titillation provided by looking at women "dressed to be undressed" (at least in thought) establishes contact with the infantile fantasy of the forbidden *and* durable; it involves no obligations, requires no performance. Thus is established one of the pillars of masculine attraction to feminine clothes, especially since the familiar child's excuse is offered, "I didn't do anything, I was just—looking."

Besides the two reasons mentioned, hiding man's fear of comparisons of the size of his sex organs and clinging to the "situation of the forbidden" in sex, there is a third reason, also not included in the existing literature on the subject, that leads to the requirement of sexual privacy. This has an intimate, though repressed, connection with the *infant's autarchic desire to be the center of the universe*. The first relation of the infant includes only one other person, his mother. Attentions from anyone else are considered by him to be "unwanted intrusion." This, in turn, produces the fantasy of a duality that is not to be disturbed by the environment. Later the duality-unity is repeated in sex.

The problem of male modesty and shame can be studied from

The Visual Drive

another angle—the simple physiological one. Too little attention has been paid to the fact that the process of erection and the experience of being, literally, shamefaced both involve an accumulation of blood. Of course, analysts long ago learned from analyses of blushers that these neurotics shift "from below upwards," blushing having the symbolic meaning of an erection. In superficial layers (see no. 2, following) it is also a denial of castration executed exhibitionistically, though on unsuitable—and sexually unusable—organs, the cheeks.

Summarizing, one can say that female modesty, in clothing and attitudes, is a masculine "invention," [43] secondarily enforced by man in woman's conduct, for the purpose of protecting the he-man from:

(a) recollection of the unfavorable comparison between his miniature organ and the "enormous" breast;

(b) recollection of hopeless attempts, in the oedipal period, to win his mother sexually;

(c) recollection of the sight of the "castrated" and bleeding female genitalia (menstruation);

(c) recollection of the "complex of the small penis," with consequent fears of ridicule because of impotence, faulty technique, etc.

The irony is that exhibitionism with a *negative* connotation is smuggled in in "shy" people; their shyness makes them conspicuous too. Here the masochistic-exhibitionistic component enters the picture.

2. BLUSHING (ERYTHROPHOBIA)

In a paper read before the Fifteenth International Psychoanalytic Convention in Paris in August 1938 [44] I pointed out that poor analytic successes with pathological blushing can be ascribed less to the tenacity of the patient's neurotic involvement than to poor understanding of the dynamics on the part of the analyst. I singled out four errors in the interpretation:

a. The symptom is typically interpreted as hysterical conversion,[45] whereas the shifted and symbolic penis exhibitionism is a late defense covering pre-oedipal vicissitudes centering around the mother's breast.

b. The exhibitionism in the symptom is not genuine but is a defense against more deeply repressed voyeuristic tendencies.

c. The pseudoparanoiac ideas of these patients, frequently adduced to explain therapeutic failures, correspond to an inner defense: "Other people peep; I don't." Thus voyeur pleasure finds a surreptitious satisfaction with a moral alibi, while at the same time the erythrophobe "makes use of others as a mirror in order to look at himself with a clear conscience."

d. The spiteful, defensive aggression unconsciously included in the defensive exhibitionism is masochistically elaborated and therefore cannot be taken at face value. An example can be found in a detailed case history in my original publication. Here the pronounced exhibitionism of the female patient also evidenced an unconscious allusion to an ironic caricature and imitation of her coquettish mother, symbolizing a masochistic, whining reproach: "You showed yourself to strange men without restraint but not to your own child."

Since the date of the first communication I have observed a series of other cases. Time and again the original findings have been confirmed, notably the visual defense: "I do not want to peep; on the contrary, I want to show myself." Moreover, the pre-oedipal substructure (breasts and cheeks) of the whole conflict seem to me to be now established.

As already stated (p. 201), in my 1950 studies on depersonalization I concluded, on the basis of clinical material, that buttocks exhibitionism is in inner reality breast exhibitionism. See also case history reproduced on pp. 292 ff.

Here I should like to draw attention to some additional facets in the neurotic symptom of blushing:

1. There exists a peculiar *"anticipation tendency" of punishment* in these patients. Cheeks are unconsciously identified with buttocks, and the redness of the former demonstrates the injustice of having the latter beaten.

2. With great regularity repressed or even conscious *beating fantasies* (even realities) could be ascertained in these cases.

3. It has been repeatedly reported, though never explained, that some people (and especially erythrophobes) blush when they are "caught red-handed" or are confronted with allusions to real or

The Visual Drive

imaginary transgressions for which they feel guilty. An attempt will be made to explain this phenomenon.

a. *The Anticipation Tendency of Punishment*

This statement appears in the above-mentioned early paper ex 1938: "The organ defensively displayed is the entire body, but particularly the penis, the cheeks, and the *buttocks* (p. 44, italics now added). Further observations have led to the belief that this buttocks exhibitionism should be stressed more emphatically in the sequence of shifts, breasts-buttocks-penis-cheeks. There are two reasons for this additional emphasis. The child unconsciously uses the buttocks to negate his lack of breasts (breast envy); also *the "red buttocks" symbolically displayed in the blushing cheeks are at the same time a masochistic demonstration of how unjustly the child has been treated,* for the buttocks are red after a beating and the child's *shift upwards exhibits exactly these "mistreated" buttocks.*

It is therefore unprecise to use the designation "defensive buttocks exhibitionism." This description is more to the point: *demonstration of reddened buttocks after a beating.*

This mechanism was first observed by me on a series of dissimilar cases. ("Anticipation of Punishment under the Disguise of 'Senseless Involuntary Actions'," *Diseases of the Nervous System,* 16:22-23, 1955.) Here are a few examples:

Mr. S., a writer cured of writer's block, had remained in analysis exactly eight months. Precisely four months after starting treatment, he began to write again. Eight months after treatment started, the amount of money he had earned from the sale of stories written after he became unblocked was $1000 over and above the cost of therapy. He considered this a major triumph and could not be convinced that certain aspects of his psychic masochism were unresolved and that it would be advisable to continue treatment.

A few years later, while I was on my summer vacation, he wrote to me asking my opinion on a specific problem. For the past twelve years he had been employed by an institution on a part-time basis. The job paid extremely well and left him a good deal of time for his literary work. He had now written a novelette about this institution, and there was the possibility, he said, that he might lose his job by publishing the piece. Among other things he was pathologically money-conscious, and he did not relish the idea of losing his high salary and convenient working conditions. On the other hand, he considered this piece his best work. I was asked to read the story and tell him my "candid" opinion. The letter was signed "Sincerely," though in numerous previous communications this expression had never appeared. Generally his letters closed with "In gratitude" or "In friendship" or "Best as always" or "Cordially."

I read the story; it sustained the obvious suspicion. Publication of the venomous attack would invite dismissal. He wanted his salary *and* his right to attack—a clear-cut masochistic action. It was evident, too, that he was aware of this; otherwise he would not have asked for my "opinion."

In reconstructing the man's psychic situation before writing the letter (a subsequent inquiry proved that he did not remember the "Sincerely," and actually denied that he had used it) it can be assumed that he knew exactly the import of my answer: shut up or put up. In other words, he was either to tear up the story and keep his salary or resign and publish it. To publish the story and keep the job was out of the question. Any attempt, therefore, to delude himself constituted a preparatory masochistic action leading to an even greater masochistic fiasco.

Superficially the ominous "Sincerely" was simply an unconscious aggression against me: "You are not my friend but rather an enemy under your disguise of a representative of the 'reality principle'."

In a deeper layer the "Sincerely" *pertained to the letter of resignation he would have to write to the institution employing him.* He thus *anticipated punishment* by preferring an imaginary resignation to the renunciation of his masochism. By projecting his superego upon his former analyst he *declared his masochistic independence* at the price of punishment!

Miss T., a remarkably pretty girl of twenty-two with "tendencies towards blushing," entered analysis because of chronic headaches, for which a host of diagnosticians and neurologists could find no reason. When questioned about her sex life she used a good deal of circumlocution until it became clear that she was somewhere on the verge of nymphomania of a *specific* type: she remained completely cold during the act, deriving her pleasure from disparaging the man.

The Visual Drive

Her favorite phrases during intercourse were: "You are just a flop like all the others," "Give me a cigarette to kill time," "How long is this silly jumping around going to go on?"

After some time in treatment she became more outspoken. It was then that she confessed to the phrases above. Two things transpired, one mentioned by the patient and the other observed by the analyst.

The patient said, "I *always* have my headache except when I give one of these fools a piece of my mind."

"What do you conclude from that?"

"Apparently my headaches mean not enough anger is discharged."

"You consider yourself a hyperaggressive person?"

"Could be."

"A few facts contradict this assumption. First, your sex routine is completely self-damaging. Second, in your appointments, every time you repeat one of the derogatory remarks you've made in a one-night stand *you rub your cheek, just as if you had been slapped in the face.* Just observe what you're doing right now."

She was caught red-handed. For a moment she was taken aback, but she quickly regained her poise and said, "That doesn't mean anything."

"On the contrary, it could mean a good deal. I suspect that you provoke these men only to be slapped."

"Nobody's done it so far."

"Too bad for you. And here is the connection with your headaches: You suffer from an accumulation of too much undischarged psychic masochism, and not—as you believe—too much undischarged aggression."

"Why don't I have headaches when I abuse a man?"

"You are taking the blame for the lesser crime. You are trying to convince your inner conscience that you are the opposite of a masochist, namely, highly aggressive. Since you present your proof under self-degrading conditions, the bargain is accepted—for the duration of your self-degradation. One lesser form of masochism exchanged for the other, bigger one."

After the headaches gradually and "mysteriously" disappeared and nymphomania was given up (the change took months, of course, with the usual ups and downs) Miss T. consented to analysis of the infantile precursors and received the explanation with some measure of understanding. Previously she had refused to "fall for that trap," as she expressed it. The story was banal: beating fantasies were behind it.

During her analytic appointment Mrs. U. reported a peculiar "mishearing" that had puzzled her. On the preceding day she and her husband had been discussing, in a detached way, the marriage of a couple who lived near by. The husband claimed that it was a good marriage; the patient was rather sceptical. In actuality she had had a clandestine affair with the man. The discussion was "purely academic." It took place just after they left their apartment to drive to the theater. While opening the door of the car the patient seemed to hear her husband saying, "Get *out*"; he had really, of course, said "Get *in*." She retorted sharply and *with a gesture of defiance,* "What do you mean?" His answer, naturally, was a surprised look. In thinking about the scene later she definitely excluded the possibility that her husband might have said "Get out." Her "mishearing" *anticipated a good deal: "My husband will find out about about my affair and tell me to get out!"*

These and similar examples use an elliptical technique: anticipation of punishment.

In more superficial though also unconscious layers the punishment anticipated pertains to aggressive actions, which are only a blind for more deeply repressed masochistic wishes.

These masochistic neurotics cannot wait until punishment strikes; in their eagerness for punishment they act it out in anticipation.

The "anticipation tendency" seems typical for erythrophobes.

b. *Beating Fantasies*

In previous publications,[46] one of which goes back to 1938, I have pointed out that the preliminary pre-oedipal vicissitudes have been neglected in the literature of the subject or have not been built into it. In beating fantasies the origin is an unsolved conflict directed against the mother's breast and secondarily masochistically elaborated and shifted to the child's own buttocks. The execution of these "cruelties" on the unconsciously willing victim has in the meantime been shifted from mother to father.

The Visual Drive

This is illustrated by a detail that came to the fore in a case described later in this chapter (see pp. 292 ff.), that of a French-Canadian woman in whom blushing, depersonalization, writer's block, and drinking were combined. The complex connection between beating fantasies and depersonalization is also explained in this case history.

c. *Blushing When Caught Red-Handed*

It is a familiar observation that some people blush when proved guilty or even when listening to a discourse or sermon dealing in a general way with their real or fantasied "misdeeds." An excellent example of this was provided by a patient, the son of a minister, who would blush in church when his father preached against sin.

These people anticipate punishment and misuse the beating not yet administered by turning it into a masochistic demonstration of the parents' injustice: they exhibit their "buttocks reddened by beating." This amounts to a defensive "negative exhibitionism"—demonstration of a "bleeding wound."

3. FEAR OF CONFINED PLACES

In a series of cases with fear of elevators and subways I found that the most primitive repressed ideas concerning certain sectors of the "septet of baby fears" were mobilized. Especially the fears of being smothered, choked, and crushed by the mother image were predominant.[47]

Mrs. V., aged twenty-eight, was, as she claimed, "obsessed with fear." She was afraid of everything, from elevators to subways, from leaving home to visiting friends, from street fear to worries over health. She lived and dressed "for an emergency." For a long time she never took off her coat or her fur in winter—in her own apartment. "I must be ready to leave at a momen't notice." Asked what she was afraid of, she claimed that her heart might fail and then "I must run to the physician." Asked whether in such an emergency (her heart was, by the way, completely normal) calling in a specialist would not be preferable, she said that she had three telephones installed—"just in case"—but could not trust mechanical devices. When she was asked whether her belief in physicians was not exaggerated, she said that she was well aware of the "stupidity of her fears." "Still," she added, "here they are."

Her inability to undress became so intolerable that, having slept one night fully dressed and in her mink coat, she decided to enter treatment.

Her "heart attack" represented unconscious identification with her mother, performed out of inner guilt. This aggression covered but thinly the deeper layer of masochism. She also had to cope with strong exhibitionistic wishes, covering voyeuristic tendencies.

4. STREET FEAR (AGORAPHOBIA)

In 1930 [48] I analyzed a case of street fear in which a previously not described connection between voyeuristic and exhibitionistic components became visible.

Miss W., a woman of thirty-five, entered analysis because of severe street fear. She could not, except on rare occasions, leave her house unaccompanied. A pretty though rather colorless woman, she had attached herself while still quite young to a tubercular man. Over her mother's objections she had nursed him devotedly until he recovered. Once he was restored to health she left him—for no particular reason—and shortly afterwards announced a new engagement to another tuberculous man. Her requirement of illness in a fiancé was clarified during analysis. Her father, an "amiable man," had become a "changed person" when he was about fifty and the patient five or six years old. He had begun to drink. At home he was noisy, and he exhibited before the patient and her twenty-five-year-old sister. Their puritanical mother started divorce proceedings. In the last few months before the marriage ended (it had lasted for twenty-six years) the patient was the only member of the family capable of "handling" the father when he was (they put it delicately) "sick." The family established a routine: when the father came home, the mother and older sister would withdraw, leaving the six-year-old alone with him. In other words, the desperate mother pushed the child into the role of Florence Nightingale and oedipal mother-substitute. Analysis revealed no indications that the father had attacked the child sexually; he had, however, urinated, perhaps defecated, and exhibited before her.

The patient had repeated this infantile situation in choosing each

The Visual Drive

of her fiancés. She attached herself to these sick men, not in spite of their illness but because it furnished a guilt-diminishing factor.

Her infantile crime had been peeping and psychic masochism. Her neurotic symptom, agoraphobia, was a dramatized denial—not of the real crime but of its opposites, exhibitionism and pseudoaggression, which constituted the lesser intrapsychic crime she had admitted to. This five-layer structure was discernible:

Layer I: Masochistic wish to be attacked by father (earlier, mother) and peeping at father's body and organs, exhibitionistically displayed by the drunken man.

Layer II: First veto of the inner conscience, objecting to both psychic masochism and peeping.

Layer III. First defense: pseudoaggression against mother as competitor; admission of exhibitionism also as lesser intrapsychic crime, partly excused by identification with the father.

Layer IV: Second veto of the inner conscience, rejecting both parts of the first defense.

Layer V: Second defense: street fear. Conscience money paid in suffering for substitute crimes of pseudoaggression and exhibitionism. Guilt further diminished by use of pseudomoral connotation: "Didn't Mother ask me to be with Father?"

A succession of details bore out these conclusions. Here is a typical dream dating from the beginning of the analysis: She is sitting on the toilet; a man is looking at her; the door in front of the toilet is missing; the man's eyes are injured. In this dream the father is the peeper and she the exhibitionist—a reversal of the infantile situation but with the crime (peeping) unchanged. In another typical dream a mother is murdered in the doctor's office; a young girl bursts into the waiting room proclaiming her innocence. The figure of the mother is a cross between the patient's mother and the analyst.

In the transference neurosis Miss W. projected the mother image on the analyst, seemingly admitting murderous wishes pertaining to the oedipal mother. But more deeply repressed pre-oedipal fantasies could also be discerned, as in dreams portraying the mother as the dreaded castrator: An unknown woman is cutting meat, while the patient looks on with a feeling of disgust.

Another pseudomoral connotation was embedded in the neurotic symptom. The mother had forbidden the child any contact with her father after the divorce; the only possibility of meeting him would have been by chance, in the street. Thus a dictum pronounced by the mother and preserved over the years further bolstered the symptom, for in childhood the street was forbidden sexual territory (prostitutes, chance acquaintances, mating dogs, and so on).

The patient's identification with her drunk, "sick" father (and especially with his exhibitionism, though this was subsequently warded off) was of a protective nature. ("I reel about as though I were drunk," she would often say in describing her symptoms.) Behind the oedipal structure could be found the unresolved pre-oedipal fear of the mother, a frightening figure until "neutralized" and immobilized by the agoraphobic patient's constant watchfulness. Miss W. never left home; she kept her mother always with her. This reversed the childhood situation when she had been left alone with her father, anxiously on the alert lest her mother enter the room. At bottom, the aggression against her mother—though accepted as the lesser crime in guilt expiation—provided a covering cloak for more deeply repressed masochistic vicissitudes antedating the oedipal rescue station.

When attacked by the superego the patient "made a stand," attempting to fight it out. She chose as battleground, in preference to the voyeuristic and masochistic layer (layer I), the stratum of exhibitionism and pseudoaggression (layer III). And here too a pseudomoral connotation was built into the structure. This secondary pseudomoral prop proclaimed that she merely repeated the actions of an educational authority, her father.

5. FEAR OF HEIGHTS (ACROPHOBIA)

The familiar symptom of acrophobia (recently seen in the modification of *fear of airplanes*) has not so far been singled out for special investigation; it leads a summary existence in our literature, being "also mentioned" when neurotic fears are discussed. Fear of heights deserves a better fate; it is characterized by a series of special features.[49]

Although generally subsumed under phobic-hysteriform mechanisms, acrophobia is, in my experience, encountered only among orally regressed neurotics, and then only when there are disturbances in the voyeuristic-exhibitionistic sphere. It is not surprising, therefore, that the situation most often met with is that of a patient with street fear who also complains of fear of heights. However, it should be said that fear of heights is not the exclusive prerogative of the agoraphobe; it may appear independently of agoraphobia. The presence of a *voyeuristic-exhibitionistic disturbance does seem to be typical.*

Fear of heights unconsciously dramatizes two inner conflicts:

1. "Bad mother will let the baby (the fear-sufferer) drop from her arms."

2. "It is not true that I'm exhibiting my genitals to anyone who stands below looking at me up here. The truth is that I'm not an exhibitionist but just a person who came up to this height for the perfectly reasonable purpose of getting a better view of my surroundings."

3. "My fear proves that I want to avoid both dangers and that I'm not attracted to either of them."

All three features call for elaboration.

a. *Ascription of "Bad Intentions" to the Mother Image*

In cases of acrophobia a specific modification of the "septet of baby fears" is preserved, and the mother is accused of "malignantly dropping the child from her arms." Often this infantile fear is combined with other constituents of the "septet." The irony of the situation is that the mother took the child into her arms, walked around with him and rocked him, in order to soothe him and stop his crying. An old-time patient of mine, a nurse, once told me that children who cannot be appeased by being picked up and held are the most "difficult" of all; those who do not stop crying when carried in their mothers' (or nurses') arms developed into "difficult" people, she claimed. An interesting, though so far unconfirmed, observation.

The fact remains that when these fears are worked out in analysis the fear of height disappears—provided the voyeuristic-exhibitionistic element is analyzed too. At first I was not familiar with this strange combination and analyzed only the "bad intention" ascribed to the mother of infancy; my results were not too impressive. Later

I learned of the other component (see b, below); this did the trick. Once, experimentally, I began treatment of a patient by taking up the voyeuristic-exhibitionistic component; the fear was diminished but not eliminated. Having experienced both varieties of partial therapy—the first because of ignorance, the second as an experiment—I came to the conclusion that each of the *partes constituentes* was indispensable.

b. *The "Voyeuristic-Exhibitionistic Exchange Mechanism"*

I became aware of the visual elements in fear of heights in the analysis of an advertising executive and later confirmed my observation in a series of cases. Mr. X., the advertising man, suffered from compulsive infidelity, which brought him into constant marital and professional conflicts. During his analysis his wife tried to console herself by successfully prevailing on him to sell the suburban house in which they had lived for many years and to buy a more luxurious one. She chose a house perched on a steep hill. The patient violently opposed her choice. Discussing the matter in analysis, he confessed for the first time to a fear of heights. In analyzing this fear we came across a recollection dating from his sixth year. He was at that time living in the country. He persuaded several girls who lived near by to climb an apple tree, allegedly because of the ripe apples; his real purpose was to peep under their skirts.

After this recollection came to the fore Mr. X. promptly reached the conclusion that a connection with his acrophobia was involved. He suspected that he unconsciously identified with the exhibiting girls. He thus took the blame for "the lesser intrapsychic crime," admitting to *feminine identification*. Gradually, however, other recollections were unearthed. These revealed that while watching the girls hanging from the branches of the tree he toyed with the possibility that one of the girls might lose her hold and come crashing down. The real, great crime—the more dangerous one—was *masochistic identification with the daring, endangered girls*. It is probable that this masochistic identification was in itself a second edition of the original fear: "Mother will let the baby drop from her arms."

So forbidden was peeping in his infantile lawbook that he disguised and attenuated it defensively twice in his symptom of acrophobia. First he used feminine identification; identifying with the allegedly exhibiting girls, he could claim that the people below him could peep at his genitalia, but he could not. Second, he made voyeurism harmless by "looking at nature," meaning the surroundings visible from a height.

An interesting connection could be established between this infantile peeping ("I'm not doing anything; I'm just looking") and the patient's professional activity. Although highly successful in his business he had difficulty in thinking up new ideas. In working out a new advertising campaign for one of his clients, he would follow a standard routine. First he would go through his files; candidly he admitted that he did so not only for the practical purpose of finding out what his competitors were doing but also in order to modify ("steal," he once said) the ideas of others. Once more, appeasement of passivity.

The strange feature in voyeurism and exhibitionism is the fact that, as I believe, only voyeurism is an original drive and exhibitionism only a defense instituted when voyeurism led to conflicts. In the clinical picture, however, both voyeurism and exhibitionism can be used for defensive purposes. In comparing street fear with fear of heights, for example, one finds that in street fear voyeurism is warded off with exhibitionism and later defensively warded off again, while in fear of heights exhibitionism is warded off with voyeurism (also in identification with the alleged spectator, corresponding to double identification as postulated by Freud for "Schautrieb") and made harmless by "looking at nature."

c. *The Denial of Points "a" and "b" in Fear*

Freud's original theory of anxiety assumed that libidinous id wishes are directly transformed into fear; later he modified his early formulation, stating that a warning signal produced by the unconscious ego is involved. The analytic literature has frequently emphasized the fact that Freud did not propose that his second theory should supplant his first but rather viewed the two theories as valid descriptions of the identical process as seen from different vantage points. In the original theory the vista is that of the id; in the modification it is that of the unconscious ego.

As we also know from Freud, the prevailing tendency of the unconscious ego is the maintenance of low tension in the psychic apparatus. The unconscious ego's anxiety signal is like the automatic whistling device of a boiler that goes into action whenever pressure reaches a critical point.

In my opinion, as elaborated in THE BASIC NEUROSIS, THE SUPEREGO, and LAUGHTER AND THE SENSE OF HUMOR, neurotic fear pertains exclusively to the inability of the unconscious ego to handle *one* particular situation: an over-large accumulation of cathexis of psychic masochism. Judging from results, the unconscious ego's forte is in transforming id wishes into defenses acceptable to the superego; it is considerably less effective in handling the punishment emanating from the superego. Its customary resource is to change such punishment into psychic masochism. If too much of this transmutation has taken place the application of this remedy threatens to conflict with the low-tension principle. Frantically, then, the unconscious ego gives the anxiety signal as S.O.S.

The signal of anxiety is in itself proof that the unconscious ego has been unable to fulfill its program. In this desperate situation the best the "inner lawyer" can do to rescue its "client in distress" is to resort to three subterfuges ("triad of fear"):

First the unconscious ego effects a change of locality by projecting inner fear outward. Now the danger appears to be external and the neurotic fear takes on the apparent attributes of "reality fear." (This shift obtains in phobic and paranoid cases; in hypochondria an organ is chosen as malefactor and treated as if it were a Greek gift, so to speak, which another person, mother, had by trickery inserted into one's body.)

Secondly, in a cunning shift the unconscious ego detaches the neurotic fear from its masochistic basis. The crime of inner crimes, psychic masochism, is warded off with pseudoaggression, and blame is accepted for the pseudoaggressive transgression. Whatever the specific contents of the neurotic fear, it always includes apprehension pertaining to a childhood violation of some educational command.

Thirdly, a change is effected in the libidinous contents of the fear. The "admission of the lesser crime" also governs this shift. In acrophobia, for example, voyeurism is warded off with exhibitionism and secondarily warded off subsequently with "harmless" peeping at "nature."

The Visual Drive

The primary purpose of all these shifts is to provide a smoke screen that will divert the superego's punitive attention from the basic masochistic conflict. This purpose is defeated, however, when the libidinous wish has also been masochistically imbued. One has the impression that the unconscious ego would not have to resort to the desperate measure of an anxiety attack if merely a libidinous wish and the defense against it were at stake. No other conclusion fits the observable fact that diminution of the neurotic libidinous contents of a symptom does not automatically spell diminution of fear.

Translated into colloquial terms, the sum total of the defenses put forward by the unconscious ego when confronted with the "triad of fear" reads as follows: "I did all I could for you—I changed both indictments (libidinous and aggressive) from felonies to misdemeanors and substituted an external for an internal enemy. Now run for your life!"

6. FEAR OF EXAMINATIONS

In general, the fear of examinations is equated in our literature with phallic castration fears. There is more to it. It is also a demonstration that one has not *successfully* mastered the ability "to suck on wisdom's breasts," to use Goethe's phrase for acquiring knowledge. If the exhibitionistic defense is burdened with "undigested" oral-voyeuristic conflicts of a primitive nature, masochistically imbued, the demonstration of knowledge, acquired through learning, is made impossible.

In an old case history, published thirty years ago, in 1932, ("Psychoanalysis of a Case of Examination Fear," *Zentralblatt fuer Psychotherapie,* 6:65-83.) I described a patient who refused to take a harmless examination. In his infantile history a peculiar fear of a "fixture" was found. This fixture, a lamp which was endowed with magic qualities and could make things disappear, could be traced to an observation of his father's penis. I added that

> the phallic castration fear had an oral substructure. In analyzing the magic attributed to the lamp the patient remembered a fairy tale that had impressed him greatly as a child. It was Grimm's "Mary's Child," in which the Virgin Mary takes a three-year-old girl, the daughter of poor parents, into heaven. When

the girl is thirteen Mary hands over to her the keys to the thirteen doors of heaven, permitting her to open twelve but forbidding the thirteenth. The girl oversteps the interdiction, touches the Trinity with her finger, which turns to gold. As punishment she is sent back to earth, where she marries a king and bears him a boy. Mary appears to her at night and requests a confession of the old, denied sin. The queen denies it again, and her child is taken away. The courtiers claim that the queen —who as added punishment is stricken dumb—is a cannibal. She is condemned to die at the stake but confesses, and the tale has a happy ending. (Masturbation fantasy, orally-cannibalistically elaborated.)

It is also interesting that this patient had complicated difficulties in photography: "I have photographed animals, plants, landscapes, but hardly ever a person. When I photographed the Sphinx in the Belvedere (in Vienna) I took it from such an angle that the breasts were half-hidden." In childhood the patient had an eye tic.

In another study, also published in 1932, "The Problem of Pseudo-Debility," l.c., I pointed out that, besides self-damaging tendencies, the refusal to learn (or reproduce learned knowledge) contains a spurious defiant aggression: by identifying learning (taking in, K. Abraham) with oral intake an old wound is reactivated: "Previously they (the parents) refused; *now* they want me to absorb!"

7. JEALOUSY, PATHOLOGICAL CURIOSITY, AND LOGORRHOEA

In a study written more than twenty years ago entitled "Contributions to the Psychology of Jealousy" (published in *Internationale Zeitschrift fuer Psychoanalyse und Imago,* as it was then known, London, 24:384-397) I drew attention to the fact that the frequently observed but not scientifically elucidated phenomenon of a jealous person imagining a love scene between the allegedly unfaithful mate and the presumptive lover has a voyeuristic-masochistic basis. In my book FASHION AND THE UNCONSCIOUS (1953) I pointed out that this voyeuristic component is subsequently warded off with defensive exhibitionism. At first the jealous person is secretive about his unconsciously libidinized self-torture, which he executes by means of the "visual imperative." In later stages he abandons this secrecy, discussing the matter freely with others. His purpose is to win agreement for his interpretation of events, to arouse compassion, and also to turn his confidants into witnesses who will attest to the injustice done him. The result is not at all as he intended; the cuckold of either sex does not cut a heroic figure.

The "visual imperative" in jealousy has a complex "case history." It is by no means "simple" peeping, but the result of infantile resignation to the situation of being excluded from the sexual activities of adults (the parents). The initial "I want to participate" is changed into "at least nobody can prevent me from looking." Later that "looking" is masochistically elaborated through the misuse of early pre-oedipal vicissitudes. Still later, looking in reality is changed into looking in fantasy; this change accounts for the typical phenomenon of a jealous person "imagining" the scenes he dreads. Needless to say, this "I'm only looking" has a guilt-diminishing effect. Allegedly, only overt acts are punishable, and every educator is familiar with the child's standard excuse when caught peeping: "I didn't do anything; I was only looking."

To complicate matters, the *starting point* of the whole procedure is not voyeurism, but *infantile megalomania.*

Unavoidable offenses to infantile megalomania are *the* real tragedy of childhood. The fate of the individual depends to a large degree on whether or not he can inwardly come to terms with these blows to his most cherished fantasy.

This becomes clear when one thinks through the genesis of the most damaging defense mechanism installed by human beings—*psychic masochism.* As I have pointed out in numerous publications and restated in the present book (Chapt. 1), it is especially important to distinguish between the *genetic* and *clinical* pictures in psychic masochism.

It should be remembered that the resultant "injustice-collecting" in the clinical picture—the percentage of profit accrued from the capital of the "pleasure-in-displeasure pattern"—contains a peculiar combination of all three inborn drives: aggression, libido, megalomania. Aggression turned against the ego is libidinized—but only under *megalomaniacal safeguards.* Unconsciously the psychic masochist knows only too well that he engineered the whole nexus himself. Therefore, while he is being externally humiliated, this neurotic unconsciously reasons: "That fool believes he is kicking me, but that's only what he thinks! By my initial provocation I *made* him kick me!"

It is exactly that infantile megalomania that plays a decisive part in jealousy's "visual imperative," masochistically imbued. *The decisive point in jealousy is an offense against megalomania, resulting in masochistic stabilization of the wish to be rejected.* Secondarily there is a shift to the pseudoaggressive defense of aggressive peeping (aggressive because it transgresses educational commands). This explains why jealous people so frequently—unconsciously on purpose—create their own private hell by choosing coquettish and unreliable partners and thus indirectly playing procurer, or at least cultivating an atmosphere of uncertainty. *Officially* these neurotics want exclusive and uncontested possession; *unofficially* they want to re-enact the "rejection game."

This factor explains a curious phenomenon, observed but unexplained: every jealous person begs for "the truth." His motto is always the same: "If I only knew." On the other hand, confessions never help. Why?

The jealous person's cruel superego is attacking him on two counts: first, for the major intrapsychic crime of re-enacting the masochistic rejection game, and second, for the lesser intrapsychic crime of pseudoaggressive peeping. As in all psychic phenomena, the neurotic follows the standard procedure and attempts to "hold the line" on the diversionary front. He accepts guilt for the lesser defensive misdemeanor in order to prevent the superego from attacking the true felony, the real masochistic basis (see p. 79 ff.). The jealous person's "thirst for knowledge," which leads him to prod his partner for confessions, will, if satisfied, diminish the guilt felt on the misdemeanor front. With this knowledge, he can with some justification prove that his imaginings were not "infantile peeping," as the superego's indictment claims, but an objective reconstruction of an objective reality.

On the other hand, these confessions do little good, simply because all of the jealous person's peeping is merely diversionary, and the real core—the masochistic elaboration of the real or fancied rejection game—is not even touched.

The jealous person accepts no data as certain. A patient, Mr. Y., told me:

"I suspected my wife of having seen our so-called friend during my recent business trip. She immediately produced a postcard from him postmarked Chicago and addressed to both of us. That was supposed to prove that he had been in Chicago while I was out of town. Sounds convincing, but does it prove anything? How can I be sure the card wasn't mailed for him by a friend? The alibi was just too pat."

"If your wife hadn't produced the proof you would have argued that she had no proof and you had a right to suspect her."

"Haven't you ever heard of cleverly constructed false alibis? The prohibition-era gangsters used that technique expertly to keep themselves out of reach of the law."

"Why not admit that your deduction is erroneous? First you have your inner need to be jealous; second, you prove that every proof to the contrary can be disproved."

"I just want to be absolutely sure. That's all."

"That's not all, nor even the beginning of 'all.' If you were even partially honest with yourself you would face the fact that you carefully avoid certainty and at the same time—unconsciously—artificially cultivate uncertainty."

"That's preposterous!"

"Less so than you think. Suppose you assume, for the sake of the argument, that my premise is correct: the first situation begins with the inner need to be jealous, and you then look for hitching posts to which you can tie your jealousy. Wouldn't certainty prevent you from playing the inner game you are dramatizing in your jealous scenes?"

"But your premise is wrong. Jealousy isn't a game; it's real torture!"

"Now you are nearer the facts. You used the correct word: torture. Within yourself, unknown to yourself, lies an infantile, unconscious pattern of self-torture that is activated by the smallest provocative factors."

"Nonsense. I hate self-torture."

"You mean consciously. Agreed. But I spoke of an unconscious pattern of torture. There's quite a difference. It explains why jealousy so often appears when there are no grounds for it. Do you remember the dialogue between Desdemona and Emilia in OTHELLO?

"Desdemona: Alas the day! I never gave him cause.
Emilia: But jealous souls will not be answered so;
 They are not even jealous for a cause,
 But jealous for they are jealous; 'tis a monster
 Begot upon itself."

In psychological language we would put it this way: first comes the torture pattern; then comes the cultivation of uncertainty, so that the game of self-torture can continue."

"And these are the only ingredients needed to prepare a dish of jealousy?" the patient countered sarcastically.

"No," I replied, "the witches' brew of jealousy requires a third ingredient, peeping."

"This gets more and more fantastic," said Mr. Y.

"Let's see if it does. What tortures you most in jealousy?"

"When I imagine my wife—"

"Stop right there. You have proved my point. 'When I imagine,' you said. Isn't imagination mental peeping?"

"You are just confusing me! I have a problem of real jealousy; you make it into an unreal succession of cultivating uncertainty, an unconscious torture pattern, mental peeping. In this discussion I'm representing reality; you are representing fantasy."

"Not quite. I'm suggesting that you look at your jealousy through the analytic microscope, to see whether it is really as simple a thing as it appears to the naked eye. But you are refusing to look through the lens on the theory that the naked eye can see all there is to see."

Psychoanalysis attacks the *basis* of jealousy. The attempt must invariably cope with the greatest resistance on the part of the patient. There is no logic in this resistance. The sufferer clings with all his might to the torture he complains of, while the analyst tries to diminish (and ultimately eradicate) his pain. After a period of resistance an impasse is usually reached. The patient is convinced that there can be only one solution to his difficulties: his wife must be persuaded to "tell the whole truth."

Mr. and Mrs. Z. were both in analysis with me.

"Her damned analysis complicates my life," complained Mr. Z. "First you insist that I stop asking her 'embarrassing' questions. Second, she wears a permanent smirk of triumph on her face; I'd like to wipe it off with a smack. If I so much begin a pertinent remark she cuts me short with a cold, polite 'Tell it to the doctor tomorrow.' I must say you have trained her well."

"In spite of your bitterness I take that as a compliment. Can you give me one reason for continuing these morbid discussions with her —that is, one reason besides enjoying them?"

"If I just said I wanted to find out the truth you would tell me for the fiftieth time, 'You don't want the truth; you want to cultivate your uncertainty.' What can I say without getting some analytic double talk in return?"

"Why not admit that analysis is debunking your pseudo arguments?"

"Because I don't see it. All I see is that you're complicating my life."

"That translates into 'neurotic pleasures are being diminished'."

Mr. Z. took the period of "abstinence" badly; he became sleepless and depressed. It was pointed out to him that he was projecting upon the analyst the "killjoy" of his childhood, the image of the "cruel mother." The next day he suggested that his wife's analysis be interrupted; the situation was "intolerable."

"I have two questions to ask," I said. "First question: what right have you to interfere with her treatment? Second question: what will you gain from halting her treatment?"

"I'll have the upper hand again, that's what I'll gain. Are you satisfied?"

"Your answer makes sense if you've decided to play the jealousy game permanently. How do you reconcile that with your admitted desire to change?"

"I simply can't stand the fact that you and my wife have secrets behind my back."

"Once more, you are repeating the infantile situation of the excluded third party."

"I can't win, that's obvious."

"More injustice-collecting."

A few days later Mr. Z. announced that he had spent a sleepless night, arising from his bed at three in the morning to work out a memorandum. He handed me a sheet of paper on which he had written:

WHAT I MUST DO

1. Accept the fact that my wife has had sexual affairs with other men.
2. Accept the probability that her brand of "love" was involved in one or more of these cases.
3. Accept the fact that deceit permeates her personality to the extent that she was capable of withholding this information for over eleven years, under constant pressure.
4. Accept the fact that I knew this "unconsciously," which was the decisive point in my part of the marriage.
5. Accept the fact that I got what I wanted: *an untrue woman.*

"If this goes on," I said, "your diagnosis will have to be changed. You will be classed as a case of jealousy paranoia. Did you show your work of art to your wife?"

"Of course. She said, sarcastically, 'Well, if you have to learn this, just do it.' Can I live in peace with this woman?"

"What kind of answer would have satisfied you?"

"A confession of her crimes."

The crisis ended shortly afterwards in a typically masochistic solution:

"I have come to the resigned conclusion that I'm just a cuckold who has to accept his fate and keep his mouth shut. I have even —just for a minute—accepted the idea that I could live *and* accept my wife's past."

The Visual Drive

"Just for the record: you know, of course, that you haven't a shred of evidence to back your charges against your wife."

"Only circumstantial evidence," Mr. Z. retorted.

Fantasies die hard. A few days later Mr. Z. asked:

"Assuming everything goes well and I change as you expect me to, am I entitled to the full truth after both of us are out of analysis?"

"You seem to think of analysis as a means of coddling your neurosis. If you were an adjusted person you would not ask for the impossible, an invasion of privacy."

"I knew you would say that. The way you put it, a normal person is just a dope anybody can push around."

"Why not say a person who does not want to suffer?"

Mr. Z. had not given up yet. A few days later he came up with this ostensibly harmless question:

"What do you want to change in my wife?"

It was not quite cagey enough; I answered: "Do you really want an enumeration of her symptoms—which you already know—or is this a trap?"

"I just wanted to find out whether you would mention one decisive symptom—her deceit."

"Do you know the story of the two enemies who were persuaded to make peace on a religious holiday? They shook hands, and all was well. Then one of them took his leave, saying, 'I wish you for the coming year all the good you are wishing me.' The rejoinder was, 'Are you starting in again?'"

It was not easy to catch it, but a flicker of a smile did appear on Mr. Z.'s face.

There exist other cases in which the popular conception of jealousy as an offense to exclusive possession seems to be totally reversed. As paradigm I am adducing the case of a homosexual man, Mr. AA., who reveled in jealousy and visual self-torture, had his lover observed by detectives, etc. However, if his partner confessed to some homosexual escapade, Mr. AA. was *immediately pacified:* "The poor fellow could not help himself." To prove their "bisexuality," Mr. AA. and his partner would sometimes have intercourse with the same girl in each other's presence, without any traces of jealousy. The decisive factor for Mr. AA. was seemingly this principle: "Nothing should happen without my knowledge." In this case subservience to alleged re-establishment of infantile megalomania by knowledge seemed to help.

Superficial defenses in the torture of not knowing were of course included. When Mr. AA. was asked how it would "help" him to receive a compromising report on his partner from a detective, he answered, "Then I would get the goods on my friend." He said that with a straight face, although his protracted jealousy scenes habitually ended with his begging for forgiveness—psychic masochism was always victorious.

Here an additional element enters the picture: the unconscious and ironic distortion of the educational precept calling for truthfulness. H. L. Mencken has written of the attitude he thinks people really take towards this precept:

> No normal human being wants to hear the truth. It is the passion of a small and aberrant minority of men, most of them pathological. They are hated for telling it while they live, and when they die they are swiftly forgotten. . . . The average man avoids the truth as diligently as he avoids arson, regicide or piracy on the high seas, and for the same reason; because he believes that it is dangerous, that no good can come of it, that it doesn't pay. . . . The man who boasts that he habitually tells the truth is simply a man with no respect for it. It is not a small thing to be thrown about loosely like small change; it is something to be cherished and hoarded, and disbursed only when absolutely necessary.

In a previous publication ("Insistence on Truth-Telling," *The Quarterly Review of Psychiatry and Neurology,* 7:141-143, 1953.), I pointed out that the professional truth-tellers so sardonically dissected by Mencken are obviously not the norm. The average person learns in the course of ordinary life experience that it *sometimes* becomes advisable to tell a white lie, or is polite to tell a white lie, or compassionate to suppress an unpleasant fact when no purpose would be served by revealing it. Between the professional truth-teller and the professional liar stretches the domain of the average person, who (as far as one can observe) is no expert at either attitude.

Both the pathological liar and the pathological truth-teller have been repeatedly reported on in the psychoanalytic literature. At bottom, both manifestations are the result of specific elaborations of the infantile conflict in the "battle of the conscience."

A specific sub-type in the field of truth-telling also exists: this is the person who vehemently insists that *the other fellow* always tell him the truth. The stickler for veracity in others is by no means a paragon of virtue himself; he has no qualms about telling white or not-so-white lies, or making hypocritical gestures, which are a usual part of the daily routine. However, he is by no means a liar on principle. If it is possible and not too disadvantageous, he will stick to what is more or less the truth. One can rate him as about average, as far as the truth-lie balance sheet is concerned. He is peculiar in only one specific foible: he insists that the other fellow tell *him* nothing but the truth. Oscar Wilde's aphorism pertains to him: "Duty is what we expect from others." One could call him a *"truth-fanatic for others."*

The individual who belongs to this sub-type presents very banal rationalizations whenever he attempts to explain the fury and indignation with which he reacts when a lie is told to him. These rationalizations range from "He insulted my intelligence" to "I just can't stand silly lies" and to more intelligent admissions, such as, "I don't know why, but when someone tells me a lie I just see red." Sometimes, these people are conscious of the farcical discrepancy between their own not too strict standards of truth-telling and their rigid insistence on absolute veracity from the other fellow.

The psychological approach is at first clouded by an unwarranted expectation: the fanatic requirement that the other fellow tell the truth at all times is only a projection of inner reproaches directed against oneself; accused of lying, the defense is shifted to the outside. Thus, this reaction is sometimes observable in everybody, but it contributes nothing to the type under scrutiny. The underlying problem is more complex.

Mr. BB., a high-ranking business executive in his early thirties, made a rather mixed impression of partly shy-detached, partly friendly-ironic apathy. He described himself as a "quiet fellow," who became excited only when someone told him a lie. When, where, and by whom the lie was told was immaterial; in a nearly compulsive manner he would berate, debunk, and unmask the "liar."

He was quite aware that this attitude of truth-fanaticism for others was slightly ridiculous, at times dangerous, and at the very least, "impractical." After discarding a few rationalizations, he said ironically, "You tell me the reason."

The reason could be detected when analyzing Mr. BB.'s *inner* elaboration of his relation to his overpowering father. The latter, a tyrant of the old school with a "terrific temper," was an intimidating educator. *Superficially* the son had identified with his father, an identification which had cautiously been kept within bounds but which was sufficiently evident to prompt the frequent comment: "The image of his father!" *Inwardly, the son used most of his inner energy for the purpose of satirizing his father.*

This became obvious when one particular recollection came to the fore. As a very small child the boy had been playing with another child in the cellar of the family house. In these games matches were used. One fell upon some combustible material and started a fire. Seeing the smoke, a neighbor called the fire department; the firemen came and put out the small blaze. The father investigated and then punished the boy—not for "arson," but for "not telling the truth," since the boy stubbornly persisted in his refusal to admit that he had been in the cellar, despite evidence.

Inwardly the child elaborated on this moral precept by reducing it to absurdity. The specific instance was generalized. When the father insisted on truth in this *specific* case, the son became an adherent of truth in *any* circumstances. Since truth proved to be unusable and impractical quite often, and often was not even expected, the son's intolerance came to include even harmless white lies. He was beating the—by now—introjected image of the father with the father's own stick; hadn't father insisted on "truth"?

The irritability and fury with which the man reacted to the other fellow's lies were dramatizations of the original situation in reverse. He acted the father, reducing the other fellow to the image of his infantile self. This was in no way a normal identification. On the con-

The Visual Drive

trary, under the disguise of identification *the ego ideal was ridiculed—via exaggeration.*

The technique used by Mr. BB. was that of the "pseudomoral connotation" (see pp. 130 ff.). By magnifying a reasonable precept and applying it formalistically at the wrong time, in the wrong place and wrong context, he arrived at a defense. The defense, it is true, involved him in other difficulties, but that was another story, related to his deeply rooted psychic masochism, which had been acquired in the pre-oedipal phase and had been only secondarily shifted (in the oedipal period) to the father.

To return to the "visual imperative": One arrives at the conclusion that *two types* of jealousy can be observed: the typical and atypical. Each of these subdivisions contains mixtures of both elements, but the preponderance of ingredients makes the difference:

Type I, the typical case, wants re-enactment of the masochistic rejection game of infancy, covered up with peeping.

Type II, the atypical case, wants the same but places inordinate importance on the "pseudomoral connotation," inwardly subjecting to an ironic interpretation the educational precept of "telling the truth."

In Type I, confession does not help; in Type II, confession does help—temporarily.

The jealous person claims that jealousy is merely a reaction to tender love. Psychologically this cannot be entirely excluded; jealousy is a possible postscript to the inner process of tender love, which—as already defined (see pp. 151 f.)—is an emotion based on projection of *one's own* ego ideal on the beloved. The beloved must satisfy two emotional requirements. One is to fit into the lover's "type" and in this way fulfill the lover's infantile wishes. The other is to disarm the torturing daimonion, accomplished by the acceptance of the lover's self-created ego ideal as fact. The discrepancy between ego and ego ideal, between aim and achievement, which has enabled the daimonion to exact the payment in the form of guilt and depression, is thus wiped out. An Eden of guiltlessness and megalomania follows.

This type—*the submissive type*—of love is characterized by psychic dependence upon the beloved object. The results include the temporary inability to exercise the critical function and the extravagant overvaluation of the beloved's charms and abilities. Overvaluation seems to be a method of increasing the effectiveness of this antidote to guilt and depression.

Less commonly encountered is the *protective type* of love, in which the lover plays the part of the grand seigneur, guarding, tending, and championing his entirely dependent "baby." The psychic origin of this type of love is again the mechanism of projection, but here the lover projects his *ego,* not his ego ideal, on the beloved, unconsciously playing the role of his own ego ideal. Although the roles seem to have been reversed there has been no change in either aim or result.

The rarer protective form of love, curiously enough, tends to appear in highly narcissistic but at the same time essentially passive individuals. For in defeating the daimonion by means of submissive love the lover has placed himself in the position of meek and passive dependence on the beloved object. Inevitably the inner conscience reproaches him for that passivity. If the ensuing guilt feeling is strong, and the individual is sufficiently narcissistic, the defense against the accusation of passivity may be a revolt against submissive love and an assumption of the grand seigneur role in subsequent love episodes. An example of this shift in type may be found in the life of the poet Heinrich Heine.

When very young, Heine fell in love with the daughter of his well-to-do uncle; her utter indifference to his feelings was, as he put it, "a stab in the heart." Considerably later Heine married a primitive and uneducated Parisian grisette. She was his "creation" in every way. He sent her to school in order to make a lady of her and even changed her name from Crescentia to Mathilde. In Heine's unhappy youthful love affair he had been the poor boy disdained by the "queen"; here he reversed the roles and smiled down from his eminence at the presumably grateful grisette. This was clearly a "magic gesture." On the surface he was demonstrating how he wanted to be treated—kindly; on a deeper level he really wanted exactly the opposite—mistreatment. The surface demonstration was a defense to conceal the inner masochistic wish. The masochistic wish supposedly routed by this move sprang to the fore soon enough. Mathilde tortured him soundly.

Only the self-assured man can experience submissive love without subjecting himself to reproaches of passivity from the superego. The inner choice of the weak man is necessarily the protective type of love; he must play the super he-man in all his relationships to counterbalance his inner passivity and provide a defense against it.

What happens when the lover of either type is faced with the beloved object's infidelity or lessening affection?

Jealousy can become conscious only after the groundwork for its appearance has been laid. The beloved's behavior is not the signal for jealousy; the progress of the battle being fought within the lover's unconscious is what matters.

The lover's unconscious ruse of projecting either ego or ego ideal on the beloved object deprived the daimonion of its main weapon. But the daimonion is not totally disarmed. Shifting its point of attack but not its technique, it continues to contrast fantasy and reality, pointing out the big and little defects of the beloved in an attempt to regain control.

The lover is handicapped in his defense. Unconsciously he has never been certain that he succeeded in cheating the daimonion. The human psyche is capable of a slave revolt against its inner torturer, but it is so lacking in the ability to win that even successful revolt is viewed with suspicion.

This is the atmosphere in which jealousy thrives: the lover's lack of confidence in his own weapon and the daimonion's renewal of attack.

Jealousy is the conscious expression of the unconscious battle between the daimonion, desperate to wipe out its defeat, and the unconscious ego, already doubtful of its ability to maintain its freedom. And as soon as the ego's doubts become serious the battle is as good as lost. For the ego swallows the enemy's propaganda whole. This is why, in Iago's words (OTHELLO, III, iii),

> Trifles light as air
> Are to the jealous confirmations strong
> As proofs of holy writ.

One gets the impression that the daimonion's tactics at this point are both ironic and revengeful. In jealousy the daimonion is in the ascendant though not yet restored to power; the slave revolt, though not yet a failure, is no longer a success. The daimonion's attack on the beloved is a barrage of trifles and flimsy complaints, sardonically echoing the "flimsy grounds" on which the beloved was chosen in the first place. And it is on this note of poetic justice that the episode ends.

Jealousy is subjectively so painful because it is a by-product of the greatest of intrapsychic defeats; the lover's own narcissism, deposited in the ego ideal, has failed him. The lover has been his own executioner, though he is not aware of it. Neither does he understand that his real purpose was to maintain his freedom from inner guilt and not to regain the beloved object. In all this he has been the daimonion's dupe as well as aide. When he swallowed whole all the "trifles" and "little signs" that proved his beloved to be untrustworthy, he was trapping himself into jealousy and eventually into renewed servitude to the daimonion. All this is under the surface; consciously he merely suffers.

The ego's revolt against the daimonion by means of tender love begins with a brilliant victory and then goes on from defeat to defeat. Jealousy is the final, and therefore the most painful, defeat in this hopeless contest. There is a "fifth column" within the lover himself, to complicate matters; it drives some lovers as far as suicide.

The last convulsions of freedom from the daimonion, the stage of jealousy, assume different forms depending on whether the lover is of the submissive or the protective type. In either case there is a violent attack, but the submissive lover will invariably attack the beloved, who is the representative of his own ego ideal, while the protective lover will attack his rival. Neither will rebel against the real torturer, the daimonion. The submissive lover turns on his own ego ideal, accusing it of conspiring with the daimonion to achieve his defeat; the protective lover's target is the third party, and the beloved is exonerated as the innocent victim of the competitor's seduction.

Both men and women of the submissive type will direct their aggression against the person of the *opposite* sex; men and women of the protective type will direct their aggression against the person of

The Visual Drive

the *same* sex. The underlying love type, therefore, can be deduced from the type of jealousy shown.

Regardless of type, two elements are strongly marked in jealousy. These are heightened voyeurism and heightened psychic masochism.

The voyeuristic component is so salient that literature's virtual failure to stress its presence is amazing. One of the rare acknowledgments of this deep-seated impulse is found in Anatole France's THE RED LILY, where the hero is so jealous of a rival of the past that he breaks off an affair with a woman he still "loves." He is incapable of seeing her "alone"; to his jealous eye "the other" is always with her.

To the jealous man and the jealous woman alike, the most painful element in jealousy is the *visualization* of love scenes between the beloved and the presumable rival. Consciously the "visual imperative" is not accompanied by pleasure—clear proof that it is forbidden. Fantasies of this type are possible only when two safeguards are used: defensive fury and self-torture.

The forbidden element in voyeurism is a combination of the infantile unconscious connotations of sexual peeping and the unconscious identification with the unfaithful beloved. In men this identification leads to the enjoyment of feminine repressed tendencies; in women it leads to the enjoyment of masculine repressed tendencies. The whole procedure is thoroughly masochistic.

There is a famous example of the combination of all three factors in a scene from Stendhal's life. His great love, Angiola Pietragrua, had an affair with another man, and through the indiscretion of her maid Stendhal surreptitiously witnessed a love scene between them. The victim's first reaction was an outburst of laughter. His friend Mérimée states:

> Stendhal told me that the peculiarity and ridiculousness of the situation provoked convulsive laughter in him at first. He went to great pains to smother his laughter so that he would not alarm the sinners. Only after some time did he become aware of his unhappiness.

Through Freud's work on the psychology of wit and laughter we are familiar with the fact that laughter is produced when a certain amount of psychic energy, otherwise used for holding down repressed material, becomes free. The conserved psychic energy must have represented something infantile and forbidden, for instance the observation of parental intimacies.

Another characteristic manifestation in jealousy can also be traced to the voyeuristic component. This is the initial tendency to conceal the feeling and the subsequent willingness to parade it in an appeal for commiseration.

Byron's observation in Don Juan,

> Yet he was jealous, though he did not show it.
> For jealousy dislikes the world to know it—

is accurate only for the early stages of jealousy, where voyeurism is unconsciously put into operation and enjoyed in the "visual imperative." Later on, when guilt is present, the guilt feeling itself transforms voyeurism into its opposite, exhibitionism. This self-display takes various forms, such as confiding in friends, asking for their sympathy, making a show of one's affairs in sensational divorce proceedings, etc.

Jealousy is an intrapsychic conflict, in which the beloved is not the cause but merely the vehicle of expression. Jealousy can exist only when the individual possesses marked, though repressed, masochistic and voyeuristic tendencies. It is proof that the individual is lacking in normally functioning narcissism. Contrary to the claims of minor poets and minor prophets, jealousy is *not* a universal emotion.

So far, this description has been limited to the manifestations of jealousy in relatively "normal" persons, meaning individuals in whom neurotic tendencies are comparatively limited. The problem changes as soon as one enters the area of considerable neurosis. The "slave revolt" of love is beyond the capability of the neurotic; his vehicle is transference. Every emotional episode in his life is the re-enactment of an infantile conflict. The neurotic is more heavily imbued with masochism than the so-called normal individual, and his sufferings are accordingly greater.

Neurotic jealousy is met with on every level of regression. It is therefore possible in *every* neurosis. Psychic masochism is an inherent part of every neurotic conflict, and jealousy is one of its common manifestations. As already pointed out, every neurotic is essentially an injustice collector; his booty is imaginary and often unconsciously self-created wrongs. Jealousy is one of the richer sources of possible "injustice." Of course, injustice-collecting as a *general* tendency does not explain the *specific* choice of jealousy as an outlet. Individual determinants must be sought.

In any case, whether it is a pre-oedipal or an oedipal situation that is unconsciously repeated in a jealousy conflict, the fact remains that shifting the blame to the partner alone is not sufficient to clarify the picture. It is true that there are psychotic cases of jealousy paranoia, which sometimes lead to murder and suicide. Where *neurotic* jealousy is involved, however, the decisive—though monotonous and never answered—question has to be posed to the partner: "Why did your instinct not warn you to avoid that person?" The answer, "I didn't know," is correct as far as consciousness is concerned. But it makes a large detour around a vital sector: the neurosis of the innocent party, which frequently makes her or him unconsciously collaborate with the partner's neurosis.

Jealousy, therefore, is merely another attempt to provide an unconscious countermeasure against man's inner fears, defeated—like the others—by inner conscience.

Pathological curiosity also plays a part in logorrhea.

Logorrhea is a phenomenon encountered at all levels of the libidinous-aggressive development. I have published an investigation ("Logorrhea," *The Psychiatric Quarterly,* 18:26-42, 1944.) subdividing the symptom according to oral, anal, and phallic manifestations. Here I reproduce only the conclusions of the oral sections of the study.

One of the most typical complaints of a husband about a neurotic wife—and vice versa—is "She (he) talks too much." The first impression is that the quantity of words is the objectionable feature for these martyrs of abnormal talkativeness, chatter, garrulity, and loquacity. A more careful observation, however, shows that the complaint refers to a combination of the following three components:

(1) incessant talking;

(2) inconsistent talking, without transition of even a second's pause or without visible connection;

(3) preponderance of unimportant details chosen aggressively, without perception of the problem as a whole.

Occasionally it is possible to observe such neurotic—psychotic logorrhea is not dealt with here—logorrheic patients of both sexes (there are as many men as women) afflicted with that triad of signs. What are the unconscious mechanisms used by people of this type, and why are they used?

Logorrhea must be distinguished from the usual urge to communicate found in the so-called cultured human being, which sometimes gives the impression of garrulity. Of course the distinction must be made by a typical human being and not by one of the "silent" variety of neurotics. The following anecdote about the Swiss poet Gottfried Keller [50] illustrates why. Keller used to drink in the evening in the company of friends without speaking a word. One evening one of his friends introduced his grown son. After hours of drinking in silence Keller dropped his handkerchief. Picking it up, the intimidated young man said, "Here, Mr. Keller," the only words he spoke during many hours. On the way home Keller's friend asked the poet his impression of his son. Keller replied, "A nice young man, but he talks too much."

The usual urge to communicate gives the impression at first that many people are inclined to speak solely for the purpose of speaking. Listening more closely, one finds that specific tendencies appear behind the urge. For instance, small transitory "garrulity societies" are sometimes created for the purpose of ranting against a particular group, institution, or individual. Hatred binds many people closer than love. As a subgroup of this type of activity one might mention "teasing," that superficial, pseudo-witty form of making fun at someone else's expense.

On the other hand there seem to be "garrulity centers" whose only reason for being is the friendly exchange of "ideas." These are built on the narcissistic basis "I'll let you play the role of the 'big shot' if you will do the same for me." That reciprocal giving of "medals of genius," based on the idea of acceptance in order to be accepted,

The Visual Drive

is clearly narcissistic. "We give each other the clues so well—one calls that friendship," says one of Arthur Schnitzler's dramatis personae. "Mutual admiration societies" is the usual term for these groups. It is known, of course, that other elements besides narcissism are involved in such gatherings; for instance, unconscious feminine identification, unconscious defense against passive wishes, etc.

Other garrulity societies are based on self-pity. Hypochondriacal chatter of old women of both sexes is found in these groups.

Generally speaking, chronic gossipers in society impress one as being inwardly still children, who would enjoy gossiping perpetually—in the absence of a severe educator. (Talking seems to the child one of the prerogatives of adults. This misleading impression is enforced upon him since persons in authority are honored with silence and spoken to only at their request. That other elements enter the picture is clear; for instance, childish ideas of omnipotence, words used "magically" or as symbolic representation in cases where words are substituted for phallic exhibitionism.) In addition to garrulousness, another element in the behavior of the logorrheic person seems to indicate the transgression of a prohibition—the divulging of secrets in the course of gossiping. Knowledge of human nature in general confirms the old Oriental aphorism "Don't let your *friends* know what could be of help to your *enemies*." In typical gatherings of gossipers many facts are divulged which, after dissolution of the transitory groups, would be recalled if it were possible. The gossiper, therefore, must feel some unconscious tendency towards self-punishment as a direct consequence of his transgressed prohibition.

Also indicative of a feeling of guilt is another characteristic of the logorrheic—his stubborn refusal to acknowledge that he makes himself a laughing-stock with his incessant garrulity. Often he has the reputation of being "simply stupid." This assumption is incorrect, although it cannot be denied that coexistence of both tendencies—logorrhea and low I.Q.—is possible. The underlying explanation of logorrhea is more complex than that often given—stupidity. How mistaken it is to apply the word "stupid" schematically to logorrheic persons is shown in the following instance: some people are very fond of the expression "If you know what I mean." Such an introduction would seem to be preparatory to a deep revelation. Experience proves, however, that the famous phrase is instead always associated with a banality. This pompous cloaking of a banality gives at first glance the impression of stupidity and a futile attempt to appear important. In reality it is an insult to the intelligence of the listener and serves the unconscious purpose of pseudoaggression.

The outer world's reaction to, and rejection of, the logorrheic is, so to speak, part of his unconsciously calculated and sought punishment for his prohibited deed. The situation is similar to that which I have described elsewhere as being operative in plagiarism. The plagiarist steals often so cynically, stupidly, and seemingly without regard for consequences because he expects unconsciously to be discovered.[51]

The logorrheic person is blind also in another respect. Not only does he not see that he is ridiculous but he is insensitive to the fact that he irritates his environment. That scotomization and oversight is reducible to the pseudoaggressive core of gossiping.

We see that the logorrheic is seemingly full of a strange optimism; exactly the opposite can be observed in the mistrustful hyper-silent person. To quote the joke of a patient, when two sympathetic logorrheics meet, the cubic contents of each merge and are doubled. The logorrheic is, so to speak, the last optimist. That in return for his optimism he receives a "kick in the jaw" is a result included unconsciously as an integral part of his inner plan.

It is analytically known that the urge to communicate can serve other neurotic tendencies as well—such as the urge to confess (Reik), an unconscious invitation to participate in joint sexual pleasure, as described by D. Burlingham. The often encountered opinion that gossiping is simply a display of exhibitionism is, however, in my opinion erroneous; the explanation is far more complicated. Also erroneous is the view that the problem of logorrhea can be dismissed simply by pointing out the phallic significance of the tongue, whether or not in conjunction with exhibitionism.

It is difficult either to prove or to disprove that language was originally a means of expressing human needs, a theory often advanced. In any case, the present use of language is a long way from those nebulous beginnings. Consider, for instance, the cynical statement of Talleyrand that words have the purpose of disguising, not expressing, thoughts. On the other hand, let us not forget that words are the chief weapon of malice and aggression in cultural societies after direct killing has been renounced. The formula "intolerant, malicious, and gossipy" is applicable to many communities all over the globe.

Furthermore, logorrhea must be distinguished from the *conscious* use of hyper-talkativeness; for instance, to confuse the enemy by unclear and ambiguous words, to throw him off the track. In this case garrulity is simply a weapon from the arsenal of the "war of nerves." Another example is the old formula "The best way to say nothing is to talk a great deal," a trick used in politics. That conscious trick is based on the wish to please everyone and to avoid losing votes.

To psychoanalysts logorrhea has a special interest because analysts —unjustly, to be sure—are accused by nearly every patient of creat- a sort of "artificial logorrhea" in asking him to use "free associations" during his analytic appointment. The more silent and reticent patients, especially, fight this basic analytic rule, objecting to being transformed into "talkative old women." The real reasons for the resistance to using free association are, of course, completely different. The interesting fact remains that in analysis the therapist is torn by the patient's behavior between the Scylla of loquacity, which he mistakenly offers as "free association" when in reality it is simply his usually garrulity used as resistance, and the Charybdis of silence, which is a form of resistance not too simple to overcome. I have described the latter form of resistance in the paper "On the Resistance Situation: The Patient Is Silent," *The Psychoanalytic Review,* 1938.

One of my patients received the following valentine from her husband:

> The rose is red,
> Vio*lence* is blue.
> You talk too much
> But I love you.

The patient was a woman with oral-masochistic regression who unconsciously repeated consistently in life the situation of the innocently tantalized child whose mother refused her everything. Her behavior was a typical example of the "mechanism of orality." That basically masochistic-pleasure-giving mechanism, as previously pointed out, consists of three parts: unconscious provocation of a refusal, with no conscious knowledge of provoking it; a feeling of being unjustly treated coupled with desire for revenge; self-pity based on the theme "nobody loves me." Of that triad only the feelings of righteous indignation and self-pity are conscious; the provocation and the masochistic pleasure are unconscious.

This patient had severe conflicts in her marriage. She treated her husband as a malicious governess would treat a naughty child. On the other hand, the fact that, despite all his protests, her husband enjoyed that kind of behavior unconsciously was proved by his endurance of that marriage for fifteen years. The neuroses of the marriage partners were complementary. She treated him aggressively, and he reacted consciously with counter-aggression. First he had the feeling of being unjustly treated; then she enjoyed the same sensation since, from her point of view, she acted in self-defense against her husband's "malice." Her own initial provocation was repressed. Unconsciously both marriage partners enjoyed that self-provoked vicious circle, often changing roles in being the initial "aggressor." Consciously, of course, her husband was unhappy over her coldness and constant nagging. He expressed this feeling in his pun "Violence (for Violets) is blue" ("Your violence makes me unhappy"). Had the husband written "I love you because you make me unhappy," he would have expressed his unconscious state of affairs. Consciously, of course, he meant, "I love you despite your making me unhappy."

The husband stressed specifically "You talk too much." Asked to elaborate upon his statement, he made it evident that he did not allude simply to the quantity of words but rather to their application. His wife possessed the never failing ability of choosing from a general situation a detail which she could use maliciously. For example: she forced her husband to spend every Sunday with her mother, though she herself hated her. The poor victim had to drive the whole family to the country, miss his rest, swallow his fury, and, above all, pretend to be very happy. Driving back once with his wife and mother-in-law in the back seat, he used the brakes too forcibly when stopping for a red light, with the result that both mother-in-law and wife received a disagreeable jolt. Instantly his wife disparaged his

The Visual Drive

driving ability. At home she continued the attack. Her husband was furious, though incapable of formulating precisely the reason for his fury, simply complaining that she made a great story of a triviality. What he really meant was that instead of appreciating his sacrifice of the day and his endurance of her mother's company she scolded him for harmlessly slamming his brakes. (That his overforceful use of the brakes constituted in itself an unconscious pseudoaggression, hence provocation, against his wife was not conscious to him.)

Had the man been capable of formulating what he meant precisely he would have said, "I mean by the objection 'You talk too much' the way you maliciously pick out of a situation a detail and magnify it in many offensive words. You are not benevolent. I have a loquacious, malicious, criticizing enemy in my house whose specialty is enlarging harmless details to prove a case against me."

The conclusion so far is: Loquacity contains a pseudoaggressive element in addition to the superficial urge to communicate. Someone might object here that for many persons garrulity is a pleasure in itself, even without the spurious aggressive element. A more precise analysis shows, however, that the aggressive basis is always present.

What is the genesis of this type of logorrhea? No satisfactory answer is offered based on the unconscious reasons for talking. If we consider the well-known statement of W. Wundt that animals do not talk because they have nothing to say, we might come to the conclusion that human beings talk because they have important things to relate. But observation would not confirm that point of view, especially observation of logorrheics. The very few facts concerning talking clinically observed and verified are these: Words are first a gift given via imitation, and later identification, by the child to the mother—even as stool is, in the anal stage, according to the child's conception, a gift to the mother (Freud). To verify that fact one has only to watch a mother praying for every word from her infant. The child denies this gift when he comes to grief with his parent. Analysis of neurotics of the "silent" type proves this fact conclusively. (See my paper "On the Resistance Situation: The Patient Is Silent." loc. cit.) It becomes even more evident in the analysis of the use of obscene words (see no. 18, below).

The problem is complicated by voyeuristic-exhibitionistic elements; one can be used as defense against the other.

Let us apply the assumption that the two parts of the visual drive can be used in defense against each other to the specific problem of logorrhea. We see immediately that the simple explanation that the garrulous person exhibits is insufficient. Garrulity is not only exhibition; it transforms the listener into a voyeur through whom the exhibiting, loquacious person can look at himself (self-voyeurism via identification). Furthermore, garrulity extends the invitation to the listener to exchange confidence for confidence, in other words to perform in return his verbal exhibitionistic act. Therefore it offers also the opportunity of voyeurism of the other person. The problem becomes clearer if we focus our attention on the element of curiosity. Garrulous persons collect material, discuss and try to decipher endlessly the secrets of others. They are in a sense "Peeping Toms."

8. "WRITER'S BLOCK" (PAINTER'S, SCULPTOR'S, COMPOSER'S "BLOCK")

The creative writer, inhibited in his productivity, is the youngest member of the large family of neurotics who seek analytic help. So recent is his advent that analysts have not even arrived at a uniform opinion on the causes of "writer's block," a term which, as far as I know, was introduced into analytic literature and explained genetically by myself, in a long series of studies conducted over twenty years and summarized in my book THE WRITER AND PSYCHOANALYSIS, 1950, (second, enlarged edition: Brunner's Psychiatric Books, New York, 1954; originally 36 cases, now more than doubled.)

As usual, when confronted with something new and untested, like writer's block, analysts' first reaction was to take the simplest way out of a dilemma: application of the already known and tested. The result has been schematized use of phallic and anal interpretations. Since both phases—phallic and anal—can be proved in every human being, the analytic "material" produced by writers in analysis seemed to confirm the gratuitous assumption: "There is nothing new in this."

Unfortunately colleagues proceeding in this fashion have been victims of a fallacy. All artistically creative people are not only orally-masochistically regressed, unconsciously using the more superficial layers as inner defense against those which are more deeply repressed, but they also reveal, within the framework of oral regression, a series of mechanisms characteristic for them and for them *exclusively*. There is also the fact that for the majority of colleagues the term "oral regression" means "I want to get," whereas I believe that this formulation confuses *historic-genetic* development with *clinical* facts, the latter indicating that the contents of oral regression are "I want to be refused." This topic has been elaborated on at length in my book, THE BASIC NEUROSIS.

In my opinion, creative writing represents a successful episode (or series of episodes) in the lifelong "battle of the conscience." This *attempt* at sublimation, achieved in this *"self-curative alibi sickness,"* is, however, *differentiated from other sublimation by three distinct features*.

First, by its temporary and probationary character: whereas in *any* field other than that of the creative artist successful sublimation, once established, guarantees relative contentment, stability, absence of fear of collapse in that specific sector of the personality, the creative writer is haunted by the fear (and even terror) of "drying up."

Second, the painful and depressive struggle which precedes periods of productivity—and which continues even in the process of creation itself, although it is counteracted at that stage by megalomaniacal self-elevation—is absent in other forms of successful sublimation.

Third, lasting and successful sublimation and emotional health are frequently identified analytically; in the case of creative writers the artistic sublimation is an isolated island, entirely surrounded by neuroticism in private life.

Taking the depth of the writer's regression into account, one must marvel—not at his difficulties but rather at the fact that he is capable of sublimation at all, even if it is *temporary and "on probation."* With only slight exaggeration, one could say that the creative writer reminds one of Baron Munchhausen, who claimed to have rescued himself from a shipwreck by holding on to his own pigtails.

The creative writer (and I am talking exclusively about this type) is a *perpetual defendant* standing trial before the tribunal of his superego. The unconscious indictment contains two parts, and reads:

First: "You still want to enjoy, masochistically, the end result of your infantile conflict—to be refused by the image of the pre-oedipal mother."

Second: "You are still an infantile Peeping Tom."

The severe indictment is unconsciously countered by the defendant's unconscious ego, claiming, in a four-point brief (the defense doubles each point):

1. "I am not guilty of being a masochistic glutton for punishment, simply because the alleged provider of disappointments does not even exist: I *myself* out of *myself* and for *myself,* give *myself* beautiful words and ideas. I am the giving mother *and* the recipient child. Isn't it an established principle that there can be no indictment for murder without a corpus delicti? Moreover, I am *autarchic* and live on the basis of the *unification theory.*"

2. "If I am guilty at all, at most I am guilty, not of psychic masochism, as alleged, but of the opposite crime—I am frequently *aggressive.*" (Mechanism of "taking the blame for the lesser crime.")

3. "I'm not guilty because *the whole of humanity is my accomplice.*"

4. "I am not guilty of being a voyeur. On the contrary, I am an *exhibitionist:* by publishing I exhibit."

In my opinion, the work of art, unconsciously, is only the dramatization of these denials and "taking the blame for the lesser crime." Hence, I believe, the writer *never expresses his unconscious wishes directly in his work; only the secondary defenses are represented.* The choice of the "lesser crime" is of course not arbitrary and corresponds to the specific elaboration of more superficial individual infantile conflicts. It is the latter which make for the variety of topics in literature.

To exemplify: Years before his analysis Mr. CC. wrote a novel of moods, centering around a sketchily described affair between a loving girl and a rather depressed man. Suddenly the hero feels that he must leave the girl and wonders about the reasons. He cannot blame the girl. He merely feels, without warning, that he is "through" with her. No feeling is left. There is only a great emptiness, indifference, and the conviction that he is impelled to leave her. In a flash of insight the hero of the narrative understands that he is in-

The Visual Drive

capable of real love. The next instant, however, he represses his understanding and begins to pursue another woman. The reader is left with the impression that the neurotic hero will endlessly repeat the same pattern: imitation love, disappointment without obvious reason, and so on.

During the preparation of this novel Mr. CC. found himself faced with the following conflict: his wife, the victim of a chronic incurable malady, had just suffered another relapse. Although he desired to leave her, he found this plan unacceptable under the tragic circumstances. The marital conflict, however, was in no way connected with his wife's relapses; he had been informed of her illness before their marriage by her family doctor, acting on behalf of her family. The patient showed me the entry made in his diary on the day this revelation was made. It reported the facts and the patient's decision: "I decided to gamble with destiny." This wish to overtrump destiny was a masochistic action of the patient's unconscious and had exactly the results inwardly intended. Every time his wife had to enter a sanitarium for some months—and this happened with regularity—he complained bitterly about the injustice she had done him. That he had unconsciously provoked the entire situation by marrying her was of course not consciously evident to the patient. These complaints about self-created ill luck were supplemented by self-commiseration.

As can be imagined, Mr. CC. did not understand his real conflict. He believed that he stayed with his wife *in spite* of the suffering she caused him. In unconscious reality, he remained with her *because* of this unconsciously self-created and inwardly sought-for unhappiness. Psychic masochists revel in situations of this type.

The hero in Mr. CC.'s novel leaves a woman without any reason for doing so. This is exactly the patient's inner alibi: "If there are men who leave their wives without adequate reasons, I can certainly do it, for I have every justification."

The neurotic hero of the story, therefore, played the part of *appeaser of my patient's conscience*. This also explains why a less important component of his neurosis—his inability to love—was permitted to become conscious, although typically repressed. Actually, Mr. CC.'s main conflict was induced by the opposite wish, which was to remain with his wife despite logical reasons to the contrary, because she gratified his neurotic-masochistic tendencies. His conflict is *seemingly* an aggressive one—to leave or not to leave his wife—and against this reproach of conscience, defenses and alibis are produced. The pseudoaggressive conflict, however, covers the dynamically decisive one: the masochistic wish to suffer. Similarly, the guilt is shifted from the masochistic to the pseudoaggressive problem.

Another subterfuge can be noted, namely the flash of insight revealing that he is incapable of love, hence neurotically ill. The fact that no explanation is given for his inability to love is significant. It denotes an alibi, too. The inexplicable means for the patient: "Neurosis is not under conscious volition, hence I cannot be held responsible."

In this example, we can observe the elaboration of the four points of the inner defense, which were previously enumerated. First, the writer denies his masochistic attachment; his problem is seemingly an aggressive one, whether to leave or not leave the wife (girl). Second, for the shifted "crime," he accepts the guilt, after the principle of "taking the blame for the lesser crime." Third, what becomes visible is the old formula of Hans Sachs, to the effect that by letting the reader or spectator partake of the author's crime via identification and approval, the writer diminishes his own guilt. But the crime for which an accomplice is so desperately sought is but a *substitute* crime. Fourth, the accusation of infantile voyeurism is negated, and exhibitionism, as "lesser crime," substituted. Before the writer can write, he must have a "plot." Products of imagination are but modified aborigines of infantile peeping. By working out the plot, and publishing it, the writer exhibits before the potential reader.

Writer's block sets in the moment the unconscious conscience does not accept, or no longer accepts, the described set of elaborated inner alibis and defenses. If creative writing is a victorious episode in the battle of the conscience, writer's block represents a defeat in that battle, which, although not recorded in history books, is the decisive one in the history of mankind and in the personal history of the individual.

The Visual Drive

There are mainly four hurdles which, either singly or in combination, constitute the impediment to creative writing.

1. The Hurdle of Oral Refusal as Defense

The writer inwardly accomplishes an amazing tour de force: he refutes the accusation of psychic masochistic attachment to the image of the pre-oedipal mother by setting up shop autarchically: "I give *myself*, out of *myself*, to *myself*." If that "magic gesture" within the inner household is challenged, two things happen: a stronger defense is instituted, and the autarchic position is relinquished. The superego's accusation is, "You want to be refused"; the strengthened defense against this accusation reads, "*I* refuse." Thus, refusal of words and ideas sets in, for the purpose of furnishing the defense. But that new alibi makes the writer—sterile. Moreover, by establishing the futile defense of refusal, the writer descends from the autarchic position, falling back into the duality situation, mother-child. And productivity thrives *exclusively* on autarchic grounds.

2. The Hurdle of "Too Little Distance" between Repressed Wish and Defenses

To quote a representative example: Time and again one writer published books in which the action was centered around an exaggerated he-man. Critics objected, declaring that his supermen were lifeless. In his last book he humanized the hero. The result was a best seller, and—writer's block. Humanizing his hero proved too much for the writer—repressed masochistic wish and defense nearly touched, and that in turn forced him, unconsciously, to institute a stronger defense, as described under "the hurdle of oral refusal as defense."

3. The Hurdle of Scopophilia

Successful writing presupposes a *"voyeuristic-exhibitionistic exchange mechanism."* Products of imagination are camouflaged as exhibitionism, as is visible in the sequence of events in creative writing, which begins with the imagined idea and proceeds to the working out of a plot and finally to writing it down, thus exhibiting before the reader. That inner defensive exchange presupposes that the superego has given its blessing to the process, or at least has been hoodwinked into giving consent. If the defensive exchange cannot be accomplished, specific types of writer's block develop. Depending on individual unsolved conflicts originating in early childhood, either the voyeuristic or the exhibitionistic ingredient is affected. The writer may find it impossible to think up a plot (voyeurism), or to work it out on paper (exhibitionism). Modifications are: overemphasis on details, inability to "find the right expression," proceeding to horror at the prospect of even approaching the typewriter.

4. *The Hurdle of Increase of Neurosis*

Oral regression covers a multitude of clinical pictures; in THE BASIC NEUROSIS I enumerated not less than twenty-seven. All have in common masochistic stabilization on the rejection level; what differentiates them is a *specific additional factor*. In blocked writers either previously observable difficulties increase (alcoholism, sometimes homosexuality), or personality difficulties subsumed as "injustice-collecting" sap the whole cathexis.

The four tributaries to writer's block produce the *"grand block."* To be distinguished from the latter is the *"abortive block,"* which lasts only a few weeks and disappears without any treatment. That type is mainly a short-lived depression and inhibition with the identical "ingredients" mentioned above, although in quantitatively minor amounts. "Punishment is one of nature's natural therapies." The depression and despair accompanying the "abortive block" consume the guilt. On the other hand, a series of "abortive blocks" may represent only precursors of the "grand block." It is worth while to mention, also, the fact that "pulp" writers, and writers for the "slick" magazines, are less subject to the "grand block" than "literary" writers. The reason is simple: whether admitted or not, the "writer with the commercial formula" considers his work in some way—degrading. Hence he uses psychic masochism in *dosi refracta*.

In general, one can say that the writer is a slave to his payments of "conscience money," expressed by typical masochistic moods.

Analytically, writer's block has an excellent prognosis; if the above-mentioned mechanisms are applied in the analytic transference and resistance situation, it is possible to remove the block in approxi-

The Visual Drive

mately eight months; the solution of the complicated personality neurosis takes, of course, more time.

Regarding psychoanalytic treatment of writer's block, there are two possibilities. One is that the analyst is familiar with the oral-masochistic substructure of the writer, in which case the patient will be unblocked.

The other is that the analyst is not acquainted with the theory and technique; in this case he will treat the patient as an oedipal-hysterical case. If this happens, the writer-patient will not be damaged; neither will he be changed—for the writing block will persist.

There are two exceptions to this rule. One is that in unusual cases even an incorrect and dynamically ineffective interpretation will result in the writer's becoming *temporarily* unblocked. In these cases the writer projects his own omnipotence upon the analyst in the transference repetition, erroneously assuming that the analyst's "X-ray eyes" will penetrate to his deeper, repressed conflicts. Frightened by that (imagined) possibility, the writer then tentatively sacrifices his symptoms in order to keep his neurosis. This "success because of unconscious fear" has been discussed in Chapter 1 (pp. 54 f.).

The trouble with these spurious successes, which can be achieved in every type of psychotherapy, is the empirical fact that they collapse after some time.

The second exception to the rule is that of the still productive writer (but one on the verge of developing writer's block), who enters analysis because of personality difficulties. Here the writer projects upon the analyst his intrapsychic image of the "bad, devouring mother."

The analyst, misunderstanding what is going on, interprets the oedipal repetition, with the result that facts and interpretation are at odds and the whole analysis goes off at a tangent. The patient plays a diabolical joke on the innocent in the easy chair and at once becomes creatively sterile. I analyzed a first-class writer who had previously been analyzed in this manner; his writing ability was restored (and even improved) in four months.

The conclusions presented here are based on *clinical* analyses of more than seventy writers. I am of the opinion that the time has passed for theoretical discussions of the "guess" type, illustrated by *literary* examples. This was quite appropriate for the first decades of analysis; at that time works of great writers were adduced as tangential evidence, further attesting to the existence of mechanisms which Freudian psychoanalysis had discovered in patients. These applied studies were useful and should not be deprecated; since I myself wrote a book of psychoanalytic biographies (TALLEYRAND-NAPOLEON-STENDHAL-GRABBE, Vienna, 1935) and later published biographical-analytical studies on Heine, Richard Savage, Hart Crane, Ruskin, Millais, et al., these remarks cannot be taken to indicate a deprecatory attitude, per se, on my part. But—and that "but" is decisive—study of *literature* and study of the *clinical case* are not identical. *Nor is circumlocution at its worst identical with solution of a clinical problem.* I seriously believe that *today* no analyst has the legitimate right to talk or write on psychoanalytic studies on literature without paralleling his *literary* examples with *clinical* ones.

A comparison with a rule prevailing in the French Chamber of Deputies is to the point: no deputy was allowed to propose an expenditure without mentioning the source of revenue which would cover it. Mutatis mutandis: it is in my opinion necessary to substantiate *clinically* what one subjectively chooses to promote as theory on writer's creativity. Colleagues who fail to do this railroad themselves into a situation ironically criticized by Freud after listening to a paper by an unproductively theorizing colleague: the paper, said Freud, reminded him of a painting he once saw in Munich's Pinocothek, representing a devil carrying stones to the top of a mountain, while a dignitary in full panoply of office, quite comfortably standing at the very peak, graciously gave his benediction.

The same applies to the problem of *talent*. Writers always want to convince us of their lack of neuroticism. True, their work represents a sublimation, but one built on shaky foundations (probationary sublimation), as stressed above. The convenient excuse that psychoanalysis has nothing to contribute to the problem of talent, since talent has a biological x as basis, is credited to Freud. We can indeed find early statements to that effect, most succinctly expressed in his study on Dostoevsky (1928): "Unfortunately, psychoanalysis must lay down its arms before the problem of the artist." However, a statement of Freud's made two years later (1930) in CIVILIZATION AND ITS DISCONTENTS is gratuitously overlooked. The statement reads:

> Another technique of fighting mental pain uses shifts of libido which our psychic apparatus permits, and which renders its functions so much more elastic. The problem to be solved consists in shifting aims of drives in such a way that these cannot be hit by the outer world. The sublimation of drives lends its help in that endeavor. One achieves the most if one is able to increase, sufficiently, the pleasure stemming from psychic and intellectual work. In this case, Fate can harm that person but little. Contentment of that type, like the *pleasure of the artist in creation,* in the personification of his fantasies, or that of the scientist in the solution of problems and finding of the truth, carries with it a *specific quality which—one day—we will surely be capable of characterizing metapsychologically.* (My translation, my italics.)

Whether or not this quotation proves that Freud's pessimism with respect to the analytic inaccessibility of artistic creation was of a tentative nature becomes immaterial when we remind ourselves that Freud always believed in scientific progress. Hence people who dismiss the problem of elucidation of psychic mechanisms of "talent" through the simple technique of quoting selectively from Freud fail to live up to a basic Freudian tenet, that of scientific progress.

Personally, I believe that we are able to define the biological *and* psychological x which produces the phenomenon "the writer." Biologically it consists of a quantitative *increase of oral tendencies,* including the derivations of orality—voyeurism. These two biological factors do not per se make a writer. In addition there is a specific psychological elaboration: the defensive *"unification" tendency,* denying infantile fancied disappointment experienced at the hands of the pre-oedipal mother by autarchically setting up the "mother-child shop" in oneself and unconsciously claiming that no disappointment could have been experienced since "mother does not even exist." That strange unconscious defense is *encountered exclusively* in the artistically creative person who acts a "magic gesture" on himself and out of himself. Added to this is the previously stressed "voyeuristic-exhibitionistic exchange mechanism."

"Talent" in writers reduces itself to a palpable biopsychological entity. The relation of "talent" to sublimation is this: "talent" is a combination of biological increase of orality and voyeurism, *plus* psychological establishment of the "unification tendency" and the "voyeuristic-exhibitionistic exchange." Sublimation, on the other hand, is the defensive technique of coping with libidinous-aggressive material.[52] The difference in talent in writers can also be formulated: *it corresponds to the amount of compromise the unconscious ego can wrest from the inner conscience.* That amount can be analytically increased—at least in some cases.

"Wresting the maximum from the superego"—meaning ability to establish a defense against the subjugation tendencies of the torturer—also accounts for the fear, encountered in every artist, that he may "dry up." The "fluid" phrase directly denotes the identification of the "flowing" of talent with the lactational precursor.

The artist's main conflict centers about his psychic masochism, acting as a constant "magnet." To avoid the latter, the defense—the creation of the "work of art"—is instituted. The artist's fear of unproductivity denotes fear of being submerged in the maelstrom, no longer capable of rescuing himself by means of his only denial.

Strangely enough, the theory of neurotic writers to the effect that they produce out of normality has recently been taken up by psychiatrists: Karen Horney in a lecture before the Academy of Medicine (triumphantly reported in *Newsweek* of March 20, 1950) and Daniel Schneider in his recent book THE PSYCHOANALYST AND THE ARTIST seem—on that point—to have accepted writers' rationalizations.

Summarizing, we are able today to explain the unconscious process in artistic creativity, hence its metapsychology; we can cure writer's block; we even have a good idea of what constitutes "talent." It is superfluous to state that analytic investigations pertain to the metapsychology of creativity and not to "secondary elaboration." Hence the naive objection of literary critics to the effect that analysis tries to explain the writer's aesthetic abilities with "mammary biting and womb plundering" is sheer ignorance. There is only one point on which we can contribute to the understanding of the *technique* of "secondary elaboration," and that is the writer's overemphasis on finding "the right expression."

It is *phenomenologically* a well-known fact that every writer creates his private hell plastered with "perfect" words. The search for the latter seems of prime importance. Viewed *analytically,* the writer's overestimation of stylistic and verbal artistry is but a by-product in his lifelong "battle of the conscience." Infinite care in finding the "right" word and a constant feeling of guilt because he has not succeeded in "perfectly" expressing the inexpressible are as characteristic for the writer as his exaggerated pride and boasting about precisely these achievements. At bottom, *an unconscious mechanism of shifted guilt is at work: guilt pertaining to the defense of the repressed masochistic problem is shifted to the technicality of expressing the defense.* In this shift the inner problem is magnificently camouflaged, and even more magnificently rationalized—who can object to verbal artistry?

Hence words absorb a great deal of inner guilt, belonging *re vera* to the warded-off problem of psychic masochism. The substitution, of course, is only partially successful—the writer tortures himself, despite his shift, with his verbal substitute. But now he toils on a reality level—and that compensates for much. At least something palpable is substituted as his daily and hourly instrument of torture.

My original deduction in 1950 was based on two decades of work with "blocked" writers; at that time it comprised thirty-six cases. That figure has more than doubled in the intervening years. A number of psychiatric colleagues have made use of the technique, reporting very favorable results. Now, a decade later, I am reaffirming my conviction that writer's block is a psychiatrically curable neurotic difficulty. Only one exception should be noted. Schizoid personalities cannot (on more than a temporary basis) be restored to productivity. In schizoid cases (there have been five among approximately fourscore writers treated) the masochistic regression is so deep that it is beyond repair. The trouble is that the diagnosis of a borderline case between neurosis and psychosis cannot always be made in the beginning. These unhappy people, unaware of the real diagnosis, become bitter and active propagandists against psychiatric treatment.

In purely neurotic cases—which are the great majority—writer's block has an excellent prognosis, provided the mechanisms outlined above are used and worked through for eight to ten months in psychiatric-psychoanalytic treatment.

9. "BLOCK" IN SCIENTIFIC, PHOTOGRAPHIC, JOURNALISTIC ENDEAVORS

The mechanism of "sublimation with renunciation" has already been mentioned in Section II. It consists in rescuing the sublimatory "right" to peep at phenomena and even to use imagination *provided* the alibi is maintained that one did not "create" these phenomena and restricts oneself to observation and deduction. The "responsibility" is that of the observed phenomena or people.

In this category belong scientists, photographers, journalists. Compared with the imaginative and creative writer, sculptor, painter, composer, one could say that the group of scientist, photographer, journalist is—half-creative. It is clear that no derogatory meaning is implied.

Photography is given as a paradigm.

Mr. DD., a once famous, now deceased, French photographer (fractionally analyzed many years ago in Vienna; he had to interrupt treatment repeatedly) went into a state of panic every time he had to attend a gathering or party or deliver a speech or lecture of an informal nature about his special field of endeavor. His explanation that "he had absolutely nothing to say" was easily reduced to absurdity; when it was pointed out that he was obviously better informed on his own subject than his listeners, he had to admit that he "simply couldn't do it." He practically lived in fear of testimonial dinners, lectures, and the like and even of social gatherings.

His analysis brought to the fore a massive layer of exhibitionism, which he could show in *substitution* only: in his work, in his choice of strikingly attractive women, in the splendor of his studio. Personally he was extremely shy, as if apologizing for his mere existence.

He was an inveterate experimentalist, never satisfied with what had already been achieved, always on the lookout for a new slant. This attitude, advantageous for his professional career, made for constant and severe personal unhappiness. It was this self-torture, combined with masochistically self-constructed "woman troubles," that pushed him into sporadic treatment.

When Mr. DD. had to deliver a speech, or even appear in public, his exhibitionism was forced into the open and could no longer be hidden behind a model (*"she* exhibits"), a photograph, or a situation. In short, bereft of his defensive cover, this man was helpless.

Undoubtedly a good deal of his voyeurism was sublimated in his work. How had he been able to convince the inner conscience that infantile peeping was no longer involved, aside from the obvious argument—the deliverance included in social approval (sublimation)?

First of all, what he found most offensive in infantile peeping at others (mother) was the element of passive dependence; whether or not anything would be displayed was another's decision and not his own. In his work he acted out the *active* reversal; he transformed his models into his *creations*.

Second, one could also say that in looking at his artistically "arranged" models he was making use of a subterfuge and actually looking at *himself,* his work! Thus, in a roundabout way, he half re-established the infantile narcissistic position that preceded peeping at others.

The two subterfuges, added to the guilt-resolving sublimation, made it possible for this man to be "all eye." Superimposed on this was the exhibitionistic defense. Here, however, he was confronted with difficulties, for he could exhibit in substitution only. In spite of its superficiality, it was to the exhibitionistic defense that he had fastened his inner guilt. In the usual way, he was fighting his inner battle on a spurious front. He had made the rescue attempt typical for every boy in the visual sphere—"I don't want to peep, I want to display myself"—a denial prompted by the mother's ban on sexual peeping at her. It worked poorly in his case, an outcome that can be explained by his *oral regression*. It seems that the prerequisite for the success of this scopophiliac defense mechanism is the *boy's acceptance of his penis as full narcissistic restitution for the breast envy*. If the shift is not accepted, or is only partly accepted, the child becomes masochistically attached to the enshrined mother image, and his pattern becomes that of masochistic injustice-collecting. As the typical defense, pseudoaggressive mechanisms are brought into play.

In the case of Mr. DD., a series of such mechanisms could be detected. In his work he treated women contemptuously; as a rule he made them into caricatures. For example, he would "deprive" them of their breasts by shooting pictures at an angle that concealed all contours. One of his recollections was particularly revealing. At the age of three and a half, at the beach with his mother, he came out of their cabin stark naked. When his mother told him to cover himself, he obeyed by putting a towel around his neck. Here we still see attempts at compensatory penis exhibitionism, later brought to nothing.

The decisive proof that he was still running away from the disappointing *living* subject for peeping—mother—was found in his poorly developed ability to photograph mass scenes. A "mass" scene for him meant one including more than two people. In photographs of this kind he had to deal with *real* people, whom he could not manipulate at will as he did his models. His elaborate inner hoax, therefore, could not be used to hoodwink conscience, and his work consequently suffered. This was also a clue to his compulsion to "experiment." Hidden behind rational factors was the old reproach: *"Mother* didn't show every part of her body, everything there is to look at." This was shifted to: *"I* haven't created anything new!"

With only slight exaggeration one could say that Mr. DD., although he worked with living people, treated his models as if they were *inanimate objects*. Besides its fear-diminishing effect, amounting almost to negation of his mother's very existence, this expedient also served to correct another childhood disappointment. Instead of infantile *furtive glances* he could now impose on others the *"hold still"* attitude.

It was this amazing string of compensatory narcissistic and pseudoaggressive recompenses that made the man a great photographer.

Curiously enough, there were rare occasions when he did not mind exhibiting—when he would play the witty clown and tell of an amus-

The Visual Drive

ing experience. Here the defense would run: "I'm only joking; don't take me seriously."

Scientific workers are peculiar in that *creative, confirming, and nihilistic types* are distinguishable. It may be a mystery how a scientist can work for decades in his specific field *without* observing or publishing *one* little new phenomenon. This can only be explained by a voyeuristic inhibition. But if someone else comes out with a new idea, the sterile types are immediately vociferous. The "nihilistic type" ignores, rejects, attacks everything new, whereas the "confirming type" confirms, hiding behind the innovator's "responsibility."

Of course this does not speed up scientific progress, but the human element cannot be excluded. As the old saying has it, "That's the way people are."

An amusing example—for posterity, that is—of the nihilistic attitude is a recently disclosed report on how Darwin's theory was received by his colleagues (quoted from the *New York Times* of July 2, 1958):

> London, July 1—Darwin's theory of evolution was nearly overlooked by the British. When the famous paper on the subject was read to the fellows of the Linnaean Society of London one hundred years ago today, Prof. Thomas Bell, the society's president then *ignored it*. In his report for the year he regretted that 1858 had 'not been marked by any of those striking discoveries which at once revolutionize, so to speak, the department of science on which they bear.'
>
> It was a pity, he thought, that no new Bacon, Newton, Wheatstone or Daguerre had arisen among them.
>
> This classic example of what a fellow called 'putting one's foot into posterity' was disclosed to hundreds of famous biologists who gathered in the Linnaean Society's rooms today to honor the name of Charles Darwin and Alfred Russel Wallace on the centenary of the historic announcement.
>
> A plaque commemorating the date was unveiled and a celebration dinner was held in the great Draper's Hall of the City of London tonight. The International Zoological Congress, schedduled to be held here later this month, also is being dedicated to the names of Darwin and Wallace.

Research has shown that Darwin learned that Wallace had written a paper almost exactly the same as his own only twelve days before the two communications, as they still call them, were read at the Linnaean Society.

Darwin developed the theory that nature selected for survival only the fittest during a voyage around the world in the Beagle between 1831 and 1836. During that time he noted that while nearly all the plants and animals seen in the old and new world were different, the larger groups to which the plant and animals belonged were the same. This gave him the idea of evolution, "unfolding" of species from simpler common forebears.

It took him twenty-two years to put his ideas on paper.

Before he finished on June 18, 1858, he received books, papers and a letter from Wallace, who was studying the distribution of species in the Malay Archipelago. The parcel contained an abstract of a theory explaining the evolution of species and their adaptation to environment by a process known as natural selection.

Darwin was startled. In a letter to his friend, the great geologist Sir Charles Lyell, he said that the originality of his ideas had been "smashed" overnight. "I never saw more striking coincidence," he added.

Sir Charles advised him to finish his own paper and present it with Wallace's to the Linnaean Society. Both papers were solemnly read July 1, 1958, by the society's secretary, James J. Bennett.

The public did not react until Darwin published his ideas, with an abundance of examples, in book form in 1859. This was the classic *Origin of Species*. It was sold out the day of publication and raised controversies between emotion and reason that still rage.

One could adduce more recent examples—*en masse.*

10. DEPERSONALIZATION

The theory has already been explained in Section I of the present chapter. Only a few addenda:

Mrs. EE., a Canadian woman of French extraction, aged thirty-six, entered analysis because of severe depersonalization. The symp-

The Visual Drive

tomology was typical; she said she was *"constantly"* suffering from "quite severe feelings of unreality." What was even worse, she was "constantly" frightened "to death" of a "great attack" of the unreality feeling. A "great attack" had been experienced by the patient for the first time ten years before, when she left her husband (after five years of marriage) allegedly to visit France and other foreign countries (attempt at sublimation of voyeurism) and to write a book. In reality she had been unhappy in her marriage; she was frigid, and her discontent had recently been aggravated by the presence of her mother-in-law, who had come for a short visit but had stayed on and on. The attack, which was a state of sheer panic —"I'm losing my mind, am completely unreal, I feel as though I had broken loose from everything, a swimming feeling"—sent her back to her husband a few days after she had left him.

A few months later she again started out to explore foreign countries. She entered upon a friendly relationship with a ship's captain whom she had met on her short-lived first trip. For no apparent reason she returned to her husband six months later, although the attachment to the captain continued for another three years. The break came when the captain insisted that she divorce her husband and marry him.

During the following years she felt only "mildly" depersonalized. However, a year before entering analysis a sudden and "full-fledged" attack had set in. She had been "drinking moderately as usual" one day while reading a dreary English novel about two unhappy spinsters. She got up to turn the radio off and "couldn't believe in the reality of the radio." Her panic lasted half an hour, subsiding slowly, only to return shortly afterwards at the dinner table. Feeling unable to fight off further attacks, she underwent psychotherapy and later spent six months in a sanatorium, where insulin shock and superficial psychotherapy were employed. Finally she started psychoanalytic treatment.

Mrs. EE. described her childhood situation as one in which she was completely dominated by a malicious, irrational, petty, and sponging father. Her mother was submissive to her father's whims. She had only one confidante, her grandmother. She described her grandmother in glowing terms. Her overenthusiasm seemed designed to demote her mother, who had nursed her for only four months and then left her in her grandmother's care for a year while she went to the west coast to take care of the father, who had been taken ill during a trip. The child's intimacy with her grandmother had been interrupted when she was ten years old and the family moved to another part of the country.

Her father's attitude towards her had been one of ridicule, although he was ambitious for her and wanted her to stand first in her class. She disliked him intensely, heaped all her hatred upon him, and finally severed her relationship with the family. At twenty-two she married a young man "with whom she could talk," a "friendly, shy, reticent, understanding, and forgiving person." He had been deeply attached to her and refused the divorce she wanted, condoning her peculiar behavior and her protracted escapade.

Characterologically Mrs. EE. presented the typical picture of an injustice collector. A series of facts in her case history pointed in the direction of *oral regression:* her *drinking,* her being an *inhibited writer,* her *injustice-collecting,* and last but not least, her *blushing.*

In the transference she quickly projected a series of "injustices" on the analyst. She felt "uncomfortable" and constantly looked at her watch as if trying to escape some danger. She refused to produce associations or to use the couch. She viewed both requests as evidence of personal malice on the part of the analyst. To produce associations was "impossible"; to use the couch unwise because there might be a "stronger feeling of unreality when in that position." Her refusals and a dream she had during the first days of analysis made it possible to analyze her exhibitionism. The manifest contents of the dream were: "A *cow* is bleeding from a wound in the side; I *observe* the scene, horrified, from somewhere in the *rear* until a veterinarian comes."

Attention was drawn to the fact that when on the couch she seemingly "exhibited" herself from the rear. Her refusal to associate also corresponded to a defense against exhibitionism ("revealing oneself"); while in the dream she observed the cow from the rear, and the wound also was on the side or back. Why that superabundance of direct or defensive showing of herself and of peeping?

Mrs. EE. could contribute nothing but a conscious recollection. At the age of five she had been taken to the bathroom by her mother and there watched her *father* take a bath. Thus shifting to the father, she said ironically, "Obviously I don't want to allow you all the pleasure." It turned out that her blind hatred of her father had been allowed to pass in her previous treatments; all her troubles were explained as "fixation to the father."

She was shown that her transference was truly a *mother* transference, fastened to the father image later in life. She was also told that she obviously identified herself with the "cow" in the dream. (In another layer, since the cow was the mother, the dreamer was watching her own sadistic-masochistic misconception of sex.) Attention was focused on the sequence of wish and defense—buttocks exhibitionism being warded off with peeping. In her refusal to use the couch, she "prevented" the analyst—*with whom she identified herself*—from being a "voyeur." But this of course pertained to her and not to the physician.

Interestingly enough, the material presented "convinced" the patient. She accepted the exhibitionistic-voyeuristic "exchange." In a long series of "refutation dreams" she defended herself against exhibitionism; these dreams were patterned after the formula "I am on the beach; everybody is naked; I am fully dressed." She protested against only one point; she did not want her weak mother dragged into the "story." She maintained her opinion that the real malefactor in her life was her father and adduced convincing reasons to prove his malice and irrationality. All this, however, was only a secondary shift.

Mrs. EE.'s psychic masochism had been warded off with extensive pseudoaggression. She constantly took the blame for the lesser crime, fastening her guilt to alleged aggressions against her family. That blind guilt, too, had to be discarded, and guilt placed where it intrapsychically belonged: to her psychic masochism.

What was the connection between beating fantasies and depersonalization in this case? The patient had very vague recollections of being beaten by her father. Later the recollections became clearer; she remembered her father using a leather strap, a *cane,* or a broom. Naturally she recalled only the fact that she was beaten and the pain;

the alluring pleasure was fully repressed. A small incident convinced her. Her favorite easy chair was made of woven rattan. She spent all her free time sitting in that chair. She could not explain exactly how that chair (which had previously belonged to her *mother-in-law*) had escaped the frequent "clean sweeps" of old furniture she made when redecorating her apartment. During analysis she toyed with "the unexplainable word ratatouille." After some time she recalled that this "meaningless" word was French slang for "ragout grossier," coarse stew. She pronounced the word "ratatue," which was suggestive of "tuer," the French for "to kill." I asked whether she could possibly have created a synthetic word for "ratan" and "tuer" and inquired if she knew the material from which her father's cane had been made. It had been rattan-bamboo. Thus the word meant: "The beating 'kills' me." In toying with the word, therefore, she was accusing her mother ("bad stew") *and* her father!

Sitting with her buttocks in the chair, she exposed herself to the hated—and loved—rattan-bamboo, and to an undercurrent of associations with Chinese torture techniques and beating methods.

The whole impact of Mrs. EE.'s repressed beating fantasies could be approached—paradoxically—through her erythrophobia. In two papers, published in 1938 and 1948, I have tried to prove that an enlargement of Freud's original formulation (described in his famous paper "A Child Is Being Beaten," GESAMMELTE SCHRIFTEN, V, and COLLECTED PAPERS, II) has become necessary because of Freud's own discovery of the pre-oedipal phase of development. This enlargement, covering the substructure, presumed first that the child's aggression was originally directed against the mother's breast and was only secondarily shifted towards his own buttocks under pressure of guilt—later sexualized guilt. After the "executive" has been shifted from mother to father Freud's original tripartite scheme applies: "My father beats a child whom I hate—I am beaten by my father (repressed)—a father substitute is beating boys."

On the other hand, in erythrophobia the two cheeks unconsciously have the meaning of two breasts; this pre-oedipal structure is later changed, in the oedipal phase, because of the exhibitionistic penis-connotation of the head. The sequence of events is:

The Visual Drive

Layer I, "I want to gaze at (tear, bite) Mother's breast."
Layer II, first superego reproach.
Layer III, (first defense) "I don't want to peep; I exhibit *my* breasts (cheeks, buttocks, later fantasied penis)."
Layer IV, second superego reproach.
Layer V, (second defense) "I am afraid of making a spectacle of myself; I blush."

In blushing, however, both warded-off visual wishes are smuggled in. By blushing the erythrophobe centers attention on himself, thus exhibiting, while in unconscious identification with the spectator he peeps—at himself.

Mrs. EE. used both defensive techniques. She fought the unfinished conflict (originally pertaining to breasts) with cheeks and buttocks. To complicate matters, a scopophiliac problem entered the picture, leading to erythrophobia and depersonalization.

The connection between *beating fantasies,* executed on the buttocks, and *depersonalization,* warding off *exhibitionism of the buttocks,* appeared to be this: In both cases the masochistic battle was fought on foreign territory, with the buttocks substituting for the breasts. The unconscious identification of breasts and buttocks (a well-known phenomenon repeatedly described by different authors, especially in dream symbolism) was of major importance to Mrs. EE. because, as a child, she had exhibited her breast-buttocks as a means of negating her lack of breasts—one of the possessions her mother had and she missed. The buttocks exhibitionism, therefore, was in itself a defense. It was also used as a *masochistic* invitation to be beaten.

It seems that in cases in which beating fantasies are combined with extensive scopophiliac tendencies depersonalization is used as a typical defense mechanism.

The combination of beating fantasies and exhibitionism also explains why Mrs. EE. so readily remembered the scene in which she watched her father take a bath. In this convenient recollection the guilt was shifted; not she but her father exhibited! She did not peep; her mother forced her to look!

We see in this patient a long series of desperate attempts to shift both the scene of the original conflict and its dramatis personae. The scene is shifted from the breasts to the buttocks, the conflict with her mother is transferred to her father. But it was precisely her pre-oedipal fixation that prevented the normal and full-fledged development of the Oedipus complex, which in her case was always imbued with pre-oedipal connotations. In her choice of husband she proceeded on the defensive level, marrying a kind, rather passive man in order to disprove her masochistic wish to be tortured. Even normal activity in a man was feared by the patient; every activity was identified (unconsciously, of course) with being pushed into the passive-masochistic position. Therefore she could not divorce her husband although she was dissatisfied with him in many respects. Therefore she refused to marry the captain, although their "mutual understanding" was "perfect."

In her depersonalization she partially succeeded in escaping the too dangerous territory of the breasts, since she denied their loss by exhibiting her buttocks. The blame was thus taken for the lesser crime—*exhibitionism substituting for the masochistic wish to be beaten.* (Even in the full-fledged perversion masochism the specific wished-for torture is only an attenuation of one of the seven ingredients of the "baby fears.") It was interesting that the external factor that presumably led up to the second "great attack" was the "unreality of the radio." As mentioned before, she was turning the radio off when the attack set in and made her doubt the radio's "reality." The unconscious reason was: *she* had *willfully* silenced the harmless announcer's voice; therefore action should follow. Transposed to the infantile situation; father stops shouting and starts beating. At precisely the moment when the buttocks should be exposed, depersonalization set in.

Her first attack had been preceded by a similar situation. She had just escaped a *woman's* tyranny (the mother-in-law who had overstayed her welcome), but the attack of depersonalization brought her back *in four days!* The "slave rebellion" was of short duration. The allure of mistreatment and exhibitionistic substitutes proved too strong.

The Visual Drive

All these desperate attempts to escape the original conflict with the pre-oedipal mother, and to disguise it by inner shifts, proved ineffective. In certain areas of the patient's personality even the secondary shift to her father did not work: in *drinking,* in her *writer's block,* in *injustice-collecting,* and in *blushing.*

Mrs. EE.'s drinking represented both a pseudoaggression against her mother *and* a self-damaging, masochistically tinged self-destructive attitude.

The deep *oral-passive*-masochistic attachment to the image of the pre-oedipal mother had been unconsciously fought by Mrs. EE. via two other *pseudoaggressive* and *autarchic* means: a predilection for cooking and attempts to write. She was an excellent and discerning cook, thus counteracting both culinary dependence on the mother and the reproach that she had been served poor food (see her pun on uneatable stew, "ratatouille"). On that battlefront she was both ingenious and successful. The other, the sublimated culinary battlefront—writing—was a more or less losing proposition. She had no great difficulty in imagining a plot (voyeurism). Her difficulty was with the writing and the working out (exhibitionism). She did manage to write a few stories, in fact a whole book, for children and adolescents. Here her cherished magic gesture entered the picture defensively: "I am showing you how I wanted to be treated—kindly."

It was also interesting that the "fear of being drained" (the reversal of her own draining tendencies) was very pronounced. She rationalized her retirement from her family by saying that her parents would sponge on her and take money from her husband.

Finally, her fear of being *"at any moment"* and *"without warning"* subjected to an "attack of unreality" found its simple explanation in her father's unpredictability in his beating procedures!

A piquant detail in the case history of this patient should be mentioned. After the connection between buttocks exhibitionism and beating fantasies had been clinically established in her case, she confessed: "The moment you mentioned buttocks exhibitionism I thought 'It must have some relation to Father's beatings'." "Why didn't you say so?" "Well, this was months ago!" That is paradigmatic for the "help" patients give us!

11. STAGE FRIGHT

A rather strange fact is to be recorded in the psychology of acting: popular and psychoanalytic interpretations coincide. This seems highly suspicious. Generally these two "explanations" are at odds, and the discrepancy contributes a good deal to the popular misconception that analysis is a science of spite and sophism, concerned only with confusing the layman. In the case of acting, however, the macroscopic view seems identical with the microscopic one. True enough, analysis uses more "highbrow" words in explanation, but when reduced to plain English both popular consent and analytic "interpretation" agree that the actor bubbles over with exhibitionism, this being the alleged basis of his talent and calling. Both agree that the actor is a show-off and a "ham."

The question arises: Is popular opinion so perspicacious or is the accepted analytic opinion so naive? I believe the latter.

First of all, acting represents a sublimation. Now a sublimation is a highly complex phenomenon in which the original repressed wish never comes directly to the fore. Quite the opposite; what appears as the "end product" is the result of a series of psychic detours, compromises, counter-compromises, achieved in the course of the "battle of the conscience." In my opinion, what is sublimated is neither the original id wish nor the defense against the id wish but the *defense against the defense against a conflict originating historically in an id wish.* In other words, sublimation is not the child but the grandchild of the original conflict—a grandchild made unrecognizable by plastic surgery to boot. Hence everyone who sees in sublimation a direct expression of repressed tendencies is as far off the beam as the man who confuses the grandchild, beautified by plastic surgery, with, let's say, the grandfather's brother.

The "five layers" in sublimation are: layer I, *end result* of an infantile *pregenital* and *libidinized* conflict; layer II, first superego reproach and veto; layer III, first defense of the unconscious ego; layer IV, rejection of the defense, second veto by the superego; layer V, second defense of the unconscious ego, irrefutable because couched in terms of what is socially approved and accepted.

The power behind this victory over the superego is derived from

The Visual Drive

the sublimator's *inner aggression*. Hence neurotics are poor sublimators simply because the distribution of aggression is unfavorable; nearly the whole aggression is concentrated in the superego, which uses it to flog the ego. In health, or in artificially produced health (successful analysis), the balance of power is different and the ego has (or gets) a good-sized amount of aggression, used now for two purposes: to fight the "battle of the conscience" more successfully and to achieve reality aims involved in the individual's fight for his place in the sun.

In the case of the actor the sequence of events is this. (First stated in "On Acting and Stage Fright," *The Psychiatric Quarterly*, 23:2, 1949.) His (her) wish entering sublimation is *not at all exhibitionism* but a modified end product of the opposite tendency, *voyeurism* (peeping). I have stressed repeatedly that one part of the visual instinct can be used as defense against the other. This is true despite the fact that voyeurism alone is (in my opinion) a derivative of an original drive and exhibitionism only a defense; after the establishment of both, one is used as defense against the other.

The material entering layer I of the actor's (or actress's) sublimation is *not* the "original" voyeurism. There is agreement in the literature that voyeurism is first narcissistic self-voyeurism. Only secondarily are other objects included in voyeurism. Hence the voyeurism of layer I ("I want to peep at mother's breast, body—later father's penis") is already a concession to reality—forbidding narcissistic concentration on oneself. This bears out the previous statement that the material entering sublimation is *not* a direct id wish.

Schematized, the actor's sublimation in acting shows, in slow motion under the analytic miscroscope, these five layers:

Layer I, "I want to be a voyeur of mother, father (later of intimacies between them)."
Layer II (first superego veto), "You have no right to peep at mother, father."
Layer III (first defense of unconscious ego), "I am not a voyeur or interested in being one; I want to exhibit my body."
Layer IV (second superego veto), "Transgression of educational commands by exhibitionism is forbidden too."

Layer V (second defense of the unconscious ego), "I am neither aggressive in exhibitionism nor am I a voyeur. I want to be a good boy (girl), be social-minded and give other people pleasure." This fifth layer, and *only* the fifth layer, is sublimation.

Compare the naivete of previous explanations concerning exhibitionism with this conclusion: the actor's behavior as a "ham" is *defensive*. He is, unconsciously, glad to attract attention to that fact (even to the point of being ridiculous) because exhibitionism is his inner shield and defense against the deeper repressed voyeurism. He gladly takes, again unconsciously, the "blame for the lesser crime."

What does the actor rescue of his earlier wishes? He wanted to be a voyeur; he got as a "bargain"—exhibitionism. That substitutive pleasure has, however, a slight saving grace. We know from Freud that every exhibitionist unconsciously enjoys double pleasure. Besides the direct exhibitionistic one a voyeuristic pleasure is also achieved by unconscious identification with the spectator. Through his voyeurism he peeps at himself.

One contradiction remains. How is it possible that the sublimation of acting includes remnants of the original wish *preceding* even layer I, that is, *narcissistic self-peeping?* This never happens in sublimation. Still, here it seems to happen. The contradiction is spurious, as the following discussion proves. It is true that the actor looks, by way of unconscious identification with the spectator, at himself. *But the actor does not represent himself but rather the part he acts.* Thus his peeping in substitution (via the spectator) is *not* self-voyeurism but rather peeping at others.

This ties in with the genetic aspects of the problem. In the childhood of *all* male and female actors whom I have analyzed (in the original publication, 1949, a dozen were mentioned, a figure since doubled) one specific situation was present. Although the evidence is too small to generalize, it is large enough to suspect more than a chance occurrence. *This situation involved peeping at some sexual scene which left these children so guilty and bewildered that they diminished their guilt by concluding "all this is not real but a play."* Instead of escaping into depersonalization, they escaped into active

The Visual Drive

repetition of the passively experienced "unreal." *The unreal—the guilt-diminishing alibi—became the guiding pattern.* Even that was not enough; the alibi was reinforced by exhibitionism, which was substituted for the original peeping *at others.*

This explains the usual "unproductivity" of actors. They don't create the characters they impersonate, they just act them. The alibi means: "The author is guilty, not I." The productivity of the actor shows up only in the re-creation (and there is originality in different versions) of a character. Still, the re-creation allows the actor to appear not guilty vis-a-vis his inner conscience: "Others did it."

There is irony in the statement that "for the actor the world of make-believe is real." The irony is that behind this "game" is the whole panic of the child who rescued himself from an *"unbelievable"* terror, experienced in peeping, into the devaluation of a "play." In my opinion, no analysis of a stage-fright-stricken actor is complete and secure from repeated later re-emergence of the symptoms without working out that infantile voyeuristic terror. This means that at least the "cover memories" must be retrieved.

To cite an instance. An actress had been caught by her mother when she was a child of three and a half peeping through the keyhole at the intimacies of a couple, guests of her parents. The mother severely reprimanded the child, who, after recoiling, answered, "Why, what's wrong? I just wanted to see how *they* played—don't you look at *my* play with stone blocks?" Of course a secondary "cover memory" is involved; the original voyeuristic scenes go back to the oral stage, which can be reconstructed only from oral fears.

We are seldom in a position to state *specifically* in a particular type of endeavor what *specific* situations forced its members into that *specific* self-chosen profession. In the case of actors, however, we are, I suspect, capable of doing just that. Two specific experiences and their appropriate elaborations are encountered: increased voyeurism of the child confronted with a specific voyeuristic experience has a traumatic effect. To counteract that effect the observed scene is declared "unreal." That "unreality," which has been passively experienced, is later actively repeated, making the little peeper into a big exhibitionist with the inner alibi, "I am not guilty."

When does stage fright set in? *Every* actor has a good-sized package of it to bear. Superficially the fear pertains to exhibitionism, to forgetting his lines, being "stuck," making a fool of himself. Deeper analysis proves that this is a superficial mirage and a defense.

Experience with all types of fear-sufferers has convinced me that *neurotic* fear pertains exclusively to *psychic masochism*.[53] Under pressure of a veto of conscience an intrapsychic sleight of hand is executed by the intrapsychic "lawyer," the unconscious ego, to help his "client in distress." The *guilt* is accepted, but for the "lesser crime," *pseudoaggression;* and the *scene is shifted outside*. Hence the neurotic fear-sufferer behaves as if he were guilty of "aggression" and the danger were outside. All this, of course, is "manipulated" without his conscious knowledge.

We see that the stage-fright neurotic is seemingly afraid of exhibitionistic dangers; basically of *exhibiting* defeat (forgetting lines, making a fool of himself, etc.). Now in the table of sublimation we see that exhibitionism in acting corresponds to layer III, the first aggressive defense. It is, therefore, quite appropriate that, if the "retaliation" of the superego sets in in neurosis, the ego tries to fight this battle not in the inner fortress but on the outer walls—on the remote line of defense. This is what actually happens!

In other words, by taking the blame for *pseudoaggression* the main danger is avoided, the need to account for psychic masochism, the "mortal danger."

What lies at the bottom of these masochistic fears can only be discovered if one has some knowledge of infantile fears. The whole "septet of baby fears" can be mobilized: fear of being starved, devoured, poisoned, choked, chopped to pieces, drained, castrated.

All this sounds more or less farfetched. However, it corresponds with clinical facts. I once analyzed an inhibited radio actor, Mr. FF., who was afraid to face the microphone. He had given up his profession, worked at an underpaid position in a different field and was indirectly forced by his wife to enter analysis. It turned out that the flight from the microphone was preceded by flight from the stage. The patient had started his career as a stage actor and switched because of neurotic, not realistic, reasons to radio. In the theater he had developed pathologic stage fright and was afraid of forgetting his lines. Allegedly to avoid that danger he entered the radio field, where parts can be read. He dreaded the advent of television, where the advantage would be lost. Many elements in his neurosis—besides the obvious scopophiliac ones—pointed in the direction of oral regression; these cannot be mentioned for reasons of discretion. For present purposes two statements made by Mr. FF. are important. The first was a recollection pertaining to the beginning of his stage fright, or rather a flash of an "impression," as he called it—still important enough to be repressed. The thought was this: "It occurred to me one night while on stage and waiting for my cue that if one looks at the two galleries in the dark, they remind one of an open mouth ready to 'swallow you up'." The other statement, this time not repressed, was a description of learning a part during that phase of analysis in which he was able to take up his radio career once more. Said Mr. FF.: "While studying my part I had the impression that somebody wanted to force something down my throat and I resisted violently." He did not connect that observation with the fact that "digesting" his part was his "bread and butter," *forced* upon him by the "cruel" analyst in the transference repetition.

The shaky basis of the actor's sublimation explains why *every* actor and actress suffers under at least traces of stage fright. The actor (of whichever sex) is *one of the most "scary"* people to be encountered in any profession. Even his defensive exhibitionism is performed *incognito;* he has never fully recovered from his infantile terror and is *never sure whether his inner conscience will accept the defensive hoax.* Hence the frequent allegation against actors that they "have no personality," that they are "empty bags" that can be molded into any shape via hysterical identification, is unjustified. The constant hiding behind someone else's "personality" is their main inner defense. The fact that they are capable of reassuring themselves by "incognito exhibitionism" is a rather heroic example of whistling in the dark, or more precisely, in the dim stage light. Even the peeping situation is re-enacted in reverse: the spectators are in the dark as the peeping child was once upon a baby time. Hence the guilt is shifted: "Others, not I, peep."

Acting and stage fright have been, in my opinion, incorrectly interpreted as referring both to exhibitionism and to oedipal castration. Not less faulty are, again in my opinion, the interpretations pertaining to three typical occurrences in the lives of some actors of both sexes: their homosexuality, their masochistic marriages, and their psychopathic trends. All three are orally conditioned. Especially grotesque is the constant flight into divorce and "affairs." As with all psychic masochists who live under "public supervision," the masochistic actor and actress get themselves into greater trouble this way than by the stage fright that is their "private hell."

12. BOREDOM (ALYSOSIS)

Boredom, declared Casanova bitterly in his old age, is that part of hell that Dante forgot to describe in THE DIVINE COMEDY. Boredom is not simply a disagreeable mood; it is an emotional experience that tends to threaten the psychic balance of the individual. It is a universal phenomenon, in spite of the comparatively few complaints about it. Most people suffer boredom silently; it is by their hectic and almost always futile search for "fun" that they betray its presence. This constant search for fun characteristic of so many people is the inner protective device against the constant danger of boredom.

The aftereffects and by-products of boredom are dissatisfaction, emptiness, inability to concentrate on either work or pleasure, restlessness, or its converse, impassivity. These manifestations are comparatively superficial; a deeper danger is also present. Boredom may result in the feeling that all one's endeavors, attachments, and aims are senseless, and this feeling that all is meaningless merges with an intense and terrified loneliness. In not too severe cases the promptness of the automatic though temporary recovery is in direct ratio to the intensity of one's inner loneliness.

Generally speaking, boredom is an interim feeling, disagreeable enough but harmless and transitory. But a quantitative increase may render it unmanageable, and it then becomes a disease entity. I have a very personal relationship with this disease; I was the first to describe it genetically and to name it in my study, "On the Disease Entity Boredom ('Alysosis') and Its Psychopathology," *The Psychiatric Quarterly*, 19:38-51, 1945.

Boredom consists, at bottom, of absence of pleasure, but what people understand by pleasure is, of course, as variable as their particular wishes, defense mechanisms, and neurotic reactions. Everyone must find some specific remedy for the potential danger of boredom.

The opposite of boredom is the concentration of interest upon a particular field. The intensity of this interest will of course lessen at certain times, but even the layman realizes that the surgeon feels a continuing interest in his surgery, the historian in his research into the medieval period, the ship captain in navigation. In general, however, people make a very precise distinction between work and fun. The ideal situation, it goes without saying, is one in which work is also fun. Expressed scientifically, the more completely one's work serves for the sublimation of unconscious defense mechanisms, the more pleasurable one's life is. But for the majority of people, unhappily, work is only some kind of hardship, essential in order to provide a livelihood but good for no other purpose.

There are two types of sufferers from boredom, the complainers and the disguisers. The complainers are wistful and hungry-eyed; they seem to be appealing to all comers to lift them up out of the Slough of Despond. After a short time they give up hope; your remarks have been of no use, and they sink back into disgusted silence. Nothing appeals to the complainer or distracts him; he is helplessly sulky and permanently unresponsive.

The disguisers are the fun-hunters already mentioned.

The openly bored are an infinitesimal minority in the huge army of the dull. The large majority are not recognizable in their true colors without the key. Phenomenologically, they seem to suffer from an utterly dissimilar disease. They are restless and constantly on the go; they behave as if they would be penalized for sitting down and relaxing for more than a minute. They seem to be driven by some inner whip. Their slogan is "Let's have fun," but every variety of fun they propose is found wanting and is quickly dropped for a substitute brand. None of their chosen antidotes to boredom works; the only result is agitated funlessness.

What is "fun?"

Fun is an extremely personal feeling of well-being produced by concentrating psychic energy on a freely chosen, usually extracurricular endeavor. Fun is the classical antidote against the constant danger signal of boredom. A well-balanced, *fun-loving and fun-experi-*

encing person, therefore, is one who has found his particular and temporarily effective palliative against boredom. Under normal conditions the connection between boredom and fun is parallel to that between being hungry and eating one's favorite dish.

The choice of one's particular brand of fun is dictated by unconscious motives; the individual is, of course, unaware of these reasons. This factor is visible indirectly in the universally supercilious attitude towards somebody else's notion of fun:

> This world is a difficult world indeed,
> And people are hard to suit,
> And the man who plays on the violin
> Is a bore to the man with the flute.
> (Walter Learned, "Consolation")

Following the rule "where logic ends, the unconscious takes over," we can guess that the intolerant rejection of all brands of fun except one's own is in some way linked to the inner battle that preceded establishment of the temporary boredom antidote. The first impression is that the ironic rejection of the other fellow's antidote reflects the ironic rejection pronounced by one's own superego against one's own fun. That inner rejection is subsequently projected outward.

What do people use as antidotes to boredom? *Fantasy, hobbies, entertainment, work.* The first two are self-created; the others make use of external factors, pressing them into service as sources of "fun." Of these four, fantasy and hobbies are the most important.

Fantasy has first priority because people are limited in the time they can devote to their hobbies. Since most people find work a disagreeable duty they sugarcoat their working hours with fantasies. A hobby is a self-created diversion which, for unconscious reasons, becomes the rallying point for many unconscious defense mechanisms.

In my opinion, boredom is always associated with three inner disturbances. It is based on a triad consisting of weak or frangible sublimations, inner inhibition of voyeurism, and defense against the accusation of masochistic pleasure.

1. *Weak sublimations.* In all cases of inability to create sublimation, or where sublimation is weak, the individual's store of aggression

is out of the ego's reach and is taken over by the superego for use against the ego. Psychic masochism—the unconscious ego's counter-action—is the result.

Where sublimation is merely weak or unstable, boredom represents the unconscious ego's defense against the intermediary phase of the superego's attack. That attack is always the aftermath of conscious defeat, and it shakes the very foundation of sublimation. The superego seizes on external defeats as torture material and then attacks. The attack is not powerful enough to destroy the sublimation, but it does succeed in making the sublimation temporarily unworkable. This interim period has a surface manifestation: the conscious boredom that is the unconscious ego's defense.

2. *Voyeurism.* Fantasy, which is imagination in free flight, is a product of the visual instinct. It is therefore logical to expect boredom in persons having a neurotic inhibition of fantasy (and consequently of voyeurism). Observation proves that such neurotics are the most frequent sufferers from boredom. The reason for the inhibition of voyeurism is to be found in its unconscious connection with pre-oedipal and oedipal fantasies.

3. *Defense against superego reproaches of psychic masochism: Boredom is a desperate preventive measure on the part of the frightened ego; it anticipates a superego raid.* Zoology reports a comparable phenomenon, called autotomy. If an animal's leg is caught in a trap, the animal will sacrifice the leg in order to save its life. The psychic dilemma of boredom implies that the ego is weak and the superego is strong. When there is successfully maintained sublimation, on the other hand, we know that the unconscious ego has been strong enough to best the superego, for the superego is the enemy of sublimation. Aggression in that particular personality, therefore, is not concentrated exclusively in the torture chambers of the inner conscience.

This fact can be clinically observed: the psychic health or illness of a person can also be measured in the stability or instability of his sublimations. This is by no means the only yardstick; the others are the individual's adaptation to reality, his sex life, and his general contentment. (The wording "sex life" is not meant to describe only the functioning ability of the sexual apparatus; it also means the ability to love *tenderly*.)

Aside from all its other attributes, neurosis is a notable consumer of psychic energy, drawing energy away from normal depositories. Hobbies that were once enjoyed become meaningless and tiresome. The mood in general deteriorates, and depression, dissatisfaction, and inner insecurity become patent. The individual's emotional life is centered on his neurotic unrest, and the symptoms, including diminution or lack of sexual interest, become widespread. The mechanical ability to work, however, is usually preserved.

In discussing the problem of work one must distinguish between *enforced* and *self-chosen* occupations or professions. There is a difference between the man who lackadaisically went into his father's business because it "made sense" and the man who "always" wanted to be a mechanical engineer and worked his way doggedly through college in order to become one. The unconscious reasons of the man who makes sacrifices to achieve his goal, or who at least knows it and cannot be swerved from it, are analytically clear; although he is not aware of it his self-chosen profession satisfies, in sublimated form, unconscious defense mechanisms covering deep inner wishes.

Work plays a decisive role in the psychic economy. It is the normal repository of unconscious guilt and unconscious psychic masochism. By paying ransom in the form of work the typical person pays his debt to his inner conscience. Since no one is free of this inner dualism the punitive connotation of work is immensely valuable. The connotation of work as punishment is a well-known phenomenon analytically (Jekels, Reik), and it has been intuitively known to mankind since time immemorial. In Genesis we are told that Adam and Eve, expelled from Eden, were compelled to work as punishment.

There is a strange paradox in the effect of neurosis upon one's working ability: *the more pleasurable work has been in "normality," the more promptly it is absorbed in the neurotic process*. The ability to work at a job to which one is indifferent is maintained for a longer period because of its greater admixture of the punitive quality.

Boredom represents an unconscious defense mechanism created by the unconscious ego under pressure of a frantic superego attack. *It is a preventive method of proving 'I'm a good boy.' The method*

The Visual Drive

consists in clearing all dangerous and incriminating material out of the psychic chambers, leaving them empty. It is like the familiar mystery-story ruse—the corpse is removed before the police arrive. But the bored person goes a step further; he denies, so to speak, that the premises could have anything at all in them, even at some future date. He is the good boy on a promissory note.

Having unconsciously furnished his alibi of innocence, the bored person becomes obstinate in a peculiar way; he refuses every substitute for the pleasure he has renounced. His behavior, in this layer, is like that of the child who has been forbidden a particular activity. Substitutes are suggested but are sulkily ignored; nothing can amuse him now.

In *inner* reality he does not want to be amused at all. Having submitted fully to the tyranny of the superego, he stages an ironic comeback in the form of a miniature slave revolt. Self-assertion becomes essential, and it is accomplished by reverting to infantile megalomania, where the ego's place is in the center of the universe and the outer world plays the role of court fool, providing amusement. Reality having been demoted, all the substitute pleasures that reality could provide are rejected. It is as if the educational authorities of the past were being reduced to absurdity.

There are two types of reaction in boredom, as O. Fenichel observed (without explaining). These are the motoric or fidgety reaction and the immobile. The existence of these varied reactions becomes understandable when one remembers that every neurotic libidinal drive is inwardly warded off with pseudoaggressive tendencies and every neurotic pseudoaggressive tendency by a libidinal one. A passive-masochistic inner conflict that is warded off by pseudoaggression results in surface hyperactivity; surface immobility and passivity result from an inner aggressive conflict.

The type of boredom is therefore a direct clue to the underlying forces that are being warded off.

There are three groups of neurotics who are largely immune to boredom. These are obsessional neurotics, hypochondriacs, and depersonalized persons. Consciously these sick people are always worried; they concentrate all their attention on their obsessions (compulsions), imaginary diseases, and disturbances of perception, respectively. They are so rarely troubled with boredom because in all these neuroses *voyeurism remains undisturbed*. A good dose of unrestricted imagination is the prerequisite for the worrier; it is familiar to hear the worried person enumerate a list of possible dangers that would never occur to an unworried person in the same situation.

The visual instinct, as stated before, comprising inner voyeurism and inner defensive exhibitionism, seems to be of major importance in preventing boredom. Everyone indulges in fantasies at certain times; if these fantasies do not interfere with action they are good antidotes to boredom. It is only when fantasy takes so predominant a place, quantitatively, that it becomes a substitute for normal action that one can speak of it as a neurotic sign, like the fantasies observable in neurotics. Imagining action, in fantasy, is a prerequisite for normal action. "Thinking is rehearsal of action" (Freud).

One is therefore prepared to expect that in persons having a neurotic inhibition of fantasy (genetically, of voyeurism) boredom will appear more frequently than in others. This expectation is borne out by observable facts.

I am adducing a clinical case:

Mr. GG., of Dutch extraction and aristocratic descent, was an example of a bored man who was also a bore. His wealthy father was a hobby-scholar who specialized in Roman history and was fond of preaching to his family; his mother, an easily excitable person, irrational in her educational methods, at times oversolicitous about her only child's welfare, at other times entirely preoccupied with herself.

The child was left a good deal alone, developing at an early age a detached and taciturn attitude. He felt "empty," unhappy, resented his parents' interference and their "preaching." He also objected to any affectionate contact with them and especially detested the family custom that required him to kiss both parents before going to bed. "I never could understand the pleasure people get out of kissing," he commented. Although his attitude towards his parents' mode of life was one of revulsion, he accepted—and even exaggerated—their code of medieval honor, based on the tradition of illustrious an-

The Visual Drive

cestors, in which "honor" was the greatest of all virtues and cowardice "the most detestable of vices."

At school Mr. GG. had been an inattentive pupil, except for a short period during adolescence when he became interested in history. At that time he wrote a pamphlet attacking all historical writing. This scorn of his hobby was resented by his father, who was also rather startled when the boy suddenly shifted from "intellectualism" to single-minded devotion to "sport and nothing." The boy became a swimming champion; the "nothing" department referred to his boredom and boresomeness, both of which became so pronounced that they could no longer be overlooked. The boy himself finally became aware of being "inwardly dead." His long silences, when he realized them, appalled him, and he consoled himself with biographies of strong and silent heroes like Lord Kitchener. His life was empty; even swimming competitions bored him, and he lost the championship by becoming convinced that he would lose.

After a few years of aimless travel he became a reserve officer in the Netherlands army, was captured by the Nazis, and spent four years in a prison camp. This tragic interlude, surprisingly enough, made very little impression on him beyond that of monotony—but this was no change from his previous life. It was actually less boring, for he was occupied with an anxiety: dwelling on his combat fears, he asked himself why he was personally so inadequate—was he a coward? After the war the old boredom and boresomeness continued. He tried travel again and came to the United States.

In his analysis it became obvious that he was well aware of being a bore. In a detached way he complained about not being able to hold a person's interest but rarely about his boredom, even though he knew only two mental processes: worry about being a coward and "deadly boredom." He could not even depend on his anxiety to prevent boredom: "When I worry for some time I get bored."

The man had virtually no daydreams with pleasurable content. "I have no imagination for anything unreal. On the other hand, my imagination plays havoc with me about my disagreeable past. I don't just relive situations in which I acted like a coward, I build in stories that never happened."

For a considerable time his analysis made little headway. With his inner cuirass of coldness, the experience of the analytic situation was a mere intellectual exercise. His high I.Q. made for speedy understanding of the masochistic components of his personality, but there the matter rested. His own complaints bored him, his life history was quickly exhausted, his dreams never remembered. He began to ask me when I would lose patience with him, saying—not without reason—that no fee could compensate for enduring his atmosphere of boredom.

One day he remarked—still in his matter-of-fact tone—"You seem to have a much better time with other patients. I've often observed you laughing with another patient as you both left the appointment room. That never happens with us."

"Don't you see that your complaint is an echo of your childhood? True, you now make the complaint unemotionally, but in your childhood the missing emotion must have been present. It is not visible now, so it must be repressed."

"You are wrong there. I suffered from too much, not too little attention. I resented my parents' constant interference."

"That's what you consciously remember. You resented all the preaching, teaching, scolding, and exhortation you got from both parents, because you felt—obviously without justification—that their only interest in you was to mold you according to their principles."

"What's wrong with that?"

"The point is what you felt about it. You constructed the fantasy of being unloved and became masochistically attached to it."

"How can you prove my resentment? I accepted their standards on honor and cowardice. Didn't you say so?"

"I didn't. What I claimed was that your inner conscience took up their medieval tradition because it could be used for purposes of torture. You took these unattainable precepts and tortured yourself with them for forty years. It isn't even true that you accepted your parents' slightly antiquated ideas. You exaggerated these ideas and made them into a caricature just so you could reduce the code to absurdity."

"I still don't see any connection with my deadly boredom."

"These facts point conclusively to the direct connection between your resentment and your boresomeness. In being a bore you are perpetuating the irony directed at your parents' preaching attitude. You take over the role of bore that they played by preaching to excess."

"If I could laugh I would do it now. You are making the fantastic claim that I—the greatest bore in the world—am playing a diabolical joke on my parents."

"You are. But the joke is on you. You are damaging yourself."

A few days later Mr. GG. said slightly ironically, "You pigeonholed the question of my being a bore. What about my boredom? Don't forget that."

"Are you aware that you just used a dash of that precious commodity: irony? Be careful; next time you are liable to laugh and disturb nature's predetermined course! Speaking seriously, your boredom comes from a combination of three ingredients. First is your superabundant psychic masochism. The second ingredient is equally important, your lack of imagination. You must have been a Peeping Tom as a child—all children are. Your conscience is incessantly accusing you of peeping, and therefore you don't dare use your imagination for pleasant fantasies. Your imagination is productive only when you torture yourself with pictures pertaining to what you call cowardice."

"I have no recollection of being a peeper at all."

"That proves nothing. Don't forget that recollections conveniently preserve inner alibis. Let's take, for example, your aversion to kissing. Don't you think it possible that your aversion was preceded by —the opposite?"

"I doubt that. I cannot imagine finding any pleasure in that occupation. I consider the Eskimo nose-rubbing no more senseless."

"You forget that you had no experience with nose-rubbing in your childhood, though you had some experience with kissing. Didn't you say that your mother alternated between too much affection and complete coldness?"

"Are you going to tell me again that I am acting out her attitude—her coldness?"

"Perhaps. To return to your peeping. There is another proof at hand—indirect but very impressive. It ties up with the third prerequisite for boredom—shaky sublimation. Did it ever occur to you that the only sublimation you ever approached was swimming? Otherwise you weren't interested in anything. And don't you exhibit when swimming? With your body, your skill, your movements? We know that exhibitionism is only an inner defense against peeping."

"But then why didn't I shift my exhibitionism to something else when I got too old—and, as you claim, too masochistic—for swimming competitions?"

"That's exactly the point. As your neurosis [54] progressed, the defensive alibi of exhibitionism was rejected more and more."

"A good point, if true. How can you prove it?"

"Very simply. After you lost the championship you traveled through many countries and visited famous places all over the globe. Look at your meager exploits. All the beauties of a tour round the world were lost on you—because of your peeping inhibition!"

In his specific inner tour de force the bored person exercises his internal Frankenstein's monster, the unconscious conscience, by compromising with his inner inhibitions. In a situation of acute danger this may seem a good solution; on a long-term basis the solution itself becomes dangerous. As James Russell Lowell said, "Compromise makes a good umbrella but a poor roof."

The alibi of boredom is dangerous from the standpoint of the internal economy; nobody can thrive on a diet exclusively composed of "being a good boy." That is the expedient of the bored person, but he soon finds that libidinous admixtures are necessary, even for his meager meals.

It is true that his life is not so completely stripped of pleasure as it seems at first glance. Since he is a psychic masochist he derives unconscious pleasure from his conscious displeasure. Consciously he is unaware of this; consciously he is entirely miserable.

Here are a few descriptive statements from bored people:

Mr. HH.: Boredom is rather tragicomic, and still I consider it one of the most painful experiences. At first I feel ashamed of being bored—as if it were some personal deficiency. Here I am—a person who considers himself intelligent—and still I can't feel any interest in anything. I've tried everything to counteract an attack of boredom:

The Visual Drive

reading, listening to the radio, eating, drinking, even sex. All in vain. The only thing that helps, stupid as it may be, is running to a movie; it doesn't matter if I like or dislike that particular type of movie; it doesn't matter if I've seen the movie before. And when I'm in the movie, I sit there in some sort of a daze. I don't concentrate on the action on the screen, and I don't care. But looking, just stupidly staring, helps a little, at least."

Mr II.: "I get the creeps when I think about an attack of boredom. I classify them—big and small attacks The first kind takes a whole day; the mild ones last from half an hour to two hours. My big attacks are really something. *I am not exactly paralyzed, but in effect I am.* For all practical intents and purposes I am—dead. I cannot move. I have no energy at all. My head is empty. I am always reminded, afterwards, of the medieval Spanish king who, because of his religious fanaticism, spent one hour every day in his future coffin. I cannot describe the feeling precisely. I feel helplessly alone, like I was propelled into some strange planet, cut off from every living soul. It is like a full-dress rehearsal of death: utter desolation, utter loneliness, utter nothingness."

Mrs. JJ.: *"I am two people in one:* an efficient publicity director and a *bored idiot.* The 'bored idiot' part of me comes on me unexpectedly, like fever. When it hits me I'm no good for anything: dull, incapable of thinking or listening—even to jokes. I leave the office, go on a buying spree—and then return the clothes and hats I buy, because *even my taste deteriorates.* Finally I give that up too—go home, mope, and suffer. Would you believe that even three Martinis don't pep me up?"

I have analyzed a long series of *bores,* and I am convinced that the chronic bore is unconsciously acting out a very complicated game. Unconsciously he is making use of a mechanism that is a subdivision of the negative magic gesture. He is demonstrating, via caricature, a masochistic complaint directed at the main educator of his childhood. In effect he is saying to that educator: *"My behavior will show you how you bored me."* And he proceeds to dramatize the boring actions and attitudes of the authority in his past (see the case history above). Of course, only an overdimensional psychic masochist can go to such lengths of self-damage in order to exact revenge for the wrongs done him in the past. The bore's demonstration —"See what you did to me!"—is too little and too late for revenge, but not for self-damage.

Why is the reaction to a bore frequently one of antipathy, sometimes bordering on fury? Clearly this can only be answered by studying the furious reaction itself.

Again the key to the problem is the inner conscience. The person so easily provoked to fury prides himself on not being a bore and can even prove his contention by means of witnesses who esteem him precisely because he is "good company" and "has a sense of humor." But his own superego is not among these applauding listeners. On the contrary, it points ironically at the bore who is so intolerantly rejected and says, "That's you—at times."

When boredom is both recurrent and quantitatively pronounced, it represents a neurotic disease. The general public is largely unaware that this disease exists and that it can be psychoanalytically cured. There is no reason to assume that dissemination of this knowledge can be achieved either easily or with celerity, nor is it likely that such dissemination would induce many bored people, or bores, to undertake treatment. Both types have in their psychic make-up a good dose of psychic masochism, and psychic masochists unconsciously want to suffer.

To venture a guess, I would say that the much maligned, "stupid" bore will consult the psychiatrist of the future more frequently than the "highbrow" bored person. Regardless of whether the bore admits the fact or camouflages it successfully, he feels that he is "inwardly dead." Moreover, the bore is a nuisance to his environment, while the bored is only a nuisance to himself.

13. "NEGATIVE EXHIBITIONISM"

Exhibitionism, as it is generally encountered, consists of a parade of achievements, abilities, talents, or works, to which the typical spectator reacts with approval, admiration, anger, or envy. But there also exists a form of exhibitionism which produces contempt in the spectator. In this "negative exhibitionism," the exhibitor

The Visual Drive

flaunts typically hidden material: words, actions, organs, traits which are disagreeable, disgusting, painful. The spectator's disapproval is often strongly colored with revulsion and anger; at his most charitable, he condemns the exhibitor's "bad taste." [55]

The language possesses no word to describe negative exhibitionism, although the phenomenon is familiar enough to be covered by a stock phrase: "He made a disagreeable spectacle of himself."

One could dismiss the problem by pointing out that negative exhibitionism is obviously a product of self-damaging, or even masochistic tendencies within the individual. This is certainly true; yet there is more to the problem. If psychic masochism were its full and complete explanation, the matter of specificity—why the specific person uses this specific outlet—would remain an unsolved question.

A person who has undergone a colostomy and is left with an artificial intestinal opening; a person with an amputated leg, a deep postoperative scar, or a disfiguring wound, will not typically exhibit his mutilation to a stranger. A negative exhibitionist does exactly that.

In my opinion, the problem hinges on "taking the blame for the *lesser* intrapsychic crime." When the defendant is accused by his inner conscience of a major crime, he admits to a lesser offense. And in the cases of negative exhibitionism I have observed, the lesser crime was exhibitionism, and the greater crime which was being warded off was—*peeping* (voyeurism).

One could put forward the objection that exhibitionism frequently contains a contradiction: the organ exhibited may seem "beautiful" or reassuring to the exhibitionist and disgusting or fear-inspiring to the involuntary spectator. That is certainly partially true in phallic exhibitionism in men; in superficial layers such exhibitionism serves as reassurance against castration fears. It is also true that in the double identification always present in all exhibitionistic and voyeuristic acts (Freud), the frightened female child to whom the adult male exposes himself has to feel—in the perpetrator's active repetition of passively endured experiences—his own repressed fears. Finally, it is also known that some hysterical women use exhibition of "ugliness" of the castrated genitals as an active castrating revenge fantasy directed against the allegedly privileged male.

All these very superficial derivatives of deeper conflicts touch only tangentially on the real state of affairs. What is frequently described in our literature as "nakedness as a means of inspiring terror" is a late *pseudo*aggressive (not "sadistic," as is assumed) elaboration of earlier conflicts.

In negative exhibitionism the conflicts are *pre-oedipal,* not oedipal; the pronounced phallic castration fears are but faint reverberations of the pre-oedipal *"septet of baby fears"* (see Chapter 1).

It is also characteristic of negative exhibitionism that a peculiar compulsion to exhibit masochistically exists and that this compulsion arises *exclusively in connection with voyeuristic conflicts.* Moreover, the purpose of the defensive negative exhibitionism is not "sadistic"; the intention is to provide a masochistic, accusatory demonstration of an injustice-collecting type: *"Look what bad Mother did to me!"* As the final act, a weak superficial *pseudoaggressive* defense is installed: the involuntary spectator is made to suffer.

To adduce clinical material:

Mrs. KK. was a painter in her late twenties, a West European on a prolonged visit to this country. She entered analysis because of personality conflicts: all of her attachments, marital and otherwise, were of the "suffering type," and consistently disappointing. She had originally concluded that "all men are nuts," but as time went on (and she was exposed to the influence of analyzed acquaintances) she began to suspect that her own cooperation in choosing disappointing men was a matter which "could not be excluded." Analysis showed that she was an exquisite injustice collector, an orally regressed psychic masochist.

In the course of her analysis a problem connected with her painting came up. She had switched from the abstract to the realistic school of painting, a turn which had alienated many of her old friends. As "hypermoderns," they now considered her "an artistic traitor." The suspicion arose that this change of style had some connection with unsolved voyeuristic vicissitudes: more and more, responsibility was being shifted from imagination to the copying of reality.

The patient dreamed of a promiscuous girl exhibiting her breasts. Some material concerning her own voyeurism came out, though she al-

The Visual Drive

ways stressed her inhibition in the exhibitionistic sphere. She dressed tastelessly, left her hair messy, and was sloppy in general. She now made some concessions and began to pay more attention to her appearance. Then came a continuation of the "breast dream," as she called it.

This time the exhibiting girl appeared again, but she was blind. The dreamer herself was a spectator, attired in a new dress which "somebody" had bought her. This dress was extremely revealing, since it consisted mostly of—interstices and left many places on the body uncovered. It was clear from the start that the patient acted all three roles in the dream; she was the exhibiting girl, the peeping girl, and the spectator. Her real intrapsychic crime was peeping; the defense was exhibitionism, and, in addition to taking the blame for the latter crime, she defended herself by demonstrating, in the dream, that "somebody" had forced her to exhibit.

The important detail in the dream is the fact that the girl is punished for her voyeurism: she is blind. Of course, the dream girl did not peep, but exhibited; she—the patient—peeped. In a projective shift, the girl (meaning herself) is blind.

At first glance, the strong hints of negative exhibitionism in this case give the impression of guilt because of overdimensional exhibitionism. This impression is misleading. In every *secondary* defense of a neurotic conflict guilt is accepted for the "substitute crime" in order to conceal the real crime. When warding off voyeurism via exhibitionism, penance has to be paid for the substitute crime as well. This has been pointed out in Chapter 1.

That voyeurism (masochistically misused) was at the bottom of the patient's negative exhibitionism could be proved to her after she reported what she called "a fantastic incident." She had been working on the portrait of a young man who was an unimportant acquaintance. This young man, the neurotic husband of a friend, had been rather flattered by her request that he sit for her and had not asked for payment. During one sitting the patient was seized by "an irresistible impulse" to tell him about her most recent problem: having gone through a prolonged period of vaginal discharge caused by trichomonas infection, she had now discovered "bumps in the vagina" which frightened her. (Subsequently an experienced gynecologist pronounced the status of her vagina to be normal.) Making due allowances for the Bohemian tone of her environment, the admission the patient made to her model can only be classed as negative exhibitionism.

In analyzing the incident the obvious connotations were all examined and excluded: she was not in the least interested in the fellow, who was immature, uninteresting, and incidentally "bisexual"; she was not projecting an oedipal rivalry conflict pertaining to her female friend; she was not acting out her penis envy by castrating the male. There was reason to believe that the scene could have involved "anyone who happened to be around at the moment." It simply did not pertain to any specific person: it was a defense against the crime of voyeurism, executed—while painting a portrait from life—via a *negative* exhibitionistic act.

Of course, one could ask why she had not instead drawn attention to her painting, which would have been "nice exhibitionism," as the patient called positive exhibitionism. Obviously the masochistic element had intervened, to be only slightly warded off secondarily with a weak display of pseudoaggression, since she could expect the young man to be "disgusted." As it happened, he was not: his interests were exclusively concentrated on his conflict with his wife, his homosexuality, and his over-drinking.

A journalist in his forties was in analysis because of persistent writer's block. He had come to me after two years of psychiatric therapy with a young female psychotherapist; this course of treatment ended abruptly after he had, as he expressed it, "a tragic experience with myself." This was his deposition: "One day last week, completely out of the blue, I felt the imperative urge to exhibit my sex organ before the bewildered and rather indignant woman. I jumped from the couch, exhibited, felt very contrite. I cannot understand myself. I never exhibited in this manner before; I never even had this perverse urge before. It's just crazy, plain crazy."

The patient's "diagnosis" was confirmed by the therapist, who, in a telephone conversation with me, regretted not having spotted the "schizophrenic." It is superfluous to mention that the man was not a schizophrenic. What happened was that the voyeuristic-masochistic tendencies were not touched, and as a result the exhibitionistic-pseudoaggressive defense was inwardly emphasized. The proof is that his writing block was subsequently removed.

The third group of phenomena to be adduced as exemplification grows out of jealousy (see no. 7, above). What tortures the jealous person most is his constant imagining of the beloved person in a love scene with the rival. There is the initial tendency to conceal this feeling; later on, the exhibitionistic defense sets in. From this develops the urge to parade the injustice done him, apparently in an appeal for commiseration and as a means of mobilizing the anger of outsiders against the unjust partner. Once more, voyeurism is warded off with *negative* exhibitionism—the cuckold does not cut a heroic figure.

In the *"triad of negative exhibitionism"* these partes constituentes are discernible in unconscious microscopy:

1. A pre-oedipal voyeuristic conflict is warded off with defensive exhibitionism.
2. A masochistic demonstration is presented of the pre-oedipal mother's "cruelty," with the ego on the receiving end.
3. A secondary, very superficial though also unconscious, pseudo-aggressive defense is made by forcing the spectator to suffer, or at least by arousing his disgust.

14. "THINKING BLOCK"

Today it is more or less acknowledged that thinking is trial action, as Freud suspected. For trial action imagination is required—again one lands in the territory of the rarefied visual drive.

Though the process per se that constitutes thinking is by no means clarified, the use of thinking for the execution of various inner defenses is better known.

Combining irony with megalomania in his typical manner, George Bernard Shaw once said: "Few people think more than two or three times a year; I have made an international reputation for myself by thinking once or twice a week." This superficially effective statement stresses the quantity of one's thoughts and sorely underestimates the matter of their quality. Topping the fallacy is the implied assumption that deep thinking automatically produces profound results.

Somewhere, too, the aphorism seems to include the idea that if only the inertia that prevents thinking could be overcome, thinking per se would result in objective evaluation of objective facts. This idea is totally at variance with clinical evidence. The individual's typical thoughts are by no means regulated by such elevated principles. William James came very near to the facts when he defined the thinking of a great many people as a "rearranging of prejudices." There is wisdom, too, in Wolcott Gibbs's bland comment: "He wasn't exactly hostile to facts but he was apathetic about them." Facts as facts make little impression on the psychic apparatus.

Thinking is a *mental form of digestion:* we "digest a problem," "absorb a thought," get the "first *taste*" of a difficulty, as the language has it. This mental work does not start without an initial impetus: just as hunger is the signal for the intake of food, *discomfort at the failure to understand a problem or to master it starts the thinking machine going.*

"Discomfort" is the outward manifestation. In inner reality, what is felt is—*fear.* This fear is a revival of the infantile situation in which everything new was felt as a threat. To counteract the threat, a "solution" of the problem presented by the new situation had to be found —and it always was found. It is true that the "solution" was as far from the facts as a technical engineer's description of a motor would be from that of a three-year-old's. But any explanation—and this includes a wrong one—is better than no explanation at all.

Early in life the child learns the trick: answers must be found. *The advantage of having alleviated fear compensates for the incorrect interpretation.* The vehicle used in finding these "answers" is called thinking.

The fear that lurks behind "overwhelming external problems" is paralleled by another impelling force. In order to keep one's "peace of mind," the constant avalanche of internal reproaches emanating from the unconscious conscience (the superego) must be silenced; *everyone, therefore, lives on the basis of his specific pet defenses.* These defenses are secondarily cloaked in "rationalizations." A good deal of "thinking" is expended on bolstering these rationalizations, and it is visible in "prejudices" and "considered opinions."

Thus, "objective" thinking is *mortgaged* beforehand by two inner

The Visual Drive

necessities, which together head the unconscious priority list: whatever is "mysterious" or cannot be understood must be "explained" by hook or by crook; rationalizations, covering the specific inner defense mechanism of the specific individual, have to be supplied, also by hook or by crook.

All this presupposes knowledge of the fantastic severity of the inner conscience. The inner torturer uses every riddle or unsolved problem as the basis for a reproach: "If you weren't such a passive weakling, you would know the answer." The reproach may be quite unjustified, but that is no deterrent, for the superego is a "torture machine" (see Chapter 1).

The twin fears to be alleviated—question not answered, rationalizations not thought out—absorb an enormous part of the sum total of our thinking. A pitiful remnant remains to be used for other purposes.

Analyzing these other purposes, one finds that much of the thinking commonly classed as "objective" is still serving subjective aims. E.g., it is an accepted theory that thinking is the precursor of action. But actions are under the influence of *inner* necessities. Constructing a daydream or a fantasy or dwelling on a hope would be expressing an inner defense. Reading a book, watching a movie or television drama, would be a means of renouncing one's own thinking and substituting another's; there is a temporary identification with the other person's thought. It is known that the reader and listener is interested only if the problem dealt with corresponds to his own inner defenses. Moreover, even in thoughts centering around one's business and profession, these seemingly objective evaluations include a good deal of subjective matter. For the choice of one's profession was unconsciously determined, or (if an enforced or chance occupation is involved) inner defenses have been smuggled in.

Finally, all exaggerated and fearful preoccupation with what the future will bring, all dreary expectations, however disguised as interest in the local or international political scene, represent in some neurotics highly subjective masochistic problems.

What James so aptly called "rearranging of prejudices" disguised as thinking is but the *necessary exchange of defense mechanisms.*

Defense mechanisms wear out and become unacceptable to the tribunal of conscience; they must then be retired for a time and substitutes used.

Since the propelling reasons for the substitution are unknown to the afflicted person, he is consciously going through a long siege of "thinking." The irony of the situation is that his "thinking" has little to do with—thinking.

Mr. LL., a scientist, was bitterly biased against what he called "bitchy females." He claimed that he had acquired this antipathy during his marriage to a termagant. In this marriage, he declared, he had been the innocent victim of his wife's malice. He did not, of course, realize that he had chosen her—unconsciously on purpose —because he had "solved" his own infantile conflict with an overdose of psychic masochism. After a divorce from his wife, he went through a prolonged period in which he brooded about the evil disposition of the genus Woman. A few years later he unexpectedly reversed his thinking and began to discover that women possessed some pleasant traits. According to him, this was purely the result of "thought processes." "One has to be objective," he explained. He then married a woman whom he classified as "nice." Nevertheless, his skilful provocations soon turned her too into "a bitch of the first order." In his desperation he entered analysis.

It soon became apparent that his "change of heart" and his opinions about women had little to do with thought processes. Since he was unconsciously stabilized on the rejection level, he had needed all the humiliation and defeat he got from his first wife. Since he was not consciously aware of the "pleasure-in-displeasure pattern," he considered himself an innocent victim of outside malice, and through deep "thinking" built up a "philosophy" that fitted in with his alibi. This state of affairs remained unchanged—as long as conscience permitted. His superego, being wise to the trick, constantly and unpleasantly reminded him of his real situation. When the repeated reproaches became a danger, the unconscious ego had to switch from the old defense to a new one. This switch accounted for the sudden and incomprehensible emergence of the theory of the "nice woman." Two defensive aims were thereby fulfilled. Conscience was temporarily appeased, and an old hope materialized in a new disguise; for by making sure to choose a new wife who could be provoked into cruelty, the old diet of masochistically enjoyed humiliation would eventually be restored. In effect, the ego said: "You claim that there are nice women; fine, I'll show you that they are all alike." The superficial defenses were exchanged, but the basis remained unaltered.

In court a lawyer asking an inadmissible question often yields to the judge's adverse ruling, not by giving up his line of attack, but by rephrasing the question. The same procedure is followed before the intrapsychic judge. This "rephrasing of defenses" has its conscious reverberation in specific types of "thinking." Since the process is fully unconscious in its origin and reasons, we typically leap to extremes in order to bestow either credit or blame. On the one hand, "objective thinking" is courted and elevated to *primum movens,* and the person involved pats himself on the shoulder for the "broad-mindedness" he has achieved through thinking; on the other hand, the malefactor is held to be relatively inexperienced with thought processes: "The art of thinking," mused H. L. Mencken, "is too recent an acquirement of man for him to exercise it continuously, or with anything resembling genuine virtuosity."

15. LACK OF IMAGINATION IN PERCEIVNG EXTERNAL PHENOMENA AND LACK OF "BUSINESS ACUMEN"

"I haven't got a good head for business," is the excuse of every failure. "I just didn't grasp the opportunity that presented itself—I did not foresee the consequences," is another such statement, applying to *all* possible situations, intra and extra commerciam.

One can best study the phenomenon by observing a pathological type—the "success hunter." [56]

The "success hunter," who clinically, of course, is not identical with the typical business man, is characterized by:

1. Contempt for moderate earnings, high-pitched ambitions, and exaggerated ideas of success, combined with a drive to overwork.

2. Constant inner tension, stemming from inner passivity, regardless of the importance of the stakes.

3. A propelling impetus towards more and more success.

4. Dissatisfaction and boredom if deprived of new business excitement and resulting opportunities to show off.

5. Cynical outlook, hypersensitivity, and hypersuspiciousness.

6. Contempt for and ruthlessness towards the unsuccessful.

7. One-sided and opinionated I-know-better attitude in general.

8. Hypochondriacal worries; doubts concerning continuous flow of ideas and luck.

9. Inability to enjoy the simple pleasures of life.

10. Hidden depression, warded off with tempered megalomania and an extensive air of importance.

The success hunter in the guise of big business man is generally admired for his quick grasp of an advantage, his energy, and his mysterious affinity for luck. He is the fairy-tale hero in modern dress.

Examined psychiatrically, the story of success looks somewhat different. To begin with, success does not commence at the moment of the brilliant idea, voyeuristically conceived. Its foundations were laid in early childhood, when the end result of the infantile conflict was definitely established. This end result, in the specific case of the success hunter, is one of great inner passivity counteracted by great inner reproach occasioned by precisely that passivity.

Inner passivity plus inner reproach spells double inner conflict. The lifelong struggle with this double conflict forces the success hunter to take defensive measures: he will establish, unconsciously, a strong alibi to disprove the inner accusation. The alibi—aggression of the compensatory variety—in future will cause people to admire his energy, iron will, and consistency.

The psychic structure of the successful man differs in no way from that of the timid failure; the two struggle with an identical conflict. The difference between them is that the former *masters the defensive aggression and the latter cannot.*

An anecdote is told about one of Napoleon's generals, a man undistinguished for intelligence, who once, out of dire necessity, came up with a really brilliant idea. Napoleon was holding, before one of his campaigns, an important council of war, and for hours no one had been allowed to leave the council room for any purpose. The hitherto rather dull general, who suffered from prostate trouble and

The Visual Drive

was in urgent need of relieving himself, finally could bear it no longer —and in this dangerously pressing situation suddenly presented to Napoleon a brilliant strategic idea, thus ending the council. Napoleon was thoroughly baffled. "And I always considered him an idiot!" he remarked to his adjutant.

Substitute for the general's prostate pressure the pressure of conscience because of inner passivity and you have the genesis of the brilliant ideas in the success hunter. A not very romantic simile, but a true one. With amazing regularity I have found that the real and decisive conception of *the* great venture, the great thought or plan in this type, came after *a long spell of depression and dissatisfaction with relative lack of success. The "intuition" coincided with that moment when pangs of torturing conscience were at the high point.* The brilliant idea represented the desperate alibi.

It is interesting to observe that there is a general misconception about big business men of the success-hunting variety. Their superior mental capacity is greatly overrated. True, quickness was there when the brilliant idea was conceived, but the point here is that it was neither a conscious nor a purely intellectual process. Quite the contrary. Under the *terrific inner pressure of guilt* the last resources were mobilized, as in the case of the Napoleonic general.

What of the follow-through process in business? In this process the superior intelligence is not discernible; it is, for the most part, a banal process, following specific, long established paths. Only outsiders take this banal part of the venture as a miracle. Even business people, the serious insiders, don't brag about it.

General opinion holds that success consists of a combination of two factors—personal initiative and impersonal luck. True, the successful man exaggerates the importance of the first ingredient and the unsuccessful that of the second. If one is to believe the man at the pinnacle of success, he is reaping the rewards of productive ideas that have come to him in a "brilliant flash." The unsuccessful citizen, however, will say that such a man was simply lucky.

Stressing the element of luck and thus minimizing the part played by personal merit is the revenge of the failure. Mark Twain perfectly expressed this sour-grapes attitude in his ironic formula, "All you need in life are ignorance and confidence, and then success is sure."

The old quarrel over the quantitative admixture of merit and luck in success overlooks a *third* and decisive factor. That factor, the *absence of inner obstacles to success,* has never been stressed and could only be completely understood with the advent of modern psychiatry. Neurotic disturbance of the third and decisive part of the triad of success results in the prevention of shrewd evaluation of external possibilities, of consistency in following through, and even, in many cases, of the very emergence of the "brilliant idea" at the right moment.

It might be assumed that the person seeking success wishes himself well and hopes wholeheartedly for the attainment of the goal. Unfortunately the assumption would be false, since there exists in the human psyche a deterring element that works to prevent success. This self-retarding element is unconscious, hence not under conscious control. Call it what you will—unconscious self-damage, gluttony for punishment, or psychic masochism—this third element has been proved, by clinical experience, to be responsible for the majority of failures.

There is, understandably, a tremendous resistance to the idea that one harbors within him a strong tendency to self-damage. Confronted with failure, people in general follow a set pattern of excuses: their competitors are cruel, ruthless, mean; or times are hard. They themselves are unlucky, even jinxed. Everything from cut-throat competition, through unfortunate external circumstances, to impersonal fate is mobilized in defense. Everyone and everything is accused—except one's own self-damaging tendencies.

Let us examine one of the more common excuses for failure, human malice. This can be disposed of speedily—it is not a valid excuse. People *are* often malicious, cruel, merciless. They may be, where self-interest in involved, after another man's scalp. But that man, when he complains of the scalping, is confessing to a remarkable miscalculation: why wasn't he prepared for such a possibility? What reason had he to believe that competitors, or even uninvolved onlookers, would give him a helping hand? Harsh though it may

The Visual Drive

sound, the realistic fact is that in the business world the precept "act decently and others will be decent too" rarely applies.

Every adult over twenty who has not acquired some conception of the darker side of human nature is automatically *suspect of cultivating naivete for the purpose of being disappointed*. It is a common masochistic trick to take an overoptimistic attitude towards others in spite of past experience having proved such an attitude unjustified. In this way the glutton for inner punishment prepares for himself a greater disappointment, and then when he has got what he was after—a kick in the jaw—he whimpers that in this rotten world you just have to expect the worst, a condition which he implies is completely foreign to his benevolent nature.

It is not my intention to negate the quality of human decency. Decency exists; it is by no means an illusion. But the neurotic conscience of many people is elastic enough to permit them to behave ruthlessly and without consideration for others. It is necessary to face that fact and to recognize the situation in which one's own consideration will not be reciprocated. Psychological insight in human contact is not a luxury but a necessity.

The facts of success and failure cannot be ignored. They enter inevitably into everyone's judgment of himself and others. But the yardstick of the average man, who in simplifying and pigeonholing phenomena is warding off the threat of complications from things he does not understand and people he cannot fathom, leads to wrong conclusions.

What are the guideposts for judging success and failure? Was Hitler a success or a failure? A failure, obviously. But for years this paranoiacal gangster appeared to be a great success. The answer lies in the fact that true success contains an element of *stability*. Hitler's goal was world domination; what he achieved was utter destitution for the master race.

What about such men as Capone and Dillinger? Each had a certain initial success in amassing money and power. Apart from the moral issues involved, the Prohibition outlaws were failures; true success, in addition to denoting something of stability, is never in jeopardy through the *taking of chances that endanger an integral part of a plan.* At the height of their success these gangsters took just such chances—and lost.

After long years of failure some men achieve a week-end success, only to lose by some stupid mistake all they have won and to return to obscurity and poverty. Others, after repeated success, fail temporarily, later recouping. Success can only be judged by taking a *cross section of a man's life.*

No one thinks it strange that in times of deep economic depression even the gifted person is temporarily down. Nor is there anything odd in the fact that a man cannot become chief engineer of an atom plant without a specialized knowledge of technical engineering. In judging success and failure we must *consider a man's opportunities.*

The epitaph of the man who has worked himself to death in his efforts to amass wealth might be: "The fool! What did he get out of life?" When one utters this familiar judgment one is using the yardstick of *inner contentment.* Success means more than fame or money in the bank; it must not impair life's normal contentment, nor, for that matter, life itself. The pleasures of the average person are relatively solid and correspond to modifications of his real unconscious wishes.

Psychic masochists have many seemingly different ways of coping with their inner problem, but most of these are unproductive and may be lumped under the heading of "injustice-collecting." Of the few productive solutions, one is the at least externally successful solution of the success hunter. He is demoniacally driven to the creation of his particular defense mechanism against the reproach of inner conscience pertaining to masochistic passivity. This inner defense results in success. But he pays a terrific price for his self-cure. Often it seems a case of the remedy being worse than the disease, though this, of course, is not always visible at the surface level.

"I'm glad I entered anaiysis *after* I'd achieved business success," remarked a clever patient of mine. "Otherwise, I'm afraid I'd never be able to pay your fee. Without my neurotic defense I would be a fifty-dollar-a-week clerk."

"You are mistaken," I said. "Assuming you had entered analysis because of your potency disturbances fifteen years ago, you would

The Visual Drive

have been cured of that trouble and still have achieved your success in business."

"Aren't you contradicting yourself? If the driving power behind success-hunting is inner passivity, as you claim—the same passivity that caused my potency troubles—then by curing me you would have made me at the same time a failure in business."

"That is a spurious conclusion. You forget that your business success could constitute a *normal* sublimation of passivity. The *neurotic* passivity, deposited in your potency disturbance, could have been eliminated and the remnants of passivity used productively in business."

"How do you differentiate between neurotic and sublimated passivity?"

"You will admit that a man who is impotent does not have public backing—he is, in fact, a slightly ridiculous figure. The successful business man *has* public backing and admiration. Both your impotence and your business success are based on passivity warded off with activity, but one deposition is made under pressure of guilt and the other is not."

"I feel it's a trick—though I admit I don't see where the trick lies."

"There is no trick. Take clinical experience as a guide: every analyst can pride himself on the fact that *some* of his patients achieved great success in their specific fields *after* successful analysis. If your assumption were correct that fact would be inexplicable. You're forgetting that every man fights a lifelong battle with passivity. The problem is one of *productive and unproductive self-damaging depositions in defense.*"

"I'm still sceptical. I believe it's safer to achieve success first and then analyze the 'remnants' of passivity. It's like the story of the man who went to Europe by ship in preference to taking a plane. In a plane, he said, you're a little *too* much in God's hands."

"How would you explain, then, the fact that men who previously were failures in business have become remarkably successful after analysis?"

"I don't know. Anyhow, this is a pointless discussion because if the patient weren't already a success he couldn't afford the analyst's fee."

"Your constant stressing of the fee shows your passivity; you feel overwhelmed and defend yourself by a persistent attack."

Happiness and the exaggerated search for success are frequently incompatible. The inner guilt that was the original impelling force is insatiable. Success means short-lived elation followed inevitably by worry, tension, and uncertainty; nothing is ever enough; there must always be more and more money, fame, power. If the success hunter's reasoning powers tell him that he ought to be satisfied with what he has achieved he becomes bored. He looks frantically for new ventures, new outlets, sometimes to settle for hypochondria, latent depression, or aggravation of an organic disease. This type of inner passivity is so great that the success hunter cannot even die peacefully. He cannot accept illness with the stoicism and resignation of the average person; even on his deathbed he is tortured by the inner reproach that if he were not a weakling this couldn't happen to him.

16. TEMPER TANTRUMS

Temper tantrums are by no means *exhibitionistic* displays of "terrific aggression," but of exactly the opposite, of helpless masochism warded off with pseudoaggression. The moment one is familiar with the mechanism of "taking the blame for the lesser intrapsychic crime" (pp. 79 ff.) and the differentiation between aggression and neurotic pseudoaggression (pp. 59 ff.), that conclusion is inescapable.

I would like to demonstrate a frequent, though neglected topic: mothers who go into tantrums because their children are "feeding problems" or nail-biters.

In a series of analyses of neurotic women in whom conflicts with their children were predominant, one particular situation arose again and again: the mother's "uncontrollable" fury when confronted with a "hunger strike" on the part of a daughter who was a poor eater. These mothers were quite familiar with, and approved, the more recent principles of child pedagogy, in which the abolition of forcible and punitive measures is advocated. Nevertheless they reacted with outbursts of anger, hitting, threats. Moreover, their fury was observable exclusively with girls; the same mothers reacted with much more leniency when their sons were guilty of the same offense.

Analysis of this fury promoted the asumption that a reversal of the woman's own infantile situation was involved. These mothers were acting out a "negative magic gesture", an *unconscious* dramatization of how badly *their* mothers had treated *them* when they were children. This is not a direct repetition but an *ironic exaggeration* and *caricature,* since it is not rooted in objective observation but in the child's distorted misconceptions of reality.

This being the case, unconsciously the grandchild of the original "malefactrix" is being used as scapegoat for an unresolved inner conflict. In *external* reality a mother and daughter are on the stage; they are the *second* generation. In *internal* reality the mistreated child represents the mother herself *as a child,* and the neurotic mother represents the grandmother: the *first* generation recreated. All the fury belongs to the grandmother, who is represented as a repellent caricature: "Look—this is how I did *not* want to be treated! You are mean!"

It was also interesting to observe that the original reproach directed against the mother was in itself an elaboration (unconscious, to be sure) of an even earlier reproach leveled by these neurotic women. In the earliest formulation the reproach read, "Mother wants to starve me." Later it was reformulated: "Even if Mother gives food, she does it ungraciously and only because it is her duty." The reformulation was necessitated by the untenability of the original "objection"—mothers do not starve their children. Instead of accepting the real situation, in which the mother is generous and providing, the old anger—which covers the masochistic solution—is maintained. As a consequence the masochistic child feels victimized; this attitude results in the paradox: he (she) really eats his (her) cake and has his (her) grievance too.

Thus a sacrificial act on the part of the mother is intrapsychically transformed into malice: bad mother forces the unwilling child. Sometimes this attitude is combined with slightly paranoiac ideas: the food is rejected as spoiled, unattractive, or at the very least tasteless. Many food idiosyncrasies and hypochondriacal ideas connected with food have this point as their affective bases.

In the "mix-up" of generations (daughter, child—grandmother, daughter) described above, the old infantile fantasy of the victimized child is frantically maintained. This is an attitude which cannot change of itself because of its derivation. Accused by inner conscience of having accepted the masochistic "solution," there is a desperate attempt to avoid paying penance for the real "crime," and the victim pleads guilty to the pseudoaggressive act. There is an additional advantage to this procedure; it is possible in this way to demonstrate how "bad" the mother really was. The "basic fallacy" that one is only an innocent victim is again strengthened.

There are three tentative explanations for the fact that the situation as described is especially pronounced in mothers where daughters are involved. First, there is the seemingly irresistible allure of specific repetition (dramatis personae being identical in sex); second, the unconscious mitigating connotations of a boy (as described by Freud) are absent with a girl. Third, I have gathered the impression from some cases that the disappointment of having a girl and not a boy activated, in the mother, old injustice-collecting fantasies connected with her own mother, thus paving the way for the "negative magic gesture."

The reaction of mothers to nail-biting did not vary from aggravation to leniency in strict accordance with the sex of the child. Here blank fury was prevalent in neurotic mothers. As though they understood the meaning behind their children's attitudes these mothers fought their losing battle with determination.

In general these mothers were *consciously* naive and considered the "habit" an outgrowth of babyish thumb-sucking. There was one case, however, in which I heard a really intuitive explanation: "The boy acts as if I would starve him."

This mother hit the nail on the head. Nail-biting, so frequently described in analytic literature as a phallic castration symbol, has a deeper layer. It denotes the child's accusation that the mother starves him, so that it is "necessary" for him to *eat himself.*

At the same time it unconsciously represents both an autarchic attempt to be independent of the mother and a masochistic-exhibitionistic demonstration of the mother's "cruelty."

17. GENERAL INHIBITION IN REPRODUCING VERBALLY OR GRAPHICALLY WHAT HAS BEEN SEEN OR HEARD

A typical example has already been reported, the man who couldn't draw (Section II, above).

The inability even to repeat observed phenomena correctly is more widespread than is generally assumed. At first glance one might believe that these imprecise observers had too much "imagination"—they add and embroider. This is a fallacy; by projecting their fears, fantasies, expectations, illogicalities, they also deny having seen in the first place.

Sometimes tragedies result—for instance, in the courtroom the honest but unreliable witness is a familiar phenomenon. In a recent book, NOT GUILTY, by Judge Jerome Frank and Barbara Frank (Doubleday, 1957) the distinguished late judge had this to say:

Even with the most conscientious prosecutor and the most scrupulously fair judge and jury an innocent man may still be found guilty; for the fate of the accused depends also on which witnesses the jury gives credence to and the reliability of their testimony.

Judge Frank quotes many legal authorities on the fallibility of human testimony, with the remark that such opinions are usually expressed to other lawyers and judges, rarely to the general public, which very much needs to know how fallible legal testimony often is and why this is so.

This is Frank's line of reasoning:

The reliability of a witness depends on three different kinds of accuracy: how carefully he observed the events he is testifying to, how well he remembers what he saw or heard, and how clearly he communicates his memory in the courtroom.

A witness's belief that his observation was accurate does not make it so. Anyone's experience of what goes on around him is a blend of inner and outer reality. The act of observing is not mechanical, like photography or sound recording. Sense perceptions are interpreted in accordance with what a person's previous experience leads him to expect. Most experience becomes standardized, following an inner pattern. An observer is apt to see what he wants to see; he is influenced by preconceptions, prejudices, wishes, fears, disregarding what he finds unfamiliar or is unwilling to believe and supplementing things actually seen or heard with what he thinks should have happened. Thus a witness's experience of an event, though subjectively true, may be objectively false.

The inner forces that prevent exact observation are even more likely to have been operative when the witness was not prepared to see the event he is asked to describe and so could not give it his considered attention or make a controlled observation. Other conditions may lessen his acuity. He may be tired, or preoccupied, or badly frightened. His particular interests may affect his attention. This often explains widely varying accounts of the same happening by different people. Concentration on one aspect of a situation may eliminate all others. A man may be trained to notice one kind of detail to the exclusion of others of equal importance. Apart from actual defects of vision and hearing, illusions of the senses may cause misinterpretations of what is perceived, especially in moments of haste or excitement. Discrepancies in estimates of size, distance, and time are common.

Witnesses are seldom aware of these processes of self-deception, and if defense lawyers are also ignorant of them no attempt is made to expose mistakes that may jeopardize innocent men.

As trial testimony concerns past facts the memory of witnesses is crucial. How accurate is anyone's memory for past details? Judge Frank points out that recollection is not a repetition of experience but a new experience, in which things perceived in the past are subject to many changes and omissions ("Many a man with a pure conscience has only a poor memory"), misinterpretations, interpolations, and enlargements. Thinking repeatedly about a subject may lead one to believe that what may have happened really did happen. Remembered accounts grow by being retold many times; one becomes unable to distinguish between fact and imagination, and mistakes becomes permanent.

Pride is a subtle force in expanding and contaminating the memory of witnesses. Most people consider accuracy of memory a part of their basic integrity. In his effort to meet the challenge of cross-examination, circumstances that fit in with a witness's general impression of an event may be supplied by his imagination and then taken for fact. Or he may be flattered by the confidence placed in him and wish to seem important. Bias for or against one of the parties may color or distort the memory of witnesses. If the bias is unconscious it cannot be brought to light at the trial and the mistakes it causes corrected.

Legal opinion, Judge Frank states, coincides with the findings of psychologists in the following conclusions: that our wishes and fears transform and transpose things remembered, changing time or place, retouching details and bridging gaps, ordering our recollections and making them more logical; that the conditions, selectivity, and length of memory vary with the individual's inner make-up, state of mind, inherited abilities, and life experience; that the capacity for remembering the various kinds of sense perceptions, visual, auditory, etc., differs greatly in different people; that forgetting is an active rather than a passive process.

A witness may be an accurate observer with a good memory and his testimony may still be misleading if it is not clearly understood by the jury. There are various causes of failure of communication. The witness may speak a foreign language and have to testify through an interpreter. He may speak his own language in an unusual way, so that, though his words are understood, the private meaning he attaches to them may not be, thus giving rise to an illusion of communication and erroneous assumptions by the jury. What he says may be contradicted by his manner of speaking or his behavior. If he is nervous or timid or over-careful in qualifying his statements he may be thought evasive. If he self-consciously attempts to explain he may throw more doubt than light on the facts he tries to convey. An assertive lie often carries more weight with a jury than a tentative statement of truth.

These are hazards encountered in the honest and more or less normal person. The danger of error increases with witnesses who have seriously disordered perceptions and memories but whose abnormalities are not obvious. Some of these people seem self-possessed and accurate and may make an excellent impression on the witness stand; but their hidden fears and anxieties, quite irrelevant to the external situation, can markedly interfere with their capacity to give valid testimony.

Finally, the limitations of observation and memory, conscious and unconscious bias, misconception, inattention, apply also to members of the jury, who must determine the facts of a case from what they see and hear. They are witnesses too—of what happens in the trial.

18. COPROPHEMIA (ACTIVE AND PASSIVE UTTERANCE OF OBSCENE WORDS)

The perversion coprophemia has at its core the pleasure some men take in actively causing women embarrassment through the use of obscene language. The technique used by these sick people consists in muttering obscene words to unknown women on the street and enjoying their subsequent shame reaction.

The complicated problem of obscenity has been repeatedly attacked analytically (Freud, Ferenczi, Jones, Reik, etc.). The published papers, however, date from the early days of psychoanalysis, and as I pointed out in my study of the subject ("Obscene Words," *The Psychoanalytic Quarterly*, V, 2, 1936) four questions were not given consideration: (1) the conditions under which the ego condones obscene words; (2) the mitigation of the sense of guilt to which the use of such words gives rise; (3) the oral basis of obscenity (there was too much emphasis on the anal explanation); (4) the passive desire to hear obscene words on the part of both men and women.

On the basis of a number of case histories of orally regressed patients I showed that in the oral stage the giving of words by the child was originally a proof of love for the mother, much as the stool represents a gift in the anal stage (Freud). Secondarily there may be observed in some children a complete interruption of this giving as a result of disappointment with the mother—"oral constipation." All these individuals go through a period of obstinate silence in their childhood; only as a tertiary development is the giving re-established at a phallic level with negative manifestations, having now, however, in the form of obscene words the meaning of pseudoaggressive abuse and disparagement. Nevertheless, in this *active* uttering of obscene words the old pleasure is smuggled in. They represent a reproach addressed to the mother: "See what you have made of me."

In orally regressed men who want passively to hear obscenity spoken by women, these words are built into the total pathological attitude that results from being shipwrecked, so to speak, on the "breast complex." They belong in the symptom complex of allegedly wishing only passively to receive. What is really involved is an ironic innuendo: "See what I can get from Mother, only dirt!" At the same time pseudoaggression is displayed—Mother is forced to use exactly the words she forbade in childhood. In this way the guilt feeling is allayed, since the woman is made responsible for the sexual transaction and at the same time vengeance is exacted, since the mother image who originally forbade the words is now forced to utter them.

These words derive a pleasure-giving quality also from the economy of inhibition and repression described by Freud in connection with wit. If in orally regressed people obscene words are important only in relation to the *mother,* in compulsion neurotics there occurs a secondary displacement upon the loved and hated *father* in the form of blasphemies. Normally obscene words play a variable role among healthy people too, as an act of forepleasure, so much so that often the uttering of such words by the man is expected by the woman as part of her sexual subjection.

On the clinical side, individual cases have shown the frequently noted combination of passive-masochistic and voyeuristic tendencies and also evidence of the living out of infantile megalomania in coprophemia. The very variable means of disposition of the guilt feeling resulting from the utterance of obscene words (that is, the fantasies concealed behind them) are elaborated on in my original paper, with emphasis on the common example of the cynic. The so-called "mechanism of cynicism" is itself a means of mitigating the sense of guilt.

Here is a clinical example exemplifying the complexity of unconscious reasons underlying coprophemia: [57]

A kleptomaniac of twenty-six entered analysis at his uncle's insistence. The uncle, incidentally, also paid the initial fees. The young man regarded his pilfering as rather a practical joke and was "tickled to death that that old hypocrite of an uncle was socially embarrassed." In addition to his kleptomania the patient was a check-forger, a pathologic gambler, and a sufferer from a potency disturbance. He also had coprophemia; he would habitually approach well-dressed women on the street and whisper obscene words to them.

"It is really superb," mused the patient, "how I am able to embarrass such a high-class lady with one well-chosen word or short epigrammatic sentence. These women either blush, pretend not to hear, or are silently furious. . . . It is enough for me to see their faces redden in embarrassment or fury. *I feel like an omnipotent sorcerer with inexhaustible power.*"

Asked whether any of his victims ever denounced him to a police officer, he laughed and said that only a very few out of "hundreds of these women" ever threatened to do so and even they were too embarrassed to go any further. Once a "bitch" had denounced him, but his uncle's lawyer was able to convince the investigating officers that the lady must have misunderstood "something." In any case, no prosecution followed.

Superficially the patient presented the picture of a constantly amused psychopath. He ridiculed accepted moral standards, claimed that "bourgeois values" were good only for "idiots," and considered himself a "superior person." He quoted Napoleon: "The moral laws do not apply to me."

I asked him whether he was aware of the risk he was running with his check-forging, kleptomania, and coprophemia. He shrugged his shoulders and replied: "Until now nothing has happened. For his own protection my uncle covers me." Pressed further, he said, "One has to take chances. Take, for example, my gambling. . . ." This was the way his gambling was brought into the discussion, tangentially and accidentally. The patient did not consider his gambling a pathological phenomenon and was rather amused that I was of a different opinion. He used gambling as a "moral alibi." His argument was that gambling as compared with kleptomania was a socially acceptable way of getting money. What's wrong with that? If, as I claimed, both his gambling and his coprophemia were based on the fantasy of childlike omnipotence, masochistically colored, why not tolerate gambling, since society tolerates it?

The patient was the only and posthumous child of a short-lived marriage; his father was accidentally drowned before the child was born. His mother was an obstinate, illiterate, aggressive, and "half-wild" person. She owned a canteen near an army camp and changed lovers every few weeks. The child was frequently present during intercourse. One scene he remembered especially clearly during analysis: an "enormous" soldier forced the mother to have intercourse by squeezing her breast until she nearly fainted from pain. That incident was repressed and came to consciousness in connection with the analysis of a strange habit the patient had developed during puberty: he believed that squeezing girls' buttocks was the surest technique for seducing them. It became apparent that this "squeezing technique" represented the precursor of his coprophemia. The reason was twofold. The progress of his neurosis necessitated stronger repression (in squeezing he repeated the soldier's technique but shifted from the forbidden breast to the more harmless buttocks); and, at the same time, coprophemia represented a megalomaniacal "improvement." The soldier had to resort to an action, but he could get the same results with a word. This explains the previously quoted boast, "It's really superb how I can embarrass a lady with *one single word*. . . . I feel like an *omnipotent* sorcerer."

The word, "lady," is again unconscious ridicule of bourgeois values. Since he did not think of his mother as a "lady" he even debased those on a higher social level. Considering his mother a "low-grade type," he demonstrated his superiority and megalomania by "seducing" upper-class women. The neurosis manifested itself in exhibitionism and peeping-tom activities too.

The next step was the shift from coprophemia to kleptomania. The patient began stealing electric light bulbs, for no apparent practical purpose. He did not sell them but destroyed them in the lavatory. Later, when he began to steal other things, he sold his loot and lost the money gambling. A series of dreams proved that in the symbolism of his unconscious vocabulary the bulbs represented breasts.

We see that the patient went through a series of pseudoaggressive acts aimed at the consciously hated mother: the "squeezing technique"—later projected upon women in general—coprophemia, and kleptomania. When his mother reproached him he said that all his actions were for the purpose of "taking revenge on her." His conscious hatred was then shifted to the family; he embarrassed his uncle socially by stealing and by forging his signature.

This pseudoaggression was only a cover, however, for psychic masochism. The erotic and "sadistic" elements served as a defense against the more deeply embedded masochistic tendency. This became clear the moment this question was put to the patient: "Don't you see that you are damaging yourself more seriously than your mother and uncle?"

One could argue that all these self-damaging acts were only belated revenge aggressions, carried out under self-damaging conditions because of inner guilt. But this was not true, as proved by the fact that he later sought these self-damaging conditions because they satisfied his desire for psychic-masochistic pleasure. The perfect proof of this was his attitude towards gambling. He stated very precisely that during gambling he experienced a thrill "not comparable to any other sensation known to me. Only once, when a lady whom I'd insulted with an obscene word called the police, did I experience anything similar to that thrill. Why an orgasm in sex is nothing compared to it. After all, sex is not forbidden. . . ."

19. THE DEMONSTRATION CHARACTER OF NEUROTIC AND PSYCHOSOMATIC MANIFESTATIONS

All inner defenses are used in their end results as objects of demonstration: "I'll show you how innocent I am!" Hence the language of the inner defense is always—dramatized *exhibitionistic demonstration.*

This in itself makes exhibitionism a "big shot" in the psychic economy.

The same applies in psychosomatic illnesses. One has only to think of the skin, the "bulletin board" of the psyche.

It seems that the superego works on the principle of the sceptic who says, "Show me!" The poor unconscious ego obliges. On the other hand, the ego frequently takes the initiative in its prayer to the inner torturer, "Would you settle for that?"

20. "SHAM SHAME" AND THE FEAR OF "BEING FOUND OUT"

Everyone has some hidden corner of his life that he wants to leave unilluminated and keep a "dark secret." People who proudly proclaim

The Visual Drive

that their lives are an open book and that they have nothing to hide (not even thoughts) should contemplate Mencken's witty definition of self-respect: "the secure feeling that no one, *as yet,* is suspicious."

Sensible people think of the potential damage if the secret should become known, prepare a good rationalization, and dismiss the thought of it, if possible. Neurotic people live in constant dread of "being unmasked and found out," using the possibility as a hitching post for masochistic deposits.

This attitude is nothing to marvel at. The basis of every neurosis is an unsolved infantile masochistic conflict, as I have stated time and again—admittedly a minority opinion.

What requires an explanation is the penalty dreaded by many neurotics. They claim that, if whatever secrets they may harbor were found out, they *"would die of shame."* Sometimes one gathers the impression that for these people the penalty of shame is weightier than the realistic consequences of the denouement.

Why exactly shame? It is of course true that education uses the argument of shame ("You ought to be ashamed of yourself!") to implant cultural restrictions in the child. But why should just this educational medium score such a resounding success when, as we all know, so many others fail?

The external hitching posts to which these fears of shame are attached are manifold.[58] In order of frequency:

1. Shame connected with being revealed as a "fake," "something of an impostor," a "phony," though no objective reason exists for the derogatory judgment.

2. Shame connected with fear that an actual fact or event will become public knowledge (e.g., homosexuality, legal entanglements, details of divorce, clandestine attachment to girl friend or boy friend, etc.).

3. Shame connected with sexual, urinary, anal, exhibitionistic, peeping functions.

4. Shame connected with clothes.

5. Shame of being conspicuous (at public appearances, speech-making, speaking in general, "not knowing what to say").

6. Shame connected with fear of being ridiculous, making a fool of oneself (intellectually, socially, culturally).

7. Shame connected with being clumsy, ugly, unattractive.
8. Shame connected with the handling of money matters.

The irony of the situation is that the list is headed by an irrational fear—the fear of being shamed because of "faking." This in itself gives a clue: *shame-fear is of infantile origin and has a complex substructure, regardless of the pseudorational disguise; shame-fear always denotes something else than the officially given reason, though the reason may be presented in good faith. In this sense every shame-fear is a sham of shame (sham shame), a convenient mask for more deeply repressed conflicts.*

Shame is frequently identified with guilt. Numerous dicta of the wise of all ages agree on that score. From Aristophanes' "Shame is the apprehension of a vision reflected from the surface of opinion—the opinion of the public" to Swift's "I never wonder to see men wicked, but I often wonder to see them unashamed" to Burke's "While shame keeps its watch, virtue is not wholly extinguished in the heart" to Shaw's "We live in an atmosphere of shame; we are ashamed of ourselves, of our relatives, of our incomes, of our accents, of our opinions, of our experiences, just as we are ashamed of our naked skin"—runs a straight line of consent.

Psychologically the identity of shame and guilt is questionable (see pp. 348 f.). The best way of proving the dissimilarity is to approach the problem clinically.

In the framework of a short subchapter it is impossible to deal with all the subdivisions of sham shame. Some of the types enumerated above are described in my recent book PRINCIPLES OF SELF-DAMAGE. A few examples will suffice.

Mr. MM. was a patient of fifty, a man of independent means and a homosexual. He had been through the equivalent of a "middle-age revolt" (that peculiar phase in heterosexuals is described in my book THE REVOLT OF THE MIDDLE-AGED MAN), consisting in homosexuals in giving up casual affairs and "falling in love" (allegedly for keeps) with a young man. The grand romance regularly collapses and leads to extensive masochistic depression. Behind this seeming resurgence is some kind of panic at the idea of getting old, and, in a second adolescence, a rebellion is staged against one's (self-created) fate, a rebellion that, inwardly, is not seriously meant. After a shattering

The Visual Drive 347

experience of this kind, Mr. MM. came into treatment, having been "hit below the belt," as he expressed it, by reading my book ONE THOUSAND HOMOSEXUALS.

It seemed that he spent most of his waking hours in gloomy thoughts centering around his "shame" if some of his acquaintances should find out about his past homosexuality and see "what a phony he really was." While thinking or talking with me about his "deepest fears" he would cry convulsively. Although he had for many years been completely promiscuous and by no means cautious or circumspect, now—all at once—the whole impact of his past descended upon him. Objectively he was in no danger; his means allowed him to live wherever he wished to; he occupied no public office; he could not be financially touched by any indiscretion on the part of his acquaintances. Still, the "shame" was paramount in his mind.

To show him the irrationality of his response, I asked him which, in his opinion, was more painful for Captain Dreyfus: ten years of Devil's Island or being demoted from his military rank in a punitive public ceremony. Without hesitation Mr. MM. answered, "The latter." I objected that to the average person the ten-year prison term would be more painful.

To bear out his contention that he "had always" been a homosexual, Mr. MM. adduced this "proof": In the city of his birth there was a reproduction of a famous sculpture of a naked youth in front of the entrance to a museum, near his family's house. At the early age of four he would run to this statue and admire it. Whenever he was missing from home his mother or governess knew where to look for him, and the boy would cry when made to stop admiring the statue and go home.

As was to be expected, that recollection covered a complex "case history." Mr. MM.'s parents had separated when he was three, his mother divorcing his father. The admiration the boy felt for the statue was by no means proof of "inborn" homosexuality; it was proof of how "unjust" his mother had been in depriving him of his father. In short, the admiring attitude represented—besides narcissistic identification—the boy's *demonstration of being mistreated by his mother.* Later his masochistic attachment to, and fear of, his mother increased to such a degree that he had to flee the female sex altogether, to rescue himself to another continent, man.

MM.'s mother was a bizarre, rather peculiar, opinionated, quarrelsome woman who frequently "embarrassed" the boy (and, later, young man) by loud, hysterical behavior in company. At times he was *"directly ashamed of her."* Here was the explanation of his perpetual shame in later life, coupled with the fear of being found out as a phony: he acted out, unconsciously, to be sure, and almost exhibitionistically, the *embarrasment and shame she caused him.* But now the center was shifted; to cover up the masochistic enjoyment she gave him, he took the blame for the "lesser intrapsychic crime"— his pseudoaggressive transgression of educational dicta, his exhibitionistically displayed homosexuality. Again, as in the statue incident, a masochistic demonstration of how "unjust" the mother had been to the allegedly innocent victim.

From these glimpses, one part of the *exhibitionism* included in MM.'s fears of being unmasked by his acquaintances is understandable. Since his "proof" contained a "demonstration character," exhibitionism had to be invoked. But this demonstration still did not explain the specificity of his choice, shame.

Shame and blushing are usually associated. "O shame! Where is thy blush?" asks Hamlet, and so did the generations before and after the melancholy prince. In a series of papers (e.g. "Further Contributions to the Problem of Blushing," *The Psychoanalytic Review,* 44:452-456, 1957) I was able to show on the basis of clinical material that blushing unconsciously represents *anticipation of punishment,* accusingly displayed as already executed. The buttocks, reddened by beating, are symbolically interchanged with the cheeks and punishment masochistically and accusingly demonstrated. Language, in its intuitive wisdom, knew this relationship all the time: in some parts of England the slang term for buttocks is cheeks; and on both sides of the Atlantic a "cheeky" boy is a fresh, provoking child.

A few examples of the "anticipation of punishment" are given on pages 239 ff.

It is now possible to define the *difference between guilt and shame.* Both are the result of reproaches of inner conscience (superego), but shame is more than guilt; *guilt may lead to various forms of self-*

punishment, but shame is guilt plus punishment already executed and accordingly demonstrated externally or in the form of an "inner blush." At bottom, shame is a masochistic demonstration of the buttocks reddened after beating by "unjust" educators.

Dr. NN. was a successful internist whose great complaint in life was that he was inhibited in his scientific productivity. In the first appointment he informed me that he always had the feeling that he was "something of a fraud," though he could not substantiate his self-accusation. He stressed particularly his dread of having his friends, acquaintances, colleagues, become aware of this "phoniness."

NN. came from a family of business people. Early in life he had rebelled against their mercantile views, of which he was ashamed—as well as of his parents—and had decided on the scientific and idealistic career of medicine. He finally achieved his aim, became successful in his specialty, and made money. But his deep dissatisfaction continued, bolstered by his masochistic marriage to a difficult woman. He lived in the suburbs, where he had built an expensive house. One day in the commuter train he thought to himself that his mode of living was no better than that of a business man who keeps regular hours.

This was the clue to his shame-fear and his accusation of phoniness. It did not pertain to his actual performance as a physician but to the ironical reproach of conscience that his masochism prevented his real aim; he wasn't a scientist but a "business man."

To show the complexity of the mechanisms included in sham shame, I am adducing a third type, people who "cannot talk in company." This type is widespread.

Confronted with an audience, neurotics with this complaint are incapable of discussing any topic intelligently. This inability does not depend on their knowledge or their ignorance of the subject. They are shy; they blush; they are tongue-tied and inhibited; they confound the core of a topic with its periphery. They go off on tangents, mix up words, express themselves badly; sometimes they even confuse the issue. The aftereffect is shame, dread and depression, remorse ("Why didn't I mention the effective argument?"). This continues until the next occasion, which is only a repeat performance. The grievance is all the more bitter since "privately" (meaning with one friend, with their wives, or in soliloquies) they can be quite eloquent.

In analyzing these patients one finds that hidden behind the more superficial (though also repressed) phallic castration fear are three specific mechanisms:

1. Unsolved peeping conflicts, secondarily warded off with exhibitionism, which in its turn is warded off by accepting the blame for exhibitionism in the form of inhibition.

2. The mechanism of the "pseudomoral connotation of the neurotic symptom."

3. The masochistic elaboration.

These unconscious techniques require some explanation:

1. In analyzing the superficial exhibitionism of these patients one very soon arrives at a dead end. Abundant material can be secured from recollections and dreams without accomplishing any noticeable external change. The reason is that one is fighting the analytical battle on a spurious front; in these patients exhibitionism is not the original drive but a defense mechanism. The story reads differently when attention is focused on the more deeply repressed peeping tendencies. The sequence of events is: Infantile peeping was contradicted by education and later by the superego; as a defense exhibitionism was pronounced (this sequence of warding off voyeurism with exhibitionism is typical in all cases of "sham shame"). With this defense also contradicted by the superego, the unconscious ego creates a secondary defense; it takes the blame for the "lesser crime" and tries to alibi itself by warding off exhibitionism. Seemingly the struggle of the shy person is concentrated on exorcising the devil of exhibitionism; in inner reality the sham is magnified out of proportion to cover the "inner fortress"—peeping fantasies.

2. In Chapter 4 I pointed out that a specific additional connotation of neurotic symptoms is often overlooked. Educational precepts, enshrined in the ego ideal, are unconsciously repeated verbatim—at the wrong time, in the wrong place, on the wrong occasion, out of context, and with the wrong intention. This literal reproduction does not reflect but rather distorts the meaning originally intended. The result is a *reductio ad absurdum* of the original meaning.

The purpose of this unconscious procedure is immobilization of the

The Visual Drive

antilibidinous part of the superego, the "daimonion," whose typical torture method consists in holding up to the frightened ego the self-created ego ideal and decreeing guilt and depression for every discrepancy. Thus the ego ideal seems the final yardstick: "Roma locuta, causa finita." But the unconscious ego can turn the tables; every time it can prove that an action corresponds to an ego-ideal precept, the daimonion is stopped cold.

The therapeutic conclusion is obvious. The described resistance is by no means the decisive one, but it poses a new problem. One must, in every specific case, discover the "private moral code" of the unconscious ego. One must, furthermore, debunk the unconscious use of irony towards educational rules, the technique whereby the weak child beats the powerful educator with his own stick.

In the case under discussion—"I cannot talk in company"—this mechanism is of importance. At one time or another the child is told, "Be quiet" or "Hold your tongue" or "I don't want to hear another word from you"; in their despair infuriated parents may even resort to the lowly "Shut up!" This applies especially to situations in which other people were present.

In certain neurotics this very "Shut up!" becomes the guiding pattern. They do as they were told—at the wrong time, in the wrong place, on the wrong occasion. Ostensibly following an educational precept, they make the educator into the malefactor: "Look what you did to me!"

3. Experience proves that the technique described, when applied to being tongue-tied in company, presupposes strong masochistic tendencies. True enough, the child "triumphs" over the educator, but at what price?

Interpretation of the triad of "sham shame," when applied to tongue-tied neurotics (especially the debunking of the "pseudomoral connotation" of their neurotic balance), leads to therapeutic results. It is possible to "untie" some of the tongue-tied neurotics.

The problem of "sham shame" is complex and, even more important, extremely torturing for its bearer. The victim is always fighting with shadows; he always hits in the wrong direction. At bottom it is an active repetition of a passively endured experience in childhood—it is not by chance that all these patients subjectively were "ashamed" of their parents. This does not mean that there was reason to be ashamed; the "shame" was already a defense. Unraveling the inner interconnections produces therapeutic successes—provided the psychiatrist knows what it is all about.

21. PERVERSION VOYEURISM

Voyeurism as a perversion (paraphilia) is distinguished from either normal or neurotic visual gratification by the following three factors: [59]

1. Peeping takes the place of the normal sex act; it is not a "preparatory act" but the total of the individual's sex life, regardless of whether it leads to or accompanies masturbation, remains on the level of excitement, or produces involuntary emission.

2. The situation in which the voyeuristic act is executed is without exception connected with the "allure of danger"—in other words, legal-punitive consequences. These sick individuals derive no excitement from peeping which is condoned or permitted by the person spied on.

3. Punishment, or the threat of punishment, is no deterrent; on the other hand, there is no observable progression to other legal infractions in the sphere of sex.

This attempt to describe the essentials of the problem corresponds closely with recorded observations. B. Karpman, in his monumental THE SEXUAL OFFENDER AND HIS OFFENSES, defines voyeurism thus:

> Excessive interest in looking at genitalia, sex acts, etc., as a sexual stimulus is called scopophilia. Voyeurism is a pathological indulgence in looking at some form of nudity as a source of gratification in place of the normal sex act. Voyeurism is a crime only when the observed has not given consent. The emphasis of the law is based upon the right to privacy of the person observed. Some prohibition is a constant condition; the price of violating the prohibition is an increasing sense of guilt. Satisfaction arises from seeing when not being seen. Excitement ranges from purely psychic stimulation to compulsory exhibitionistic masturbation. (Oberndorf)" (p. 17)

Allen, Caprio, Markey have expressed similar views; Hartwell adds that voyeurs do not usually marry, that they show no marked tendency to other sex crimes, and that they are unaggressive and independent. Finally, Hartwell confirms the observation that the voyeur manifests no interest in nakedness he can witness in an acceptable way.

As to motivations, the literature on the subject mentions castration anxiety (Fenichel), incest fantasies (Karpman), masturbation conflicts (Karpman), feminine identification, desire to exhibit (Oberndorf), latent homosexuality (Karpman; London and Caprio), and modifications of early traumatic experiences.

Voyeurism as a perversion cannot be understood without a preliminary discussion of the following: [60]
1. The dynamics of perversion.
2. The specificity of the "voyeuristic-exhibitionistic exchange mechanism," as modified in the perversion.
3. The mechanism of criminosis.

1. *Psychodynamics of Perversions*

In a case of homosexuality analyzed in 1930, partly by myself and partly by a colleague (L. Eidelberg, the first analyst to treat the patient, fell ill, and during the many months before his recovery I took over the analysis; upon Eidelberg's return to health he resumed treatment of the patient), it could be ascertained that the patient's conscious approval of the perversion covered something more deeply repressed: oral regression to the pre-oedipal mother. This experience (published in 1933, in collaboration with L. Eidelberg, in "The Breast Complex in the Male") became paradigmatic for me, subject to some subsequent modifications, of which the most important clarified oral regression in neurotics as denoting "the wish to be refused." In the thirty years since first reaching these conclusions, they have been confirmed in the analysis of over one hundred twenty homosexuals. As stated previously (pp. 65 ff.), the homosexual uses a specific technique in solving the trauma of weaning. Instead of applying the typical solution which leads to normality—a fantasied identification of penis and breast which utilizes the "mechanism of unconscious repetition compulsion" (Freud) to repeat actively a passively endured experience in order to restore a lesion in narcissism—the male homosexual finds his solution in "the reduplication of his own defense mechanism." Normally, the male child negates his *passivity* as a recipient of milk by building up the fantasy of his penis as an *active* dispenser of fluid, and by identifying milk with urine and later with sperm. In adult intercourse, he *actively* pushes an oblong, fluid-"producing" object into a *passive* opening, identifying mouth and vagina, thus achieving an "unconscious repetition" of an infantile experience.

Two barriers prevent the adult male homosexual from using this mechanism. First, he needs assurance that his penis constitutes a fully adequate substitute for the breast, and seeks to reinforce his fantasy by finding a "reduplication of his own defense" in the penis of his partner; his pursuit of a partner is a search for the breast and for reassurance. Second, he is so angry with the disappointing female, and so afraid of her, that he rejects her sex entirely and escapes to another continent: man. As I subsequently learned, his anger and disappointment form the pseudoaggressive cover for his fear of his own overdimensional psychic masochism.

The whole pre-oedipal picture is unconsciously camouflaged by an oedipal blind. The exaggerated "femininity" of some homosexuals, and the "husband-wife" game they play, is a device designed to accept the blame for a *lesser* intrapsychic crime, and to cover up a *greater* inner infraction. The homosexual's real problem is his masochistic attachment to the pre-oedipal mother and her successive representatives; its surface manifestations are frequent quarrels of the "injustice-collecting" type, constant jealousy, a succession of partners, disappointments, etc. The male homosexual cannot be merely and only an "effeminate" man (feminine identification), for every "feminine" homosexual has a "masculine" homosexual as his partner. The latter type cannot be so conveniently—and incorrectly—explained.

The homosexual's inner guilt apparently pertains to his perversion, but in inner reality this guilt has merely been shifted and actually arises from his oral-masochistic regression. I have pointed out these interconnections in Chapter 2.

Perversion, therefore, is neither the "negative of neurosis" nor a

The Visual Drive 355

direct volcanic eruption of id wishes, but a complex chain of specific inner defenses.

In my opinion, this applies to every perversion, including the specific perversion voyeurism. Upon further scrutiny, the material on voyeurism proved to be less "obvious" than it originally appeared.

2. *The Specificity of the "Voyeuristic-Exhibitionistic Exchange Mechanism" as Modified in the Perversion Voyeurism*

The theory of the "voyeuristic-exhibitionistic exchange mechanism" has been described earlier in this chapter (pp. 199 ff.).

In *perversion* voyeurism, the voyeurism seems to be on the surface; nevertheless, the surface manifestations are a blind. My experiences have proved to my satisfaction that *these sick people, at bottom, are struggling with a specific masochistic conflict: every woman they surreptitiously "inspect" is unconsciously identified with a denying infantile prototype.* What they are inwardly after is *not* the sight of the woman but the masochistically tinged disappointment derived from that woman's alleged refusal to show herself. Defensive pseudoaggression counteracts this masochistic stabilization, and the voyeur "goes after" and "gets" his sight of the woman despite the refusal that would be forthcoming if she knew of the incident. This leads straight to the mechanism observed by the authors quoted above: ". . . the voyeur manifests no interest in nakedness he can witness in an acceptable way."

This mechanism of being shut out from seeing—an elaboration of the infantile-oral starvation theory from the "septet of baby fears"—seems to me the crux of the matter in the perversion voyeurism.

Tangentially, exhibitionistic defenses are included. Many of these "inspections" are so clumsily staged that detection (and inevitably, exhibitionistic exposure) should logically follow. Here, of course, the wish to be punished, once more masochistically elaborated, enters the picture. The exhibitionistic defense also accounts for Oberndorf's observation in 1939 to the effect that one of the possible outcomes of the perverse voyeuristic act is "compulsory exhibitionistic masturbation." This observation obviously makes use of the "voyeuristic-exhibitionistic exchange mechanism" described by me in 1935 and reproduced earlier in this chapter.

One can note a series of frantic attempts on the part of the voyeuristic pervert to stress his *pseudo*aggressive defense: the possibility (and even likelihood) of detection and exhibitionistic exposure; active exhibitionism per se (included in the "voyeuristic-exhibitionistic exchange mechanism"); unconscious fantasy of undressing the woman. This last element has gone through a succession of inhibitory channels: it begins with megalomania (the woman becomes the executive organ of the voyeur's alleged omnipotence), proceeds to active-aggressive thoughts which are subsequently repressed, and finally settles on total inhibition of this activity, with all responsibility shifted to the totally oblivious woman. This goes so far that many voyeuristic perverts protest that they did not peep, but that the woman "made them look" by exposing herself. This is their convenient excuse, of course, but at the same time it cannot be denied that many exhibitionistic women only too often and too regularly have these experiences.

One should also mention that in some cases "draining fantasies" are involved in the aftereffects of the perverse act: some of the voyeurs have involuntary emissions with the penis only half-erect or not even erect.

3. *The "Mechanism of Criminosis"*

In a long series of articles published since 1943 and summarized in my books THE BATTLE OF THE CONSCIENCE, THE BASIC NEUROSIS, and THE SUPEREGO, I have been reiterating my conviction that analytic investigations on criminosis (this apt term was created by A. N. Foxe) have gone astray because their guiding principle was that of analogy with neurosis taken as paradigm. This has gone so far that B. Karpman, one of the pioneers in the field, has uttered the justified warning:

> ... the psychoanalytic approach has as yet failed to contribute significantly to the solution of the problem because it gratuitously went on the assumption that the same mechanism operated in criminals as in neurotics. ... The great majority of the professional and habitual criminals must be approached by a method different from that used for neurotics. (THE INDIVIDUAL CRIMINAL. Foreword, vii)

The Visual Drive

Without going into the tragicomedy of errors and misconceptions which makes up the literature on criminosis, I will summarize in brief my personal opinions on the problem:

I believe that the criminotic is propelled by a specific modification of the mechanism of orality; I have called this modification the "mechanism of criminosis."

The primary difficulty with criminotics lies in the fact that they unconsciously act under the influence of a pre-oedipal and not an oedipal conflict.

I conceive of the criminotic as the most passive person in this world, helpless as a baby in his motorically inexpressible fury. The giant who is the mother is not even impressed with the fact that the helpless child wants to take revenge for alleged injustices done him. The motor act in criminosis is based on the inner feeling that nothing the child can do will successfully pierce through the screen of the mother's unawareness. The situation is that of a dwarf trying to annoy a giant who superciliously refuses to see these attempts. There is a direct relationship between the "herostratic" tendency in criminosis and the feeling that one is helpless to make one's revenge evident. Because the criminotic unconsciously sees himself as a dwarf, the weapon he chooses is the equivalent of dynamite—of which even the giant must take cognizance. It is true that the "revenge" harms the avenger; if it is sufficiently sweeping, he may be legally executed. But he has fulfilled his primary aim—that of forcing the giant to acknowledge the dwarf's fury.

Every criminal action has an element of the "herostratic" in it. Herostrates was the individual who, in 356 B.C., burned the famous Temple of Artemis in Ephesus in order to become "renowned." Our "herostratic" criminals unconsciously perform similar deeds for another purpose: that of forcing the image of the pre-oedipal mother to acknowledge their power to revenge themselves upon her. The deepest, and dynamically most effective, core in the unconscious conflict of the criminotic consists of this compensatory and concealed helplessness, originally turned against the mother and subsequently turned against society.

The conception of crime outlined here differs specifically from the usual schematic application of analytic knowledge, gained from the therapy of neuroses. According to the standard misconception, an Oedipus complex is "discovered" in criminals. The proud but naive authors of certain treatises flatter themselves on being very "modern" and at the same time assume that they have "discovered" the "reason" why people commit crimes. Unfortunately for these pseudo trailblazers, the Oedipus complex can be found in every human being. Unfortunately for their theory, not everybody who is burdened with this complex commits crimes.

Schematic application of neurosis to criminosis leads to still another fallacy: that of using the findings of unconscious motivations in a specific criminotic to explain the motor act. *Psychologic motivations* and the *motor act*—that is, the execution of the specific crime—are two distinct and different entities; linking them artificially as cause and effect can lead only to confusion.

The major source of confusion in criminal psychopathology, however, arises from the failure to differentiate between a *variable* and a *constant* factor in every criminal action. The variable factor is made up of the psychologic contents; it takes innumerable forms and differs from case to case. The variety of motives for a crime is as great as the variety of unconscious motives in general. The constant factor in crime is the now known "x" which explains the motor act of performing the criminal move itself. This constant and pathognomonic factor constitutes "the mechanism of criminosis." These two factors must be determined in every criminal action.

The differential diagnosis between these two factors is accomplished by keeping the following in mind: The variable factor explains the unconscious contents of a criminal action. To explain these, we must use all of the knowledge of unconscious mechanisms discovered by Freud and so successfully applied to the explanation of human conduct in general—unconscious wishes, defense mechanisms, projections, identifications, atonement of unconscious guilt feelings, etc. The constant factor, the mechanism of criminosis, does not refer to the variable psychologic contents of a specific crime, but to the motor act which executes the results of the variable factor. I repeat, the real riddle in crime is the motor act. The propelling force of the motor act derives from the criminotic's inexhaustible store of aggression, and in the act itself aggression is displayed on so primitive a level that one cannot easily determine whether it is primary or secondary (pseudoaggression, used as an unconscious defense mechanism).

What happens if there is a failure to distinguish between these two decisive factors? The answer is simple: confusion reigns. That confusion is based mainly on naivety, but sometimes on malice. A *cause célèbre* of the recent past, the case of Halsmann, provides an example of confusion arising from malice. The reactionary medical faculty of the University of Innsbruck in pre-Hitler Austria was asked by the courts to express its opinion on why a young Latvian Jew had killed his father. The defendant had pleaded innocent to the crime; his complicity had been "proved" only by extremely doubtful circumstantial evidence. The Nazi-infested faculty decided that Halsmann had an Oedipus complex which was "operative." Freud objected to this biased nonsense, pointing out the universality of the Oedipus complex. Said he: "Even if the conflict between father and son could be proved, one must say that there is a great distance between the conflict and the causative factors of such a crime." Freud illustrated this point with a joke: A man was sentenced for robbery on the basis of circumstantial evidence; he had been arrested near the pilfered apartment, and a skeleton key had been found in his pocket. Before sentence was passed, he was asked if he had anything to say. He then stated that he wanted to be sentenced for adultery as well, having that "key," too, in his pocket. . . . The "great" distance mentioned by Freud is exactly the distance between present ignorance and the determination of the "specific factor" in crime.

Obviously the eradication of a misconception is a considerable job, since it can only be done by overcoming one human fault—the reluctance to think, or its opposite: the preference for thinking in accordance with prefabricated patterns. Examples of confused thinking on this problem which are due to naivety can be found in numerous scientific journals and books. The basis is almost invariably the same: failure to differentiate between neurosis and criminosis.

The criminotic's aggression, in my opinion, is exclusively pseudoaggression of a specific type. It differs in the following ways from neurotic aggression:

1. It represents a subdivision of neurotic pseudoaggression. Proof positive is the fact that the alleged aggression damages the person executing the criminal act; he will either be caught, or remain in constant danger of apprehension and punishment.

2. It differs from neurotic aggression in both the nature of the risk taken and the extent of it. The neurotic's punishment is limited to consciously experienced unhappiness; the criminotic, however, risks jail or capital punishment.

3. Social ostracism is involved in criminotic aggression and not in neurotic self-damage.

4. In contradistinction to neurotic aggression, exhibitionism plays an indispensable part in criminotic aggression. The majority of criminals are caught because of the "little mistakes" they themselves have made. Inner guilt partly accounts for their unconsciously deliberate self-betrayal, but the pressure of the exhibitionistic tendency can also be discerned. The crime demonstrates to the mother image—shifted to society as a whole—that the child was capable of taking his revenge.

5. Infantile megalomania is more strongly represented in criminotic than in neurotic aggression. The criminal's view of himself as a unique exception to the rule that "crime does not pay" and that "murder will out" derives from his megalomania. His exaggerated view of his own power, coupled with the unconscious wish to be punished, explains all the unaccountable lapses which make the "perfect crime" impossible.

6. The criminotic inwardly accepts the fact that he will be punished. That is why one so frequently encounters criminals who phenomenologically appear to be without remorse or guilt.

At this point, one could conclude that criminosis represents a specific "solution" of a repressed infantile conflict which has its source in the earliest months of life. The criminotic act is composed of two parts: a constant (mechanism of criminosis) which explains the motor act, and a variable which accounts for differences in psychological content. This psychological content is specific for the specific crime alone.

What about the conscience of the criminotic? Why does it not prevent the dangerous act? Does the criminotic have a conscience at all?

A person without a conscience does not and cannot exist. Recent investigations prove conclusively that conscience is not at all a photographic copy of the environment, as was once assumed, but an inner institution having an intimate relation with the person's aggression. A part of this aggression is unconsciously curbed and redirected against the person himself.

To state that a person has no conscience simply means that the investigator who made the statement was unable to uncover the hidden inner "deals" the "conscienceless" person made with his conscience in order to appease it.

In the specific situation of perversion voyeurism, the unconscious expectation of legal punishment is included in the act. This goes so far that in some cases a note of disappointment (of course not conscious disappointment) creeps in when it is realized that "nothing has happened." Quite frequently the voyeur himself, or his lawyer, manages to convince the arresting officer or the District Attorney's office that a "mistake" is being made. In many cases, light sentences are imposed; in other cases, however, the aftermath is jail and its consequent damage to the voyeur's social standing and future prospects.

22. PERVERSION EXHIBITIONISM

In *perversion* voyeurism the voyeur looks masochistically for the sight-forbidding, hence disappointing, woman (basically her breast).

In *perversion* exhibitionism the same material is defensively elaborated. A *"magic gesture"* is used: "I'll show you in my behavior how I would have liked you to act." The passivity of looking at the breast is changed into the activity of displaying the penis (breast equivalent), and the masochistic element is *seemingly* omitted.

The accent is on "seemingly" for two reasons: The perverted exhibitionist courts arrest, and the "magic gesture" itself contains a fearful-masochistic accusation.

This is the structure of the magic gesture:

Layer I. Masochistic submission as end result of the infantile conflict.

Layer II. First veto of the inner conscience.
Layer III. First defense of the unconscious ego: "I am not guilty of psychic masochism, as the indictment claims. On the contrary, I *hate* my upbringers because I have so many justified grievances against them" (pseudoaggression).
Layer IV. Second veto of the inner conscience.
Layer V. Second defense of the unconscious ego: "All I want is to be loved. In my behavior I will *dramatize* how I wanted to be treated in childhood—*kindly and lovingly.*" Ironic lip-service conformity with ego-ideal precepts: "What's wrong with being kind and wanting to be loved?" "Conscience money" is paid in the form of the outer world's suspicion and the foreseen ingratitude of the beneficiary.

The unconscious dramatization of the last alibi is the magic gesture. It leads to the amazing fact that an *unimportant* outsider is chosen as beneficiary for these "good deeds." The more unimportant the beneficiary, the deeper the masochistic injustice-collecting: "You, bad Mother (Father) did not care for your own child. I care even for strangers!" It is exactly this discrepancy that makes for the choice of outsiders.

Here is a typical example from the analysis of a woman in constant feud with her family, who lived in a northwestern state. She complained continually about their cruelty and neglect, though she provoked such treatment. Both sides got a good-sized masochistic kick out of it. One day the patient heard from her mother that a bookkeeper from the family business was going to visit New York and she was asked to be nice to her. The patient reacted paradoxically; she did not complain or consider herself imposed on, her usual attitude, but devoted the next ten days to being a guide for the guest. She invited the girl out, showered her with gifts, went out of her way to be helpful, a trait otherwise foreign to her. The unconscious meaning of her action was a reproachful innuendo against her mother.

The synthetic basis of the magic gesture can be demonstrated. The beneficiary never feels secure in his elevation to favor, and there comes a moment when he is dropped, for no reason, and even becomes the object of his former benefactor's wrath. What happens is that the inner conscience objects to the unconscious trick and forces the benefactor to a new alibi. This is promptly furnished; he denies his inner masochistic tendencies by reversing his role. He now acts the "cruel" parent, reducing his previous beneficiary to the image of his mistreated self. Thus a "positive" magic gesture changes into a "negative" one, which demonstrates in caricature how cruel the parent really was.

Bitterness over alleged neglect in childhood—the masochistic misuse being overlooked—sometimes goes so far that the demonstration cannot be performed on living people, and so animals or inanimate objects are chosen.

A schizoid patient suffered from, among other things, reckless spending. This brought him into serious conflict with his penurious mother, towards whom he used this method of showing aggression. He had a curious inability to make a decision in selecting objects for purchase. Wishing to order three shirts, he went to an expensive shop and looked at hundreds of samples. Without hesitation he narrowed his choice down to about thirty. Although he could readily have separated the ones he liked from those he considered in bad taste, he was incapable of making a further choice and there was no way out of his indecision but to order the whole lot. On another occasion he went to a book store to buy a recently published book. The salesman showed him several dozen that had appeared in recent months. He rejected a number on the ground that they did not interest him. About fifteen remained, and, unable to come to a decision, he bought all fifteen.

From the history of this patient one could learn that his mother preferred some of her six children to others, and he felt that he had been discriminated against. By means of his extravagance and indecision he acted out a magic gesture. Unconsciously he performed a symbolic act designed to show her how he would have liked to be treated. His unconscious formula was: "You, Mother, have discriminated against some of your children; you have played favorites. I, however, cannot even choose between indifferent objects—shirts, books, etc. How much less would I be capable of doing so among my own children!" Behind this tearful aggression deep masochism was hidden. That defensive aggression was not the real reason for his actions was also proved by the fact that by being a spendthrift he also showed conscious aggression towards his mother, who paid the bills. His pseudoaggression was a palimpsest only, covering deep masochistic attachment to his mother.

Some neurotics choose animals as the recipients of their magic gestures. Another schizoid patient was an enthusiastic pigeon-feeder. He collected crumbs incessantly and spent hours watching the pigeons eat from his hand, with tears in his eyes the while. He did not want to be put in the category of ordinary animal-loving humanitarians. Correctly enough, he placed the emphasis, not on the pigeons but on his tears, although he was incapable of explaining their cause. Unconsciously his tears meant: "You treated me badly, bad Mother. Look how I wanted to be treated—kindly." The five-layer structure described above was fully visible under the analytic microscope, as was the specific determining factor in the symbolic use of pigeons.

The magic gesture sometimes appears—and very effectively—in literature. Dostoievsky's use of it in CRIME AND PUNISHMENT is memorable. Raskolnikov has just received a letter from his mother containing the news that his sister has consented to marry a man she does not love, for the sake of the money he would contribute to her brother's support. In a park he sees an obviously wealthy man pursuing a drunken girl. He calls on a policeman for aid and rescues the girl, although it means that he must lay out money, which he needs for food, to pay for a cab to take her home. The reader clearly understands that Raskolnikov identifies the girl with his sister, especially in view of another item in his mother's letter: the news that Swidrigailov, the man in whose house his sister was employed as a governess, has been pursuing her sexually. During the scene in the park Raskolnikov calls the unknown man pursuing the unknown girl "Swidrigailov." Dostoievsky cautiously explains even the policeman's interest in the girl via Raskolnikov's thought that perhaps the policeman had daughters of about the girl's age. He also shows the senseless shift from the positive magic gesture to the negative one: in the end Raskolnikov suddenly flies into a fury and turns against the poor girl.

Whether the neurotic uses the mechanism of the magic gesture on persons, objects, or animals, he always expresses it in an aggressive reproach, hidden behind the disguise of the superficial layer: unconscious identification with both the beneficiary and the idealized mother (father). Hidden still further, behind this reproach, is the real, dynamically effective psychic masochism, which is warded off with pseudoaggression.

My first acquaintanceship with perversion exhibitionism was made at a "small mass experiment" conducted by a court in Vienna.

In Vienna many years ago there was a judge who harbored the naive idea that psychoanalysis could cure any perversion, and therefore, for a time, he did not sentence reiterant exhibitionists to the rather long prison terms usually imposed in such cases. Instead he passed a suspended sentence and remitted their punishment if they could prove after six months that they were under psychoanalytic treatment. Five cases were sent to our clinic, where they were to be treated free of charge. Of these five people who faced the alternatives of imprisonment or psychoanalysis, one began analysis with one of our colleagues, but gave it up promptly a few days after he had received the written confirmation that he had begun treatment. Two others did not appear after the first interview with the head of the clinic. With the two others I spoke once or twice. After receiving notice that they could start treatment, they withdrew, giving the most threadbare excuses, and all four allowed themselves to be imprisoned.

How can this grotesque situation be explained? Even the fear of the alleged unpleasantness of the treatment cannot be used as an excuse for the behavior of these four individuals, since they had no idea what the treatment consisted of. There could not have been any antipathy for the particular physician since these five people spoke with three different physicians on the staff of the clinic. Nor was there a conspiracy, for there was no proof that these patients even knew each other. From the discussions I had with two of them, I received the impression that imprisonment from time to time was inseparably bound up with their psychic equilibrium. It offered them the opportunity of atoning for their inward feeling of guilt. The prison term gave them, so to speak, the ticket of leave for the next perverse action. It was also striking how awkwardly they acted when they were caught. They actually provoked arrest. One of them, for instance, was threatened by an old woman during his exhibitionistic act with a child. The woman saw his exhibition from the window of the third story. The man ran away but returned after a few minutes, giving as rationalization that he wanted to see whether the old woman was still there. She was exactly where he suspected she would be, but she had a police officer with her, to whom she reported the case, and our man was arrested.

Not only was imprisonment preferred by these two sick people, but it became directly a part of the routine of their lives. One of them had a small business delivering packages by car; he told his family from time to time that he had to make a business trip into the country, whereas in reality he spent the time serving out a prison sentence. Another worked in his brother-in-law's print shop, and he was able to convince him that he occasionally had to take a trip to the mountains in order to keep fit. The "mountain trip" was carried out in prison. One could not but feel that treatment would obviously have disturbed the vicious circle of the unconscious self-provoked punishment, followed consecutively by permission from within to practice the perversion.

Later I analyzed five cases in which the structure was always the same: the tearful "magic gesture" was acted out. The innuendo: "I show myself—under danger!—to strangers; you, bad Mother, didn't show yourself in *safety* to your own child!" [61]

IV. THE UNSUSPECTED IMPORTANCE OF THE VISUAL DRIVE

Having passed in review twenty-two neurotic manifestations directly connected with the visual drive and its shielding duenna, exhibitionism, we can proceed with an attempt to establish this psychic orbit in its proper place.

Everything related to "taking in" is of basic importance for the child. Today there is no longer any doubt in psychiatric circles of the importance of the *"oral" drive*. Voyeurism, *one of its subdivisions, rates high*—exactly because of this relation to orality—*on the psychic priority list*. Strangely enough, its importance has been greatly underestimated—so far.

Above and beyond the oral connection, there are two other determinants that make the visual drive, with its two unequal con-

The Visual Drive

stituents, even more important. One is the *"demonstration character"* in all neurotic and normal *defenses*. As already stated, the inner conscience (superego) constantly forces the unconscious ego to find ever new defenses. And each new defense is—to express it drastically and almost in caricature—built on this principle: *For crying out loud! I'm not guilty of the infraction you accuse me of, but of something else! I'll show you what I really did, or want!* This defensive "showing" of the *"lesser crime,"* or the alleged, though really only defensive, "wish," is executed—*via exhibitionism.*

The other determinant making for the importance of the visual drive is its *early connection with psychic masochism*. Parallel with the *normal* solution of the interdiction of peeping—defensive exhibitionism negating the disappointment at the breast—goes a *neurotic-masochistic* elaboration in which the "meanness" of the sight-refusing mother is stressed; and it is exactly to this fantasy that the child becomes masochistically attached. Thus the universal fantasy of "the mother (later, woman in general) as seductress," attracting with the forbidden sight and then refusing it. The mother is accused of a "cat-and-mouse" game in projection: "By half exhibiting she *made me* look!" Projection has its value as a guilt-diminisher.

Now psychic masochism is *not created* by visual disappointments; it has a different genesis (see Chapter 1). But once established, it is *strongly reinforced by voyeuristic vicissitudes,* or, more precisely, fantasies.

Three factors, therefore, contribute to the importance for the psychic economy of the visual drive and its elaborations:

1. Connection with orality in general—the visual drive being one of its subdivisions.
2. "Demonstration character" of all neurotic *and* normal unconscious defenses.
3. Reinforcement of psychic masochism.

The whole problem of the visual drive is incomprehensible without clarifying for oneself the *all-pervasive power of the inner conscience.* I have devoted three books to the subject, THE BATTLE OF THE

Conscience (1948), The Superego (1952), and Principles of Self-Damage (1959).

It can be said that the visual drive plays an indispensable part in our lives *day* and *night*. By day each and every one of us, without being aware of it, displays his exhibitionistic badge of inner defenses. By night—we dream. Whether or not one accepts B. Lewin's idea of a dream screen (a sort of permanent parchment made of mother's breast), certainly the images that flash through the mind, whose function of wish-fulfillment Freud so brilliantly elucidated, are exemplifying the voyeuristic-exhibitionistic technique with inconceivable speed. If one adds, as Jekels and I did ("Instinct Dualism in Dreams." Paper read at the XIII International Psychoanalytic Convention in Luzerne, Switzerland, 1934. Printed in *Imago,* 20:4, 1934, and *The Psychoanalytic Quarterly,* 9:3, 1940.), the important dreams evoked by superego reproaches with which the poor ego frantically defends itself, the scope of the visual orbit becomes even more clearly defined.

Life without imagination—the rarefied product of the visual drive is hardly to be thought of. Whether, as a wit put it, imagination was given to man to console him for what he is *not* and a sense of humor to compensate for what he *is,* the fact remains that the life of fantasy makes our ordinary lives more endurable. Moreover, the dreary world without the works of imagination would exclude no less than all the amenities and comforts, all inventions and technical conveniences; all science, including medicine, chemistry, industry; all social and political progress; all the arts, all literature, painting, sculpture, architecture, music; all the entertainments, theater, radio, movies, television; all love, foresight, thought, reverie, originality, ambition.

Though one can always counterpose Samuel Johnson's ironical reflection, "Were it not for imagination a man would be as happy in the arms of a chambermaid as of a duchess," the case *for* imagination is overwhelming. As proof of how much *normal* imagination enriches and lends color to life one could perhaps adduce the psychology of *romantic love:* [62]

The Visual Drive

Tender love is preceded by a period of heightened inner guilt. It would be naive to assume that the guilt—or its actual content—is conscious. The candidate for future love cannot be spotted by the way he beats his breast or tears his hair, crying "Mea culpa, mea maxima culpa, why am I not in love?" There are, of course, no such manifestations. What does rise to the psychic surface, in consciousness, is dissatisfaction, boredom, self-derision, and the type of complaint and doubt expressed in such familiar clichés as "life has no meaning," "life isn't worth living," etc. In some cases there is a feeling that one is living a "vegetable" existence, which indicates a mechanization of activity, coupled with depression.

Psychologically all these feelings are surface reverberations of a typical conflict in which the inflated ego ideal is compared with the ego's real achievement. The difference between the two is balanced by guilt. In this quandary the *normal* person tries the "slave revolt" of tender love, by which he can wrest the instrument of torture from his inner monster. The normal person projects his ego ideal upon the beloved, receives credit—before the event—for the achievement of all his ambitions, and thus eradicates the discrepancy between fantasy and reality. In consequence guilt is eliminated.

Without being aware of the real connection intuitive writers have described these facts correctly. True writers have this strange ability.

In Anatole France's novel THE RED LILY, Thérèse says:

> If you knew my life, if you had seen how empty it was without you, you would know what you mean to me, and you would no longer think of leaving me.

And in another passage:

> As for my past, if you knew how empty it was you would be content. I don't believe any other woman made for love as I am could have come to you as untouched by love as I did. That I swear to you. *In the years I passed without you I did not live.*

In his Letters to Eliza, Charles de Coster writes (1851-1853):

> Before I met you I did not know what love was. . . . *Only now [do] I realize the meaning of life.* . . . In emotional matters my judgment has become correct and certain, I should say unfail-

ing. And what caused this change? My loving you.... Nothing can hurt me, nothing offend me. If I gambled today I would win millions, if I had to take an examination I would surely pass.

...I have thrown off a cursed burden and from now on I shall be myself, because I love you as you deserve and because I want to make you happy....

What I now feel I have never felt before.... *I was blind and now I see.... You have taught me the meaning of living,* of thinking. I owe you everything.

Elizabeth Barrett makes an admission in a letter to Robert Browning dated February 24, 1846:

You are all to me, all the light, all the life; I am living for you now. And *before I knew you, what was I and where? What was the world to me, ... and the meaning of life?*

At bottom, what the lover loves in the beloved is himself; the beloved is the depository of a part of his own personality; the ego ideal.

Beethoven, for instance, wrote in an undated letter to his "immortal beloved":

My angel! My all! *My second self!*... I weep in thinking that you will receive no intelligence from me till probably Saturday. However dearly you may love me, I love you more fondly still. ... Oh, heavens! What a life without you!... I must live either wholly with you, or not at all.... Never can another possess my heart—never, never!... Continue to love me.... Oh, love me forever.

And Charles de Coster writes to Eliza (1851):

I know a heart belongs to me that is almost my own, that loves me more than I could love myself.... Each of us is incomplete without the other.... Now I have two hearts in my bosom, yours and mine. Your blood is my blood...you know my thoughts, ... you love what I love, and hate what I hate.

It is characteristic that "I" and "you" should be equated; additional evidence of this feeling is seen in the tender lover's emphasis on his complete absorption by the beloved object.

John Keats to Fanny Brawne (October 13, 1819):

My love has made me selfish. I cannot exist without you. I am forgetful of everything but seeing you again—my life seems to stop there.... *You have absorb'd me....* I could die for you. My Creed is Love and you are its only tenet.

And Keats again, in May 1820:

I am greedy of you. Do not think of anything but me.... I see *life* in nothing but the certainty of your love.... If I am not somehow convinced I shall die of agony.

Natalie Sacharin wrote to Alexander Herzen in 1835:

I remember the day we ... said adieu.... My heart was so heavy at the time that I could not possibly express myself in words, and yet, I felt as if I had everything, *as if my soul had joined yours, secretly.* Then I forgot the whole world....

Elizabeth Barrett wrote to Browning, in the same letter quoted above:

I am a great hero-worshipper.... By two or three half-words you made me see you, and other people had delivered orations on the same subject quite without effect.... Then, when you came, you never went away. *I mean I had a sense of your presence constantly....* Your love has been to me like God's own love, which makes the receivers of it kneelers.

Gustave Flaubert expressed his profoundest wish in "Novembre":

Oh, if I could hug something, smother it with my warmth or *become two myself,* love this other thing and *become one with it....*

An unconscious fantasy of the lover is secondarily amalgamated with the love object. The narcissistic basis of tender love explains why lovers so frequently claim that they have known each other all their lives.

Elizabeth Barrett to Robert Browning:

I had loved you all my life unawares, that is, the idea of you. ... Women ... love such and such an ideal, seen sometimes in a dream and sometimes in a book. ... One's ideal must be above one, ... it is as far as one can reach with one's eyes (soul-eyes), not reach to touch. And here is mine ... even to the visible outward sign of the black hair and the complexion, ... if it had been red hair quite, it had been the same thing. ...

Since one's ego ideal—a part of oneself—is loved in the beloved, the beloved is idealized.

Sir Richard Steele to Mary Scurlock, August 14, 1707:

The Vainest Woman upon Earth never saw in her Glasse half the attractions which I view in you. Your Air, Yr. Shape, Your every Glance, Motion and Gesture have such peculiar Graces that you possess my whole Soul, and I know no life but in the hope of Your approbation.

Claire Clairmont to Lord Byron in 1816:

You bid me write short to you and I have much to say. You also bade me believe that it was a fancy which made me cherish an attachment for you. It cannot be a fancy since you have been for the last year the object upon which every solitary moment led me to muse.

And Henrik Ibsen at sixty-two wrote to eighteen-year-old Emilie Bardach in 1889:

Well, for the time being I must do without your photograph. But I prefer it this way, I wait rather than have an unsatisfactory picture. And besides—how vivid is my memory of your charming, most serene appearance! I still believe there is a *mysterious princess* behind it. How about the mystery? Well—*one is free to dream about it and adorn it poetically*—and that I do. Anyway, it compensates somewhat for the unattainable and—unfathomable reality.

The Visual Drive

Ibsen put the lover's motto very well: "One is free to dream" about the mystery "and adorn it poetically."

Bourrienne, in his MEMOIRS, quotes Napoleon as saying about 1801, "The human race is governed by its imagination." In 1884 John Fiske said, "All human science is but the increment of the power of the eye" (THE DESTINY OF MAN). And as recently as 1929 John Dewey stated, "Every great advance in science has issued from a new audacity of imagination" (THE QUEST FOR CERTAINTY).

That imagination *per se* is but one of the two ingredients of science (the other being the checking of data) is acknowledged. "Put off your imagination, as you put off your overcoat, when you enter the laboratory," Claude Bernard said in 1865, "but put it on again, as you put on your overcoat, when you leave" (INTRODUCTION À LA MEDICINE EXPERIMENTALE). Only a few years later Oliver Wendell Holmes, independently of Bernard, maintained: "Science is a first-rate piece of furniture for a man's upper chamber, if he has common sense on the ground floor" (THE POET AT THE BREAKFAST TABLE, 1872).

As far as neuroses are concerned, I am convinced that the twenty-two clinical entities elucidated by the deeper structure of the visual drive are only a preliminary sample. More and more material will probably be found belonging to this orbit. Let us also not forget that all scientific progress in the field of psychotherapy means restoration of happiness for innumerable sufferers.

CHAPTER 8

HOW CAN ONE PROVE THAT THE SUPEREGO IS THE REAL MASTER OF THE PERSONALITY?

MANY informed people, including many colleagues, have difficulty in making it clear in their own minds that the real troublemaker, hence the "real boss" of the personality, is not the id, the reservoir of "repressed desires," but the forbidding inner conscience, the superego. In a long series of books I have tried to point out that the tragicomedy of the situation lies in the fact that the human being is dangling by a thread from twin alibis while the *superego reigns supreme*.

Whenever one makes the point that some action or reaction is a "defense mechanism," one is alluding—unwittingly—to this fact. All inner defenses are built for the benefit of the inner conscience. And of all these numerous defense mechanisms the most important is psychic masochism. The belabored ego accepts punishment, meted out on a twenty-four-hour basis, but changes it (by unconscious sleight of hand) into an unconscious pleasure.

In PRINCIPLES OF SELF-DAMAGE I gave this summary of the human tragedy:

A megalomaniacal philosopher of the last century (who, to counteract his own overdimensional inner passive-masochistic deposits, created the "superman" concept that was subsequently exploited for political purposes) numbered among his minor defensive efforts the statement that man's suffering was so excruciating that he was driven to invent laughter.

Is Superego the Real Master of Personality? 375

The suffering to which Nietzsche referred pertains to shortness of life, disease, misfortune, inequities, disappointments, but his observation also—and decisively—pertains to incalculable, unconscious, self-inflicted mental misery. It is a terrifying thought that each of us, in earliest childhood, installs an internal "misery machine" in his superego and thereafter must—in self-defense—learn to enjoy suffering, again unknowingly and unwittingly. On the other hand, life might possibly be unendurable without a certain amount of psychic masochism, though one should distinguish between productive and unproductive depositions.

The purpose of science is not to deplore but to investigate. And in investigating psychic phenomena one finds that the real responsibility for human misery must be ascribed to that impersonal factor biology. Biology decrees both the long maturation time of the human child and the fact that the newborn, helpless human child is endowed with drives that are potentially as strong as those he will have at his disposal as an adult. The three inborn drives rebel helplessly from the first moment of life: megalomania is offended, aggression rebounds against the ego, and libido sheds its saving grace on the unfortunate solution known as psychic masochism. In psychic masochism self-aggression is libidinized and megalomania artificially satisfied by provoking, and thus allegedly decreeing, punishment.

The majority of analysts avoid as unpalatable the fact that psychic masochism is universal; they show even more distaste for the fact behind this fact—the unremitting cruelty of the superego. But science cannot be converted to the program of happy endings adhered to by the slick magazines. Even distasteful facts must be swallowed when their accuracy has been demonstrated.

Biologically conditioned unfavorable depositions of rebounding aggression in earliest infancy result in the installation of the superego. Again in earliest infancy unplaceable megalomania, coupled with libido's rule of thumb, the pleasure principle, which tries to make the best of an impossible situation, results in the installation of the only possible defense against constant torture emanating from the superego—psychic masochism.

Unlike contemporary politics, where "too little and too late" is the main trouble, human biology presents the problem of "too much and too early."

"All humanity is pathetic," was Mark Twain's summing up, and not the least pathetic aspect of humanity deals with the fact that people forge their unconscious happiness out of conscious misery and are aware of the misery alone.

To prove how universal is the dualism of superego triumphant and *unconscious ego making the masochistic best of it,* I am collecting in this chapter a dozen or so *purposely unconnected* reactions. The common denominator is the dualism, plus the devious ways used by the ego in attempting to cling to its infantile megalomania, now masochistically (at best pseudoaggressively) tinged.

1. A NEW APPROACH TO THE OLD PROBLEM OF MASTURBATION

In my monograph, COUNTERFEIT-SEX, I gave the following summary of the general analytic experience concerning the near universality of masturbation among adult neurotics:

> There are male neurotics who avoid having any sexual contact whatsoever with a woman. Others marry as a sort of alibi, and even have intercourse occasionally without experiencing pleasure, while parallel with this "official" sex life there runs another "unofficial" one, devoted to masturbation (page 22).

The same applies, of course, to female neurotics.

It seems to be generally agreed in the analytic literature that adult masturbationists are unconsciously chained to their Oedipal fantasies. It is also acknowledged that adults who prefer masturbation to intercourse are neurotics.

Independently of each other, Jekels-Bergler and Nunberg arrived at the conclusion that the minus of satisfaction and surplus of guilt in adult masturbation has connection with insufficient discharge of aggression in the procedure. In "Transference and Love," [63] Jekels-Bergler stated:

> Why does normal man not stick to masturbation, which has been familiar to him since childhood? . . . There is not enough possibility in the subject's own ego of discharge of the so important

aggressive elements, which in part form the substratum of these tendencies, such as revenge, hostile feelings, etc., *unless one chooses the masochistic and hence neurotic way out.* It is practically the stigma of neurotics, with their insufficient and inhibited directing of aggression from their own egos upon objects, that they have to be contented with masturbation. The insufficient discharge of aggression in masturbation seems to us a circumstance of which the importance should not be under-rated. It is one which seems important to us for two reasons: first, it explains the inadequacy of satisfaction through masturbation; second, it makes highly questionable the frequent allegation that masturbation in adults is harmless—indeed, it may contradict it (pp. 349 ff., my italics).

H. Nunberg, in ALLGEMEINE NEUROSENLEHRE (Hans Huber, Berne, 1932), states that the reason for guilt feelings accompanying masturbation "is not quite clear." It cannot be the educational interdiction alone, because that guilt is visible even in cases in which that interdiction in childhood cannot be proven. The author suspects that puberal masturbation revives infantile guilt connected with Oedipal fantasies. Moreover, "in the inhibition of satisfaction of sexual drives also the aggressive drives cannot find cathexis outside, hence are turned inside and are changed into guilt. Never is there full satisfaction in masturbation, at least not in the sexual sphere, since the real object is missing. The aggression, connected with libidinous tendencies, changes into need for punishment" (p. 168).

That masturbation fantasies do not represent direct id-eruptions, but *modified inner defenses,* was first pointed out by myself in 1934. In my study, "Some Special Varieties of Ejaculatory Disturbance Not Hitherto Described," [64] I adduced the case of a man who practiced "coitus incognito," forcing the girl to describe in obscene words experiences with other men. This man's masturbation fantasy had the background of direct repetition of an observed intercourse of the parents. It was this masturbation fantasy which pushed him into analysis. The question arose: why had the patient retained in consciousness a fantasy otherwise repressed? The answer was that he was hiding behind someone else (when he attempted intercourse "in his proper person" the erection collapsed immediately), and that the fantasy also served as unconscious camouflage for feminine identification. Specifically, the text states: "Other determinants of his peculiar wish were *a tendency to masochistic abasement* . . ." etc.[65]

Summarizing the literature, one can state that adult masturbation is based on being chained to Oedipal fantasies, and the minus of satisfaction and plus of guilt (as compared with normal intercourse) is reducible to insufficient discharge of aggression outside.

In the already quoted extract from "Transference and Love" (which Jekels and I wrote in 1931) will be found the dictum: ". . . unless one chooses the masochistic and hence neurotic way out." In the intervening thirty years, recognition of the masochistic component has become more and more important clinically.

As stated repeatedly in these pages, I believe that the masochistic solution, based on oral regression, is *the* basic neurosis. All later stages are unconsciously used either as rescue stations from the oral danger, or as camouflages (expressing on a higher level in the language of these stations) of old, never-relinquished oral-masochistic conflicts. Nobody denies the existence and reality of higher developmental levels in the libidinous-aggressive development of the child; the question is solely whether or not these are subsumed and "reformulated" under the direction of the oral-masochistic "solution."

Not enough attention has been paid to the baby's many and powerful fears; the more superficial phallic castration fear has been overrated. The precursors of castration fears are decisive. In THE BASIC NEUROSIS I described the *"septet of baby fears,"* comprising such fantastic (to the adult, that is) entities as fear of being starved, devoured, poisoned, choked, chopped to pieces, drained, castrated.

Every unprejudiced analytic observer who scrutinizes the contents of masturbation fantasies of adult male neurotics will attest to the fact that seemingly sadistic features (or at least situations embarrassing to the woman) dominate; these are covered by conquering heroic feats. One small exception can be noted: actual masochistic fantasies in which the masturbationist is either the direct victim or a spectator.

In adult masturbating women, fantasies of being "forced," raped or victimized are just as frequent as idyllic, covering love-fantasies. Even the naive Kinsey claimed (on the basis of statements made by his neurotic volunteers, whom he mistakenly took to represent a cross-section of normality) that women are aroused by fantasies connected with reading romantic novels, seeing love movies, and— by being bitten. That the first two parts of his triad could constitute an inner defense against the third did not occur to Kinsey.[66]

To my surprise, it turned out that—regardless of the camouflage— *all adult masturbationists unconsciously live out masochistic fantasies.* Those who half-admit to this substitute a more attenuated, "harmless," masochistic fantasy for a more deeply repressed, dangerous one, connected with one of the participants from the "septet of baby fears."

What does this mean?

In my opinion, the allure of masturbation to the adult neurotic does not rest on Oedipal and/or pre-Oedipal fantasies. These are subsequently adduced (unconsciously, to be sure) as "admission of the lesser intrapsychic crime." The main *unconscious* attraction is that "something is done to me." Although the masturbationist seemingly plays an active role—he produces the accompanying fantasy, handles his sex organ or moves it on the bed sheet—the underlying propelling fantasy is *passive* in scope. In this repressed fantasy, some *partes constituentes* of the "septet of baby fears" are invoked, with the masturbationist on the receiving end. As defense, pseudo-sadistic and narcissistic covering illusions are put in operation.

In cases in which masochistic fantasies dominate outright, a strong attenuation is discernible. Beating fantasies are relatively harmless, compared with any of the *partes constituentes* of the ominous "septet of baby fears." There is also the known fact of double identification even in sadistic fantasies (Freud), where the official torturer also unconsciously identifies with the victim.

One could add that *"doing it oneself to oneself"*—which is what masturbation actually is—*reproduces in a watered-down and diluted form (with the addition of greater safeguards) what the child imagined as forcefully and with malicious intent done to him by the Giantess of the Nursery. That transformation of an acute inner danger into a self-produced game is the strongest allure of masturbation.*

Thus, *masturbation is a sanctuary of masochistic passivity,* regardless of the "package wrapping" of superimposed, alibi-providing secondary defenses.

The best the male neurotic can do in intercourse is to place passivity —in a process that requires activity—by unconsciously identifying with the allegedly passive woman. These attitudes have been connected with the negative Oedipus (feminine identification in the man), a conclusion which overlooks the fact that the negative Oedipus has an oral substructure.

In previous years, many authors stressed the fact that many men, after a satisfactory intercourse, dream a homosexual dream. This was taken as positive proof of bisexuality. I believe that homosexuality is but a defense against oral-masochistic vicissitudes (see ONE THOUSAND HOMOSEXUALS and HOMOSEXUALITY: DISEASE OR WAY OF LIFE?). Hence, these dreams are, once more, a disguise of passivity. In short, homosexuality had been misunderstood.

There is a connection with homosexuality, however. It is a well-known fact that homosexuals are constantly eager for new sexual experiences. Since masochistic passivity is the basis of homosexuality, the need for an alibi (of conquering "sex") must be constant as well.

Masturbation is the faithful duenna of every adult neurotic for the following reasons:

1. Masturbation is the sanctuary of earliest, dangerous masochistic passivity, now converted into a "harmless" game; instead of being cruelly manipulated by the pre-Oedipal mother image, the masturbationist handles himself in a "repetition in reverse" (active repetition of passively endured or fantasied passive experiences).

2. In men, masturbation as depository of the "septet of baby fears" is defensively covered by narcissistic-conquering, woman-embarrassing fantasies. In woman, the original supposed cruelties of the mother image are diluted and attenuated into more superficial fantasies of being raped, mishandled or forced, or into superficial, secondarily defensive romantic fantasies of unending love.

3. An added inner allure in masturbation is provided by elements of the forbidden and uncanny, with their promise of dangerous self-

damage. These are faint reverberations of the original dangerous masochism.

4. Guilt because of masturbation pertains to the masochistic substructure, and is secondarily shifted to the pseudo-aggression in the act itself or the fantasy (Oedipal, pre-Oedipal).

5. Normal intercourse is no substitute for masochistically tinged masturbation; the normal satisfaction accruing from placing normal aggression in the sex act does not allure the masochistic neurotic; his major problem is the inability to place a superabundance of masochistic passivity.

6. Oedipal and pre-Oedipal repressed fantasies are not the motor power of neurotic masturbation, but the half-admitted (though also unconscious) "lesser intrapsychic crime." These fantasies cover the "crime of inner crimes"—psychic baby-masochism.

The conclusion from the thesis—masturbation in adults covers exclusively a masochistic substratum—is inescapable: analyzing the sexual-aggressive cover fantasies alone *cannot* destroy the masochistic basis. The opposite technique is necessary: these fantasies have to be discarded as camouflage and the hidden oral-masochistic basis analytically attacked.

2. THE UNIVERSAL, THOUGH UNDERESTIMATED, IMPORTANCE OF PASSIVE BEATING FANTASIES COVERING DEEPER FEARS.

In a long series of studies and books, I have been pointing out for a quarter of a century that the earliest fears of the infant, baby, small child, can be subsumed in a "septet of baby fears" which comprises such "improbabilities" as fear of being starved, devoured, poisoned, choked, chopped to pieces, drained, castrated. Later in life these fears are repressed and secondarily included in the *psychic masochistic solution.*

The interesting fact about these early fears is that *none lends itself either to daydreams or to masturbation fantasies.* However, in all neurotics and half-neurotics beating fantasies can be unconsciously ascertained, and all neurotics and half-neurotics masturbate, drawn by the unconscious allure of the uncanny in masturbation, which consists entirely of an attenuation of "something is done to me." (For elaboration see No. 1 of this chapter.)

The question arises as to why beating fantasies are expressible, and all constituents of the "septet" unusable for defensive—though pleasure-giving—fantasies, regardless of whether or not those lead to masturbation.

In my opinion, the answer lies in the extremity of fear connected with the original "septet" and *the veto of the superego*. Assuming this to be the case, how and why is the attenuated expression in beating fantasies (passive, or defensively "sadistic") possible. What singles out beating fantasies?

The first approach to the solution of the riddle could naively point out that traditionally most corporal punishments imposed by educators are executed on the buttocks (less frequently on the cheeks). There are obvious advantages: the anatomic locality chosen cannot reveal marks of beatings to outsiders because it is covered with clothing; the harm possibly done by spanking is minimal; the pain which results is sufficient to be felt by the culprit. In short, practical considerations dominate.

That "practical" explanation suffers from a series of drawbacks. To start with, it overlooks the fact that even children who have never actually been spanked or threatened, and who live in comparative isolation, produce the fantasy of being spanked on the buttocks. Second, it is unlikely that so universal a psychic phenomenon as the fantasy of being punished by such a spanking should arise in the absence of *all* psychic reasons.

The whole analytic literature, following Freud's study, "A Child is Being Beaten," labors under a time restriction. When Freud published his study in 1919, the pre-Oedipal phase had not yet been worked out by the creator of psychoanalysis; that task was incompletely accomplished in 1931 in "On Female Sexuality." I attempted to build in the precursors of the beating fantasy in my study, "Preliminary Phases of the Masculine Beating Fantasy" (1938),[46] showing that the infantile aggressions directed against the *maternal breast* are shifted because of guilt (*secondarily libidinized*) towards *the individual's own buttocks* (*an identification also unconsciously presented as "proof positive" that the child has "breasts," too*), where

—on higher developmental levels—Freud's tripartite scheme on Oedipal beating fantasies applies. So far, I have never read a refutation of that obvious conclusion, backed up by clinical material.

Moreover, in a later study [67] I was able to show that in cases in which beating fantasies are combined with strong voyeuristic-exhibitionistic ones, depersonalization is used as typical defense mechanism.

A clinical example of recent experience may help clarify the issue.

A man in his late forties, a writer of high achievement in a specific field, spent a great deal of his time in fantasies centering around one single theme: A naked girl (or a number of girls) was forced to undress, then bound and flogged by a "mean older woman." Unending variations were imagined and executed in fantasy.

The patient had been happily married for twenty-six years, retaining good potency. This part of his life was totally split off from his *masochistic fantasy life,* although the circumstances under which he met and chose his wife provided a significant link. He had been visiting a Southern city. At the suggestion of an acquaintance, he looked up a family which included two presentable girls. The acquaintance described them as "one nice, the other bitchy." He attached himself to and married the "bitchy" girl. As it turned out, the acquaintance's "diagnosis" happened to be wrong, because the girl was actually kind and loving. Since he had originally approached her convinced of the wrong diagnosis, he certainly had an ulterior, masochistic motive, as he freely admitted later, after coming to understand the interconnections.

The term, "masochistic," was deliberately used in describing his fantasies, despite their pseudo-sadistic disguises. It became clear in analysis that the patient identified himself with these mistreated girls, admitting to feminine identification as the "lesser intrapsychic crime" in order to disguise his real crime: masochism.

The highly intelligent patient was decidedly astonished when another of his traits—the constant expectation of external threats, disasters, doom—was connected in analysis with his passive beating fantasies, in inner identification with the mistreated girls. He interposed a reasonable objection: The "sadistic" beating fantasies (as he erroneously called them) gave him pleasure; his expectations of danger, ruin, collapse of existence gave him "only displeasure." If he were as all-pervading a masochist as I claimed, why would he miss out on the opportunity to "libidinize" this apprehension?

My answer was simple: *Passive, though disguised, beating fantasies were the maximum one could rescue, in fantasy, from the libidinized terror of the "septet of baby fears."* The actual components of the septet, the seven passive fears of babyhood and their elaborations, are too frightening to be used directly for pleasure in fantasy or action; moreover, the superego's veto is too stringent to be defied. The beating fantasies would disappear, I told the patient, when his analysis had progressed to the point where the original terrors hidden behind the beating fantasies had been emotionally digested and become conscious. Politely the patient reserved the right to be skeptical.

He described his childhood situation as dominated by a stern, puritanical, domineering mother and an ineffectual father. He openly admitted that he had hated his mother. Later in analysis, however, he changed his opinion of his mother; he conceded that she did the best she could, though "her light was not too bright."

To show how the Midwestern "Bible Belt" philosophy of constant threat of punishment by God (the mother being the representative) permeated his childhood, he cited an example dating from his third or fourth year. His father had been fired from his job, again. The boy heard the phrase but did not understand it, and developed a fear of the outdoor privy, believing that hellfire, coming from below, would consume him. . .

In every case of beating fantasy the specific repressed fear (from the unconscious "septet") which hides behind it must be sought for. In this patient's case it turned out to be the fear of being chopped to pieces. All parts of the ominous septet are inwardly in evidence in every one. Still, in individual cases, one constituent is finally singled out. E.g., in this case, the patient settled for "being chopped to pieces." But, as the dream and associations reported below show, the fantasy of "being eaten up" (devoured) by mother was also in evidence. The usual recollections of the mother cutting meat, fowl, fish were available. This patient had also witnessed the slaughtering of pigs. All these experiences were covered by the unspoken formula: "A woman capable of *that* is capable of doing it to me, too."

Since the patient was a blocked writer, the *anti*-masochistic technique of artistic creativity was discussed. The productive writer denies his masochistic attachment to the pre-Oedipal mother by establishing an autarchy via the "unification tendency": "Bad mother doesn't even exist for me; I, out of myself, for myself, through myself, establish myself as the corrected, *giving* mother and the happy *recipient* child, giving myself beautiful ideas, words, masterpieces." (See Chapter 7, no. 8.)

A longer period of typical oscillation followed. On some days, the block disappeared (when the patient gave himself interpretation); on others it was very much in evidence, despite all interpretations. One morning, on the patient's way to his office, he found himself in a "brilliant mood" and asked himself ironically, "Who's afraid of the big bad wolf?" Result: total block on that day. Obviously his superego was teaching him a lesson in humility and modesty. The patient reported: "The night before I dreamed of a tree, some uncanny being (a woman?) with a big knife." There was only one association: wildcats were present in his part of the country; he thought of them as "she." The dream seems to represent a mixture between a refutation and a neurotic vindication dream: "The bad, devouring mother actually exists; therefore I am not playing a masochistic game with myself."

After extended periods of ups and downs the unexpected (by the patient, that is) happened: he caught himself changing his beloved fantasy. In the new version he, not the girl, was bound, and the woman had a whip ending in a *knife*. The more real precursor behind the palimpsest of the beating fantasy had emerged.

Typically, the patient could not use that fantasy for "pleasure." It merely "frightened the hell out of him." Result: increase of unrealistic fearful expectations of external threats, dismissed with relative ease by connecting the facts.

The further phases of this successful analysis are without significance here.

Whatever the "package wrapping," all neuroses are reducible to the basic masochistic conflict, elaborated on in the genetic and clinical pictures. (See Chapter 1.)

As mentioned before, one invariably comes across two facts in analyzing adult neurotics: unconsciously, they all harbor passive *"beating fantasies"* and consciously they all *masturbate*. How are we to explain these observations and in what way—if any—are they interconnected?

The language in its primitive intuitive wisdom answers the first question. Phrases like these are common: "He was leading with his chin."—"He was asking for a kick in the pants."—"He worked hard to get a kick in the jaw."—"He didn't roll with the punches." Always bodily harm is alluded to. That means that *the precursor of mental masochism is bodily masochism.*

The problem can be understood only if one scrutinizes the "septet of baby fears."

All these fears pertain to *bodily* harm. In the great majority of people these fears are transferred from reality to imagination and *psychic* masochism results. In a small minority of people the accent on bodily harm (though libidinized) is retained, and *perversion* masochism results. In both psychic and perverted masochists, however, the baby fears are eliminated from consciousness and the buttocks chosen as executive organ of "passive beating fantasies." Why exactly that anatomical location?

The maternal organ that becomes the child's greatest hope and greatest defeat is the breast. The naive argument that most babies in progressive countries are bottle- and not breast-fed, thus experiencing no direct contact with the breast, is best refuted by stating that every time the mother takes the child in her arms, the breast is felt, and modern clothing rather accentuates that organ by decreeing the firming and form-shaping brassiere. Nobody can deny that the child wants everything it does not possess—why not the breast?

The breast becomes the unachievable model. The boy finally solves the conflict by identifying penis and breast. The girl, having less illusory length at her disposal, endows the clitoris with growth possibilities, still consoling herself with the identification clitoris = nipple, and with "fluid production." The latter fantastic identification, milk = urine, is based on the fact that the orifice of the female urethra is

Is Superego the Real Master of the Personality? 387

directly below the clitoris. One does not expect from a baby knowledge that two different organs are involved. How many adult men have precise, detailed knowledge of the anatomic position of the genitalia in women?

In both sexes, however, buttocks and breast are unconsciously identified. From this stems the overwhelming importance of beating fantasies in the unconscious: the masochistic solution is at least dealt with at a consoling substitutive organ used as denial of one's own lack of the cherished organ, the breast! The inner fantasy reads: "I have a breast!"

Moreover, the buttocks are chosen as substitutive organ for another reason as well. *The buttocks include a "pseudo-moral connotation"* (see Chapter 4, pp. 130 ff.)—*the parents use them as organ for application of punishment.*

This problem is intimately connected with *the enigma of adult masturbation*, as stated in no. 1 of this chapter.

Repressed beating fantasies play an important part in blushing; see Chapter 7, no. 2.

Finally, the attenuation of beating fantasies to the universal wish to be stroked and caressed should be adduced. In a previous paper (" 'Stroke'—Neurotic Progressive Attenuation from Noun to Verb," *The Psychoanalytic Review,* XL:44-60, 1953), I pointed out that a peculiar and ambiguous connotation is attached to the word "stroke" in the English language: used as a noun, the word indicates a *blow;* used as a verb, it means *to caress.* Philologists cannot explain the duality; they merely register the contradiction. They quote, for example, Isaiah XXX, 26: "Healeth the *stroke* of their wound," and with no apparent uneasiness continue, a few lines later, with a Chaucer epigram: "Ye mote with the plat sword again/ *Stroke* him in the wound, and it will close."

Thus, to hurt and to soothe stand in close proximity, although in meaning they are exact opposites. The most that can be coaxed (off the record) from a devotee of semantics is the tentative suspicion that "perhaps" caresses developed from blows, a theory in line with the European peasants' joke in which a wife complains of her husband's indifference—"He hasn't beaten me for a whole week."

Jokes and semantics aside, there exists a group of neurotics whose whole psychic development can be summarized "from stroke to stroke," the first used as a noun, the second as a verb. They progress from the noun to the verb, at the point of "stroke." Inwardly, one could say, they cling to a curious economy in words which can be compared to Hamlet's sarcastic comment on his mother's hasty marriage after his father's death:

> Thrift, thrift, Horatio! The funeral baked meats
> Did coldly furnish forth the marriage tables.

Leaving semantics and poetry to their respective adherents, let us concentrate on clinical material.

A woman in her middle twenties came into analysis because of personality conflicts. With a few rare exceptions, she was able to achieve orgasm only after the performance of a preparatory routine in which her husband stroked her buttocks for quite a long time. During intercourse proper, she habitually imagined herself in an exhibitionistic act of one kind or another. Generally this was a strip-tease.

It developed that the stroking requirement had been preceded by fantasies which were promptly brought to the surface in analysis. These fantasies dated from a period between her tenth and twelfth years. In them, she and *a* boy were beaten by the boy's father. Sometimes merely verbal lashing sufficed.

What prompted the transition from *beating fantasies* to *stroking reality*?

The patient's further recollections pertained to a distant cousin, a young boy who had spent a few months in her parents' house when she was four or five years of age. The children shared the same room but had separate beds. The sleeping arrangement insisted upon by the patient's mother was that the children keep their backs turned to one another. "In the morning she would regularly find us sleeping in the same bed." What had "happened" was repressed. When the two cousins met again, at the time of puberty, they were both "deeply embarrassed," and both unable to explain their embarrassment.

The patient's home situation was based on the duality, weak passive father, energetic mother. Even as an adult, she remained neurotically attached to her mother; she would spend many hours at her mother's house every day. Most of the time the two women sat reading detective stories; both seemingly indulged in killing fantasies. Although the patient's parents were well-to-do and the patient and her husband lived in very restricted circumstances, the young woman was incapable of asking her mother for the slightest financial help. Both the mother and father were pathologically stingy, which embittered the patient's husband. Her own attitude was "objective." In theory she agreed with her husband; practically speaking, she was "paralyzed" when urged to ask them any favor at all.

The patient's husband was some years older than herself. She had married him against her parents' wishes. Her marriage had changed her peculiarly; she had been an intelligent and alert college student, but then became "an intellectual nobody." Intellectually, she had—so to speak—gone on strike. She never read anything but mystery stories.

The first approach to her "strip-tease" fantasies became possible. It was clear that her exhibitionism—the defense against her more deeply repressed voyeurism—was a means of "taking the blame for the lesser intrapsychic crime." She was accepting the blame for exhibitionism. She reproduced these fantasies while she was being stroked; the strokes obviously represented an attenuated beating.

The beating fantasies had a complicated substructure. Freud subdivided feminine beating fantasies into three stages: *First phase:* "My father beats a child whom I hate." *Second phase:* "I am beaten by my father" (repressed). *Third phase:* "A teacher (father substitute) is beating boys."

In continuation of Freud's basic paper on beating fantasies, I pointed out (in several published papers) and in COUNTERFEIT-SEX that the pre-Oedipal substructure is missing. The child directs strongly aggressive impulses against mother's breast; the breasts are later shifted, because of guilt, to the child's own buttocks (an identification also presented as positive proof that the child has "breasts," too); the guilt is accepted and secondarily libidinized. All this leads straight to masochistic beating fantasies. Subsequently, in the Oedipal phase, Freud's tripartite formula applies, the execution being transferred to the father.

As mentioned previously, the only retrieved recollections of the patient's beating fantasies pertained to the personality of "*a* boy and his father." It turned out that the boy was identical with the distant cousin who had shared the girl's room. What had happened between the two children could be reconstructed from two peculiarities in the patient's behavior as an adult: first, her adamant refusal to lift her legs during intercourse, for which her explanation was that she was "physically incapable of doing that"; second, her strip-tease fantasies during the sex act proper. Since these fantasies were conscious, the suspicion arose that these exhibitionistic fantasies covered more deeply repressed voyeuristic ones as "admission of the lesser crime." This was confirmed when the reason for the cousin's protracted visit was clarified. The boy's mother was suffering from paralysis of the lower extremities after the birth of a child. Since, in intercourse, the patient also acted the paralyzed person (in her inability to lift her legs), the probability arose that mutual inspection must have taken place. Later these voyeuristic acts became guilt-laden on the basis of identification with the boy's paralyzed mother. Finally, the probability could not be dismissed that the children acted "making a baby," the latter anally and masochistically-sadistically misconstrued. This would explain the patient's side-position and buttocks preference during adult intercourse.

These half-Oedipal imitations, it developed, covered a repressed pre-Oedipal layer. The latter could be reconstructed from the patient's extreme intolerance of being touched at her breasts. She was afraid of some indefinable danger, and declared that any touch—even her beloved stroking—was painful. Having missed the possession of breasts as a child, regarding these as mother's prerogative, she was inwardly afraid of endangering her most cherished possession, which she had finally achieved. There was also an attempt at avoidance of the infantile conflict on the original battlefield.

Another hint pointing in the same direction was the patient's overeating. In the last few years, the patient had put on a good deal of weight, much to the chagrin of her husband, who still saw in her the sylph of the past. Her overeating, it became clear, was the typical inner defense of the orally regressed gourmet: accused by the inner conscience of masochistically wanting to be refused, the unconscious ego brings forth the defense: "I want to get." Overeating results.

After working out and through these interconnections, the

patient changed remarkably. She lost twenty-five pounds, finding herself for the first time capable of reducing (her innumerable attempts in previous years had all been failures). In addition, the "paralysis" of her legs "disappeared."

The most tenacious resistance attached itself to two other symptoms: the inability to ask her mother for the smallest favor, and the "untouchability" of the whole breast region. Both symptoms were eventually worked out and changed. The explanation of the first symptom pertained to the patient's "basic fallacy," the latter consisting of the "proof" that she, the patient, was not being masochistic in wanting to be refused by mother but that mother was really stingy and refusing. By not giving her mother a chance (the mother did need some prodding), she maintained the fantasy which constituted her alibi. The patient at last conceded the efficacy of analysis when she asked her stingy mother for a house—and got it.

Besides being "the woman who could not lift her legs" and an industrious injustice collector, the patient presented the interesting problem of *the mechanism of unconscious attenuation:* she was capable of unconsciously changing her original, quite dangerous *beating fantasy* into a comparatively harmless *stroking reality.*

How frantically the patient fought her repressed masochistic attachment to the pre-Oedipal mother was visible in her peculiar, compulsive, "mutual detective-story session" with her mother. Here she superficially identified with the killer, unconsciously with the victim. Another facet was her intellectual drought since marriage: she renounced any improvement, since, in the patient's unconscious vocabulary, "taking in knowledge" meant taking in nourishment. As Faust had it: "sucking on wisdom's breasts."

In another layer, marriage and sex meant an attempt at dissociation from mother, and therefore no further "nourishment" (equated with mother) was allowed.

The patient described above could almost be called a hedonist when contrasted with another young woman—a deeply depressed patient, aged thirty-two, who gave herself the epithet of "a beautiful but unusable blonde." She complained that she spent her time "in constant pain." Her pain was a muscular tension around the lower part of her back. She characterized it as "a burning, tearing, fiery-tongue-like, torturing" sensation. Neurologists, internists, even surgeons were of no avail; finally she was sent into analysis.

"My whole life is concentrated on my back, and believe me, my pains are real. When I get my attacks, I scream like a wounded or tortured animal, and mind you, this goes on for hours at a time." She admitted to being frigid in her marriage. She was deeply offended when someone voiced the suspicion that she was "acting up" to torture her husband. "I don't believe that: I started having my attacks before my marriage. Too bad that marriage didn't cure the pain."

Two suspicions arose. The first was that this constant, painful self-observation was some pseudo-hypochondriacal precursor, or attenuated after-effect of depersonalization. The second was that the patient was also acting out, in a negative magic gesture, the after-effects of an infantile beating scene: "I'll show you—bad mother or father—what you did to me!"

When asked about beating episodes in her childhood, the patient recalled actual whippings given by her father. (Beating realities seldom account for beating fantasies; the first patient cited was never beaten as a child. Moreover, many a thrashing is unconsciously provoked by the neurotic child.) The patient remembered a temper tantrum which came after one of these beatings; she had refused to leave her position on the edge of the bed where the beating took place, and had cried furiously for a long time, making uncoordinated movements with her legs, burying her head in the pillow, and refusing to allow anyone to rearrange her dress. "With a naked red behind, I must have looked pretty," she remarked with some irony. Still, her manner as she reported this memory was as detached as if she were mentioning the time she had the measles—an unimportant incident from the distant past.

Her father had administered the thrashing, the patient admitted, because as a child she had been "unmanageable to such a degree that her weak father had been driven to desperation." The "real boss" in the family was mother; the child and her mother "just did not get along."

Depersonalization was well known to her as a feeling, although she had never before heard the technical term. When her symptoms first became aggravated (which was a few years before entering analysis, and after her marriage proved unsatisfactory), she had gone through a period of "mental disorientation, although I was fully oriented." Everything, including her body, seemed "strange, different, unreal."

This period of frightening unreality when she believed she was "losing her mind" was followed by heightened "back pain." This continued and gradually dominated her life. Only one remedy proved of use: "gentle massage" by a female osteopath successfully eased acute pain, but unfortunately for only a few hours at a time.

The patient was extremely reticent and taciturn. She had little to contribute in the form of associations, recollections, observations. If she talked at all, she simply elaborated on minute descriptions of her "burning" sensations. She never remembered her dreams; she merely, monotonously, complained.

One day, to break the deadlock, I asked her whether she remembered a fairy tale in which a person is punished in the identical (though slightly romanticized) fashion in which she was torturing herself.

"That's impossible; not even fairy tales record such tortures."

"Think; perhaps you can find an analogy."

"I don't remember."

"May I remind you of Snow White? Isn't the bad stepmother forced to dance at the wedding in red-hot shoes till she dies?" (American translations omit this detail, which is to be found in the original Grimm version. The patient recognized it because she had first heard the story, in all its gruesomeness, from a nurse of German extraction.)

"That's true."

"You see, I suspect that in your pains you are repeating the after-effects of thrashing, as if demonstrating to the world how your father tortured you. On the other hand, you said that your father was a weak and ineffectual man, completely under your mother's dominance. Add to this the way you described your feelings, which was not appropriate for a feeling of simple pain while being thrashed. Behind this superficial disguise there is a torture chamber, obviously attributed to infantile conceptions of mother. You spoke of 'burning, tearing, fiery-tongue-like, torturing sensations.'"

"Don't forget the rest of the fairy tale: the bad stepmother tried to choke the poor girl to death by tight lacing, to poison her with the comb and the apple. Well, I can't accuse my mother of *that!*"

"Of course. Don't overlook the fact that we are not dealing with realities, but with repressed baby fantasies. And we know that the child creates a septet of baby fears, a series of imaginary dangers, all attributed to mother. These are fear of being starved, devoured, poisoned, choked, chopped to pieces, drained, castrated. You will admit that your description is in some ways similar to these."

"But my pain is real."

"Nobody denies that, if you understand by 'real' the fact that you feel it. Yes, your pains are real, though unconsciously you are creating them yourself. Just as the relief given by the osteopath—a woman—is real enough, even though the reasons are created by you yourself."

"That's fantastic."

"Not less so than your self-created torture chamber. Isn't it possible that you are using your osteopath as proof that what you really want from your mother is *stroking,* not strokes?"— (In some other cases I have observed, the unconscious effect of osteopathic practices was based on the pain and discomfort associated with the procedures, hence appealed more directly to the masochistic sufferers. The osteopathic practitioner, of course, explains it differently, and does not adduce psychological factors.)—"In splitting off the images of good and bad mother, you are quite consistent."

"Can you prove all that?" the patient asked.

"Only by material you will have to provide."

For some time a renewed stalemate ensued: the patient had nothing to say. One day, however, she came up with a recollection dating from her third year. At that time she possessed a favorite doll; she made quite a fuss over this doll and in doing so incurred the anger of a "malicious housekeeper." In the child's opinion, this woman had burned her doll. The child accused her of having done so, even claiming to have discovered remnants of the doll in the open fireplace. The parents did not believe the aggrieved child's accusations. The child developed a peculiar fear of burning wood, and later a fear of everything connected with the fireplace. Half-burnt, glimmering pieces of coal especially frightened her; she remembered "rigidity of the whole body" at even a glimpse of red-hot coals, or of the tongs with which the coals were handled.

I asked the patient: "Isn't it possible that you identified yourself with your pet doll, and acted as if you were burnt in an auto-da-fe?"

"But this was so long ago!"

"That's exactly what neurosis means: unconsciously keeping alive anachronistic wishes, defenses, guilt—all belonging to the infantile past."

"But why should I have felt guilty? I was the injured party!"

"You are forgetting a little detail. Your fury was directed against people with the family halo, your mother in particular. That causes guilt."

"But mother didn't burn the doll."

"Didn't you say your mother didn't believe your accusation against the housekeeper? And who engaged this woman in the first place, and who left her untouched in her position? And wasn't the hatred of the housekeeper only the second edition of the original conflict with mother?"

The patient did not answer. We discussed the genesis of psychic masochism, and I explained its unconscious structure.

"According to you," the patient indignantly objected, "I'm a lover of pain, humiliation, self-defeat. I am exactly the opposite. I am a fun-loving person."

"Let's not confuse conscious with unconscious aims," I replied.

"I still don't understand. My whole environment accuses me of torturing my husband; you claim I torture myself and get unconscious pleasure out of it. How can I do both?"

"Now you are confusing wish and defense. Exactly because your inner conscience accuses you—and justifiably—of being a glutton for punishment, you put up the defense of pseudo-aggression, which was originally directed against your mother. Your husband is just an innocent substitute object. The frantic attempt to prove your aggression to yourself can also be seen in your selective memory: you remember the temper tantrum you had after a whipping, but you don't remember the beating itself."

"According to you, my terrible pains are just my way of putting my mother in the wrong, in short, *heaping coals of fire on mother's head."*

"That's correct. What makes you use exactly these words?"

"I don't know. It's a quotation from the Bible."

"I know that. The question is, why do you use it? Isn't there some connection with your auto-da-fe?"

The woman was stunned; she had not connected these two facts.

The next (rather typical) result was a "negative therapeutic reaction": her symptom flared up again. The aggravation was explained as a "slave revolt" of the unconscious, and quickly squelched. The patient's next resistance pertained to the fact that all I could tell her was at best a series of guesses, not backed up by recollections.

"What you call 'guesses' are reconstructions, based on your behavior as an adult. There are no human recollections before the age of two, and your troubles started before that age. According to Freud, recollections and reconstructions have the identical dynamic value in analysis. Speaking of recollections, I don't believe that you have retrieved everything retrievable."

A few days later the patient admitted that for some time she had been holding back a recollection, "How I improved on Snow White."

"So you do remember the fairy tale?"

As a child—"mind you, only playfully"—she had acted out an improvement on the tightly-laced girl in the tale. In these games, she would stand in front of the mirror, tightly squeezing her buttocks with a strap, "till it hurt."

"Are you now convinced that you are the manufacturer of your pains?"

"I have been for some time, but why should I give you the satisfaction of being right?"

"So in the transference you are once again repeating the 'heaping coals of fire' technique?"

After working out the connections with depersonalization, the patient was cured.

Both cases described used, to varying extents, the "mechanism of unconscious attenuation," unconsciously diluting to harmlessness the original dangerous "solution." The first patient resorted to this mechanism as a defense, claiming it was only "harmless

Is Superego the Real Master of the Personality? 397

stroking." The second patient found this means of establishing a new defense when the superego's reproaches invalidated earlier ones; she claimed that her alleged need was "being loved," and proved her point temporarily when her pains yielded to the osteopath's stroking. In each case, too, the extent of the simulated retreat from the real (though repressed) masochistic aim varied. The first patient no longer executed her beating fantasies. The second patient's defense of depersonalization, though it camouflaged her beating fantasies, remained comparatively closely allied to them. In both cases, the propelling factor prompting the reformulation of the defense was the inner conscience.

"Stroke," in its progression from noun to verb, served these neurotics well, fostering the "playful" element in masochism. Neurosis is intrapsychically perceived as deep pleasure, camouflaged as "game." Even perverted masochists, it is known, act out their practices under this guise.

The "mechanism of unconscious attenuation" sheds light on two clinical facts which have so far not been too well understood.

It explains some of the mysterious "backaches" for which no organic cause can be found, and where medicine so often loses out to —osteopathy. And it also shows why some women need so much tenderness and constant reassurance from the impatient husbands who are required to perform as stroking "tenderness machines."

3. THE MULTIPLE MEANING OF PSYCHOGENIC PHENOMENA [68]

Psychiatrists whose basic tenet is the concept of the dynamic unconscious are familiar with the phenomenon called "over-determination," which was originally described by Freud as "Ueberdeterminierung." The term has been unhappily translated; in German, it denotes "consisting of many determinants, many layers," while in English the linguistic vicinity of the word "determination" has tended to confuse its meaning. "Over-determination," as technically used, merely describes the construction of psychic phenomena: each psychic phenomenon has a specific center, surrounded by successive coats; it can be compared in structure to a snowball rolled down from the top of a mountain. In short, every symptom has many meanings.

The therapist's job is to separate the wheat from the chaff, the meaningful from the secondary camouflage. The worst that can happen is to confuse the essentials with the "also present." The result, applied to a different sphere, was wittily summed up by Elbert Hubbard, who defined an editor as "a person employed on a newspaper to separate the wheat from the chaff, and to see that the chaff is printed."

Moreover, identical symptoms may have completely different meanings. This is inevitable, because of the paucity of the organs and symptoms at the individual's disposal and the infinite variety of unconscious defenses. To reduce the problem to simple terms, there is only one penis, only one vagina. The psychogenic misuse of either can lead to literally hundreds of specific meanings, exemplified in the hundreds of forms and sub-forms of impotence and frigidity, summarized in my triple monograph on impotence, frigidity, homosexuality, COUNTERFEIT-SEX.

Here, at least, finer differentiations and "pointers" can be distinguished. "Oral," "anal," and "phallic" forms of potency disturbances can be diagnosed through the use of these finer differentiations, even though the identical symptom—impotence—is present in all cases. This is true, too, of different forms of frigidity.

To adduce two examples: The patient with premature ejaculation merely reports his failure; his intercourse consists of two to four thrusts. If we ask him, as stated by K. Abraham, whether the ejaculation comes in spurts, or flows out like urine, his answer will immediately indicate whether or not he is curable. Urine-like ejaculation with a non-erect penis spells therapeutic hopelessness, whereas spurt-type ejaculation can be cured, provided the oral-masochistic components are tapped in therapy.

The vaginally frigid patient informs us that she "feels nothing" during intercourse. We then ask whether there is lubrication (Bartholin's gland secretion). The reply provides the required pointer: severe case if typically absent, simpler case if present. And so on.

There are, however, neurotic symptoms where, at the same level of regression, the identical symptom may have thoroughly contradictory meanings. This section deals with symptoms of this perplexing type.

Is Superego the Real Master of the Personality?

By chance I treated two female pianists simultaneously. The patients were in no way connected; neither had even heard of the other. Both patients came into treatment primarily because of marital conflicts, partly because of professional difficulties. Mrs. OO. complained of being "dead" emotionally when playing before an audience. Mrs. PP. was bitter about her own failings, claiming that she could "do better, be a *real,* first-class performer" if she were not "inhibited in her practicing at home."

Both women had married severe neurotics, both marriages were rich with masochistic injustice-collecting. Both patients were regressed to the oral level.

What is pertinent here is the fact that, despite the identical level of regression in these cases, *the identical symptom (the difference between the patient's playing at home and in public) had diametrically opposed applications:*

Mrs. OO.: *"At home,* when practicing and playing for myself, with nobody around, *I play beautifully;* I have feeling, warmth and strength. *When there is an audience, I'm emotionally dead.* I become a technically perfect automaton. No feeling, no warmth, 'no nothing.' "

Mrs. PP.: *"I am a brilliant performer in public, and a silly inhibited one at home* when I'm practicing. This prevents me from practicing. After a short time, I fall into some kind of sexual reverie, frequently leading to masturbation, I'm ashamed to say. This has no connection with whether or not I'm sexually starved. I tried to remedy the situation by having someone around while I practice. This doesn't help. I need a big audience. . . ."

One can hardly imagine a greater contradiction. Mrs. PP.'s meat was Mrs. OO.'s poison, and vice versa.

A few obvious suspicions were aroused by these recitals; they were quickly confirmed. The term "playing" was unconsciously taken to mean playing sexually with oneself. This was clearly visible in Mrs. PP., whose piano-playing, when she was alone, almost invariably led up to physical self-play. It was evident that in neither case was the inner conscience convinced that the sublimation of playing the piano was not identical with masturbation. Since the hands are used both for the attempted sublimation and for masturbation, it was easy for the superego to point ironically to the inner identity of the two.

Every sublimation rests on elaborations of infantile, pregenital precursors. The problem is complicated. For our purposes one conclusion suffices: The sublimator has to convince his superego that he is acting out, in his sublimatory endeavor, *a rational activity with no infantile strings attached; if he is unable to adduce convincing proof, the sublimation is inhibited,* as in the cases of Mrs. OO. and Mrs. PP.

Experience with other "musical" patients has shown that Mrs. OO.'s difficulty—that of playing well at home and poorly in front of an audience—is the more typical, more frequently encountered inhibition. Mrs. PP.'s difficulty—playing badly when practicing alone, playing uninhibitedly in public—was rather the exception. Still, there it was, and had to be explained.

In the typical case, that of Mrs. OO., the obvious interpretation pertaining to *exhibitionism* was applied: "Your inner conscience charges that the harmless act of playing the piano still has, for you, the connotation of *exhibitionistically executed masturbation.* Your inner "lawyer" (unconscious ego) presents the defense: 'My client is innocent of exhibitionistic display: she is so much against exhibitionism that even harmless display of her approved ability to play the piano is inhibited, if people are around.' "

The interpretation was worked through—with no results.

The next step was application of my experiences pertaining to the genesis of exhibitionism. Exhibitionism is not, as previously assumed, an original "partial drive" domiciled in the id, *but is in itself a defense mechanism against peeping (voyeurism).* Once the *primary* defense has been established, voyeurism and exhibitionism can be secondarily used as defenses against each other. The following interpretation was therefore given to Mrs. OO.: "At your inner lawyer's advice, you admit to the lesser crime of exhibitionism, and even accept punishment for that crime, in order to cover up your greater inner crime, peeping." This interpretation led to analysis of Mrs. OO.'s infantile peeping, for which a good deal of confirming material could be found.

The interpretation was worked through. It was only slightly effective; the improvement in Mrs. OO.'s performance was nothing to brag about.

Obviously, something was missing. This "something" centered around two doubts:

1. What reason was there for the assumption that the exhibitionistic masturbation, symbolically materialized in her inhibited piano playing, had an adult sexual meaning?
2. Was it likely that so deeply masochistic a person as Mrs. OO. could have completely escaped those masochistic deposits in her attempts at sublimation?

The two doubts added up to one question: Was there in her playing an element representing some inner defense against masochism? The only possible defense would be pseudoaggression.

This led to my asking Mrs. OO., who was unaware of my private deliberations: "Does it make any difference, as far as publicly visible inhibition is concerned, whether you play *piano* or *forte* pieces?"

"Of course," she answered. "*Forte* pieces are impossible for me; if I play at all, I play *piano* pieces; they are easier for me—in public, I mean. Here, the trouble is that I cannot show any feelings."

"Why didn't you mention that before?"

"I didn't know that it could make a difference one way or another."

"It does. I suspect that what really causes your trouble is—a deep masochistic fantasy which you ward off by admitting to aggression (*forte*), for which you prefer to take the blame."

This suspicion led to a further analysis of Mrs. OO.'s infantile masochistic-sadistic fantasies. At first, she admitted to sadistic fantasies only, such as the torture of insects, and the attempt, at the age of four, to put a stick into a horse's anus. Much later, she admitted that during these tortures she "imagined how the animals would feel"; in other words, she identified masochistically with her victims.

Working out this interpretation "did the trick," as Mrs. OO. triumphantly stated; her playing improved to an "amazing degree" and remained on its new high level.

Some of the conclusions reached with Mrs. OO. were applied to Mrs. PP. Very similar material came to the fore, with this exception: no difference was found between *piano* and *forte*. In public, Mrs. PP. claimed, she was "first class." It soon became apparent that the masturbation fantasies so invariably produced in her when she played alone were by no means simple sexual fantasies. Little by little, and with great reluctance, Mrs. PP. described the contents of these fantasies. When she had a "piano fantasy," a man would begin to "manhandle" her "in a rough way." She would not allow him to continue till he promised "to be nice," which meant to accept "cultured intercourse without sadistic trimmings." This thinly disguised masochistic fantasy was excluded when playing in public: she could then prove that she was merely donig a rational, culturally accepted thing—playing the piano.

Working out the masochistic substructure helped Mrs. PP. to overcome her "practice troubles."

One problem remained: Why was exhibitionism the *savior* for Mrs. PP., who played *better* in public, and the *pitfall* for Mrs. OO., who played *worse* in public?

The probable answer was that in Mrs. OO. exhibitionism was so over-mortgaged with early guilt connected with masochistic-sadistic games (as a child she had been a show-off and her torturing of animals had not been secret) that secondarily it became unusable as a defense. This was not true of Mrs. PP.; her masochistic fantasies were "private" and never directly displayed.

The cases of Mrs. OO. and Mrs. PP. show how futile it is to envisage, as some younger colleagues do, a future in which all known neurotic difficulties will be catalogued and keyed so that a list can be consulted, as one consults a dictionary or encyclopedia, and finding the right column will be equivalent to finding the "right interpretation." Psychic phenomena are seemingly not constructed to make the lives of simplifiers too easy.

I doubt whether the present state of affairs—"sweating it out" in each individual case and frequently finding the individual reason different though the symptoms are identical to those previously encountered—will ever be changed.

4. "MORTGAGING ONE'S FUTURE THROUGH INDIGNANT REPROACHES"

The practice of heaping reproaches on others is a popular and favored sport without any real consequences; the bystander dissects, deplores, and disavows the other fellow's actions or attitudes, and here the matter rests. If the criticism is openly expressed, it may give offense; the target of criticism is not always meek and biddable. In such cases some self-damage is incurred.

Differing from the above are cases in which the *criticism of others leads to mortgaging of the critic's own future actions and reactions.* An equivalent situation would be that of a politician who freely dispenses criticism of an opponent and who, years later, is taken to task and forced to fulfill conditions implied in the campaign oratory he never seriously meant.

Both the politician and the bystander critic *commit themselves for the future through their criticism,* but the forum which compels this commitment is not the same. The politician is impelled by the fear that his constituents will repudiate him; the neurotic I have in mind is accountable to the forum internum: his inner conscience (superego).

Why does the critic take his own criticism so seriously? Generally speaking, he does not; he makes a fine distinction between himself and the rest of the world and is never shaken in his conviction that his own dicta apply to other people only. "Duty," mocked Oscar Wilde, "is what we expect from others." But this protective device is useless *when the specific criticism is an integral part of the "basic fallacy" upon which a specific sector of neurosis rests.* To preserve this "basic fallacy" the neurotic must then perform the action implied by his criticism. Performance of the action is an inner necessity.

A woman of thirty-six ascribed all the neurotic misery of her life to one specific factor: her mother had deserted both husband and children when the patient was four years old. "Brought up in a motherless home, you can imagine the rest," was her theme song. She had never forgiven her father for the "contemptible weakness" that had permitted her mother to leave their home. She was quite vague about the countermeasures her father could have used to prevent her mother from running away with another man.

Her own marriage was rather a caricature: she domineered over her husband, and her husband retaliated with sexual retirement. She herself was "not too interested" in sex; her complaints against her husband were mainly concerned with the "irrational quarrels" he provoked. She was quite blind to her own cooperation in these quarrels; actually she was as skilled as her husband at injustice-collecting.

After some time in analysis she came to an understanding of the neurotic tie-up. She then began to argue that the marriage should be maintained until her daughter had passed puberty, reducing the marriage to no more than a protective device designed to benefit the child. When it was pointed out to her that a bad marriage which constantly erupts into quarrels does not protect the child, she countered with lame excuses.

Unexpectedly, at this point, her husband brought matters to a head. After his long subjection to what he called "marital slavery," the husband (a few years his wife's senior) staged his "middle-age revolt," [69] attached himself to a younger woman—a domineering person, like his wife—and demanded a divorce.

Although consciously aware that her sick marriage was only a shell (the husband consistently refused to enter analysis himself), the patient started a campaign of terror. The next few weeks were crowded with threats of suicide, exhibitions of pathologic jealousy, shouting denunciations, and violence. She was in no way affected by the fact that her excuse for continuing the marriage—protecting the child—had collapsed when the neurotic husband kept her in the dark about his divorce plans until *after* he had revealed them to his fourteen-year-old daughter.

Analysis of the patient's strange behavior led to the assumption that *she was acting out her fantasy of how her father should have behaved in order to prevent his wife from leaving home.* Temporarily she regressed to the level of a four-year-old.

The phase passed after interpretation and working through; a reasonable adjustment took place.

It seems that the injustice done her by her mother in leaving home was the strongest bulwark against understanding her own masochistic elaboration of this tragic fact. Her marriage proved conclusively that its driving power was not love but masochism. On the other hand, the patient strongly disapproved of divorce—she preferred even a bad marriage to a decisive break.

The hatred she felt for her mother was a thin, pseudoaggressive layer, covering her more deeply repressed masochism. If she had admitted, as in the cases of her mother and her husband, that some

Is Superego the Real Master of the Personality?

marriages are hopeless, her own "case" against her mother would have collapsed, and she would have found herself face to face with the force she repressed all her life: her own overdimensional masochism.[70]

5. THE INNER IDENTITY OF "REFUSING" AND "GIVING UNDER IMPOSSIBLE CONDITIONS"

One of the typical tongue-in-cheek defenses of the unconscious ego is that of "giving" under impossible conditions—an action which, in inner reality, is tantamount to "refusing." [71]

A patient suffering from premature ejaculation was capable of intercourse lasting three to four *minutes* whenever one specific condition was fulfilled: intercourse had to take place immediately after he awakened, when his wife (still half-asleep) abhorred sex. Otherwise, the duration of his intercourse was three to four *seconds,* and frequently his ejaculation was ante portas.

Analysis of the patient's prematurity revealed the typical oral-masochistic substructure. The defense against the dynamic masochistic *wish to be refused* is pseudoaggressive *refusal.* Since this defense, too, is vetoed by the superego, a secondary defense is registered: "How can I be accused of refusing—I give immediately!" This "promptness" is of course inner mockery; no woman can derive pleasure from two to four thrusts and a premature ejaculation, executed by a husband who is depressed, to boot.

Outright denial is identical with giving under conditions of mockery: both spell *refusal.* This patient derived what was actually a triple unconscious defense from his ability to have "normal" intercourse in the morning. First, he proved to himself, once more, how "unjust" his wife was—she refused sex merely because she was half-asleep! Second, he proved to himself, and incidentally to her, that he did not suffer from prematurity at all. Third, he was still under the influence of his "dream girl" in these early morning encounters, and therefore the intercourse was more or less impersonal; again, this was a pseudoaggression against his wife.

These interconnections were explained to the patient; he did not accept them. I suggested that he experiment by trying intercourse on a morning when his wife awakened earlier than he did, and was amenable to his advances. The experiment was attempted. It was a complete fiasco. The patient concluded: "If she wants sex, I feel drained, forced, trapped." In short, he still (unconsciously) saw in his wife the monster of his baby days.

The complexity of manifestations of defensive neurotic refusal is necessarily great, because defenses in general are not static. When a defense is vetoed by the inner conscience, the trimmings and external expressions are altered. This is a compromise designed to maintain the substructure intact. Phenomenologically the result is a confusing array of seeming contradictions.

To name a typical contradiction: Sometimes, out of analysis, and rather typically within analysis, neurotics with premature ejaculation go through a temporary period in which they suddenly find themselves unable to ejaculate at all, despite protracted intercourse. This change from *ejaculatio praecox* to *psychogenic aspermia* is baffling only when one is unaware that the prematurist refuses by giving too soon, while the aspermist refuses by not giving at all. Both refuse defensively; both are orally regressed psychic masochists. (For elaboration, see details of "psychogenic oral aspermia," a neurotic symptom first described by me; summary in COUNTERFEIT-SEX).

The mechanism of "giving under impossible conditions" is quite apt to produce a mirage which thoroughly deludes the "giver." How frequent, for example, are marital conflicts in which the wife objects that the husband "fails to create the mood for sex," and the husband —in real or pretended naivety—replies: "You wanted sex; you got it; what are you whining about?"

The identical conflicts are carried out in the sphere of money. A particular type addicted to this technique—one of many described at length in MONEY AND EMOTIONAL CONFLICTS—is the "refusing giver." This man "goes wild" when his wife asks him for money; he shouts, curses, reproaches, complains, and slams angrily out of the house. When he has gone through the entire antic performance, he gives exactly the amount he was asked for in the first place. The inevitable result is that the wife cherishes her recollection of the disagreeable scene and disregards the fact that eventually he "forked out." Thus the neurotic fosters in his spouse the feeling that he is a refusing miser.

Consciously the man remembers that he gave the money and

forgets the row; consciously the woman remembers the row and forgets the money. Unconsciously the situation is slightly different. The husband has an easy conscience because he gave "freely," and when his wife reproaches him for his stinginess—as she invariably does—he feels terribly abused. This feeling is exactly what he was looking for, hence the opening scene of the drama. In short, the stage was set, once again, by a psychic masochist.

Some neurotic women do actually drive their husbands to desperation with exaggerated and irrational demands. We are not dealing with this situation here, however, but only with that of the neurotic type of "refusing giver," for whom the inability to *give with grace* is typical. Whether the demand is rational or not, the initial reaction is an *automatic* refusal.

A description of a psychic phenomenon teaches us little of its genesis. Symptoms which on the surface appear to be identical may have widely disparate genetic structures. On the other hand, identical phenomena may vary in their outward manifestations. For the latter, the inner identity of "refusing" and "giving under impossible conditions" is a paradigm.

6. THE DANGER OF "CARICATURISTIC RELATIONSHIPS"

> Satire is a lonely and introspective occupation, for nobody can describe a fool to the life without much self-inspection.
> —Frank Moore Colby

A "caricaturistic relationship"—between husband and wife, "girl friend" and "boy friend," two cronies, or two acquaintances—is base on the choice of a person who represents an unconsciously produced caricature of some infantile image, or of one's own unconsciously rejected traits, exaggerated and distorted. Two types, therefore, are encountered. The person chosen may unconsciously represent a caricature of mother, father, sister, or brother, or else may represent a distorted and caricaturistically embroidered "oneself"—in projection. In the former type the purpose of the choice is masochistic suffering with a slight overlay of defensive, pseudoaggressive irony. In the latter type the choice has the purpose of outdistancing a reproach of the inner conscience by dramatizing the alibi: "I hate, reject, and make fun of these impossible traits."

Both types are common and are as commonly misunderstood. When a dissolution of these impossible relationships is attempted during psychotherapy, great therapeutic difficulties are met with. Despite conscious contempt for the partner, "incomprehensible," cement-like adherence prevails for long periods, especially if the choice is also masochistically imbued.

TYPE I

Mr. QQ., a homosexual of forty-two, was attached to a psychopathic man some seven years his junior, who exploited him financially and emotionally on a grand scale. He kept this man in luxury. Mr. QQ. suffered constantly and "intensely" from jealousy, for which he seemingly had good reason, but still he clung to his "charming" friend. Although the relationship consisted only of turbulent scenes, followed by reconciliations—with QQ. always taking the initiative in both conflict and abject apology—there was no evidence that he was approaching the usual "point of no return," where even the psychic masochist has had enough of the inner wish for humiliation and mistreatment—for some time, at least in a specific situation. In this case the relationship seemed to become firmer as the friend behaved more impossibly.

It seemed reasonable to assume that QQ. was so masochistic that he would simply swallow everything. Before accepting that conclusion this reconstruction was attempted: his mother had been a "willful and whimsical" personality, to quote the patient. "She acted the grande dame, made scenes, was full of snobbish whims, neglected the children emotionally." There was reason to asume that QQ.'s masochistic propensities had been built up in that relationship. It seemed that the parasitic homosexual boy friend was fashioned after the maternal model: essentially a neurotic self-assured taker, never a giver.

Now unconsciously QQ. seemed to have created in his friend a caricature of his own mother. In this caricature, he degraded her socially (the boy friend was "scum and slum"), made an outright parasite and half-prostitute out of her (the face his mother presented to the world was that of a grande dame presiding over a large and wealthy household), subjected her to his own whims (thus, in identification, actively reversing the passive situation in childhood). At the same time, the thinly veiled pseudoaggression covered a truly fantastic attachment. QQ. took a great deal of "intolerable nonsense" from his friend, whom he loved not in spite of his bad qualities but *because* he was "rotten, unreliable, and no good."

The repetition of the infantile situation went so far that it could explain a peculiar attitude of QQ.'s. Repeatedly he broke off his relationship with his impossible friend and then started it again. This was an unconscious recapitulation of his feeling that his irrational mother had repeatedly let her child down, and then after some time resumed her loving attitude and acted as if nothing had happened.

Unconsciously every homosexual is a fugitive from, not a renouncer of women (see Chapter 2). Behind the homosexual facade, QQ. repeated an undigested masochistic conflict with the earliest image of the mother.

However, the image of the mother he created was a decidedly malicious caricature. Simultaneously, and ironically, he created a "pseudomoral alibi" for sexual attachment: by taking the blame for the "lesser intrapsychic crime" of incest, he covered up the more deeply repressed masochistic attachment. (The second camouflage was, of course, the switch from hetero- to homosexuality.)

This also explained why the patient could not reach a "point of no return." He was quite aware of his friend's "worthlessness," but he did not realize that he deeply cherished and even promoted this very "worthlessness." The boy friend's unsavory qualities provided him with an alibi for his pseudoaggression and with guilt-relieving confirmation of his opinion of his mother's "worthlessness"; provided him (under this guise) with masochistic pleasure; gave him the "moral right" to have sex with a shifted mother image.

Cases such as Mr. QQ.'s prove that recourse to quantitative factors as excuse for failure in the solution of masochistic "caricaturistic relationships" can be justified only *after* protracted "working through" of the deepest layers.

TYPE II

Mrs. RR. enjoyed an income from a large trust fund left her by her wealthy family. She married a man "beneath her station" (her words), a parasitic and neurotic fellow only out for a "good time." Their quarrels centered around money, which provided a convenient blind for deeper conflicts. Though the man was supported on a "nice scale" (his words), he felt insecure about the future and kept asking his wife to set aside some part of her income to take care of him in his old age, or in case of her death. So much "greed," Mrs. RR. claimed, revolted her. She herself, as it happened, was both stingy and demanding. In analysis it turned out that the marriage was held together by masochistic injustice-collecting *and* the fact that Mr. RR. represented a caricature of Mrs. RR.'s own trends, projected outward, distorted, and "enlarged."

Both types inwardly create a caricature: they write a satire (though unknowingly and unwittingly) and live it. Franklin's saying, "Strange that a man who has wit enough to write a satire should have folly enough to publish it," becomes even more pointed when applied to these "inner satirists" who *live* their creation.

7. TEARS OF ANTICIPATION

In neurosis the superego is meretricious and venal. Conscience money is paid in the form of constant, self-inflicted punishment. This is not all, however. There exists a strange tendency to anticipate the punishment which is to be meted out by the inner conscience. This "anticipation tendency" manifests itself in two ways.

First, before the superego's whip cracks down, *the prisoner starts to whip himself;* after having proclaimed his innocence of Charge I, he voluntarily proclaims himself guilty of Charge II ("taking the blame for the lesser crime"). The inner tormenter, being interested in punishment only, seems to accede, perhaps because the victim has relieved "him" of the task of doing his "dirty work" himself.

The "anticipation tendency" manifests itself, second, in *"preventive depression."* This phenomenon is by no means as simple as the frequent assumption—depression is the superego's punishment—makes it. This type of depression undoubtedly exists. But another type is no less common: anticipating the expected punishment, the unconscious ego produces the depression beforehand. This, of course, makes it possible for the "lesser crime" to be used as hitching post, so that—once more—the defense scores a victory over the superego.

One can hardly find a better capsule distinction between normality and neurosis than the fact that anticipatory depression is *not* observable in not-too-neurotic people. They seem to bide their time, reacting only when the inner tormenter actually strikes. Anticipatory depression is not their technique. Perhaps a naive patient of mine (a gambler) hit the nail on the head when, after coming to understand the neurotic mechanisms of his unconscious, he remarked: "The neurotic behaves like a scared and chronically beaten-down gambler who has stopped thinking of how he can win and now thinks of how to lose as little as possible."

Recently I came across a confirmation of the above deduction; the example supplies additional details to the description of the "anticipation tendency" mechanism.

The patient, a professional woman in her middle thirties, repeated her inwardly unsolved relation to the image of her pre-oedipal mother in the analytic transference situation. Everything I did or said—as well as what I did not do or say—was taken as proof of malice and "cruelty." It was possible to work out these infantile projections; as a result some kind of analytic modus vivendi was established.

During the grand scenes she constructed around the "injustice" done her the patient had cried a good deal. This was not surprising, for her entire attitude was that of an innocent, thwarted child. Skilfully, she would re-enact the masochistic situation of unconsciously provoking (or misusing) an external situation for the purpose of feeling "unjustly treated." Since her own provocation was repressed, she saw only external malice. This she fought with spurious aggression. The climax was a bath of self-pity, and again the unconscious enjoyment of psychic masochistic pleasure. (The above triad constitutes the "mechanism of orality," corresponding to the clinical picture of psychic masochism.)

The situation became suspect after the naive repetitions had been analytically clarified, worked through, and (to a great extent) discarded. The weeping continued even after this point had been achieved; it appeared whenever she had to "confess" to "tensions" or to "not feeling well."

I believed at first that this was merely a continuation of the old routine. I asked what my "crime" had been this time, and to reduce her attitude to absurdity I told her of an amusing incident in the analysis of another patient, also a woman. There had been a short circuit during the latter's appointment, with the usual startling sizzle of the burnt-out bulb, followed by darkness. The patient immediately leaped from the couch, exclaiming: "But I didn't do anything!" In enlarging on this incident, I remarked: "Do you want me to say, 'But I didn't do anything'? Why are you crying *now?*"

She conceded that "I didn't do anything"; I had merely misunderstood her motives. Her crying, she explained, had nothing to do with me. She was "just tense" because she was about to begin taking a course that would prepare her for an important examination; passing the examination would improve her professional status. Automatically she assumed that her instructor would be "mean and disagreeable." And therefore she felt "tense."

"Very well, though I do not understand what importance the instructor has in the first place. He is simply there to tell you the facts you have to know for the examination. And besides, how do you know the fellow is 'mean and disagreeable'?"

"I have been told he is."

"But you haven't checked; you've never even seen the man."

"But I'm always tense in situations like this. Even when I was a child. . . ."

Every time she had had to tell her mother that she did not feel well—and there was no exception for the occasions when the reason was legitimate enough—she had cried. There were times, however, when she "only felt tense"; the "tenseness" was transmuted into some kind of incipient transitory illness that also kept her home from school. On the other hand, she had been a sickly child.

The patient could not explain why she should have cried in these situations. She had not been punished or deprived of privileges. Her "irrational" mother had reacted with worry on some occasions, with indifference on others. The banal assumption that the child had cried for the conscious purpose of arousing pity and thus avoiding punishment was also excluded; her mother had never paid any attention to this technique. The patient specifically stressed that her crying came "from deep down," and that she had no control over it.

It turned out that the crying meant *anticipated punishment*. The sequence of events was provocation—expectation of punishment—crying over punishment received in fantasy. Of this triad the first part materialized most often; parts two and three were frequently not forthcoming. Still, she cried.

In other words, the girl was so eager for punishment that she could not wait for the actual event and react accordingly. She did not react by crying when punished and laughing (or at least feeling contented) when not punished; she cried [72] in any case, disregarding reality when it was favorable.

The technique of anticipation is by no means rare; even wisecracks take cognizance of it. For example, there is the story of the man who wants to borrow fifty dollars from an acquaintance. He makes his request, only to get the peculiar reply: "Let's be enemies immediately." The elliptic technique suppresses the transitional phrases: "I'll lend you the money; you will not return it; when I ask for it you will be angry with me. So why wait? Let's be enemies immediately."

It is superfluous to mention that people who act in the manner of the patient described are psychic masochists and "injustice-collectors."

8. THE GREATEST COMPLIMENT: "I NEVER THOUGHT OF THAT!"

> He who says he hates all kinds of flattery, and says so in earnest, simply says that he has not yet become acquainted with all kinds of it.
> —Georg Litchtenberg

The ability to smuggle one's own "I" into situations where the "you" should dominate is one of the most remarkable achievements of the human mind. Everything goes through narcissistic channels. In this respect human beings are like those children's toys so constructed that however you turn or tip them they always revert to the upright position.

This banal fact becomes remarkable only in its exaggerations. A wit's recommendation that the personal pronoun "I" should be the coat of arms of some people is living reality—especially when compliments are paid. Obviously a compliment denotes acknowledgment of the "you," provided it is seriously meant and not hypocritically uttered. Even so, no compliment fully excludes the note of "I."

Exactly this personal admixture is repulsive to some people; witness Thoreau's statement:

> Compliments and flattery excite my contempt by the pretensions they imply; for who is he that assumes to flatter me? To compliment often implies the assumption of superiority in the complimenter. It is, in fact, *a subtle detraction.*

That "subtle detraction" denotes condescension, the half-surprised acknowledgment that the other fellow can think at all, since thinking is a privilege that should be reserved for one's own wonderful self. Actually many people solve the problem by using a technique of appropriation: they have found a kindred soul, they conclude, and therefore a part of themselves. Many a plagiarism starts at this point; as C. C. Colton said, "Imitation is the sincerest flattery."

To clarify the problem, one should observe the emergence of a spontaneous compliment, at the moment when, for example, an individual is taken aback and surprised by hearing for the first time of an interconnection. Only too frequently this first reaction is expressed in the stock phrase: "I never thought of that."

In scrutinizing that reaction one must conclude that the individual takes his own ego as the sole yardstick.

To make matters more personal, the phrase, "I never thought of that," implies a negation of any real compliment. The other fellow's original thought is pigeonholed as representing merely a priority of timing; of course, the complimentary phrase conveys, the listener could have figured out the answer himself if he had devoted any time to it. He didn't, and the other fellow did—that's the whole difference. Sometimes his crowded schedule, which eats up all his time, is adduced as inner excuse; this little twist demotes the man of ideas to the status of a loafer.

One could object that many people do not use this narcissistic phrase at all; instead, they go in for shameless flattery and pretend real admiration. Experience and self-observation prove that the only difference between users of and abstainers from the ominous phrase is in expression and not in thought. *Inwardly* everyone reacts with "I never thought of that!"

This point can be proved by investigating the reaction to flattery. Most sages have expressed the opinion that susceptibility to flattery is universal:

> We sometimes think that we hate flattery, but we only hate the manner in which it is done (La Rochefoucauld).

> Among all the diseases of the mind, there is not one more epidemic, or more pernicious, than the love of flattery. First, we flatter ourselves, then flattery of others is sure of success (Richard Steele).

> I love flattery so well, I would fain have some circumstances of probability added to it, that I might swallow it with comfort (Lady Mary Wortley Montagu).

> This was really a compliment to be pleased with—a nice little pot of butter made up by a neat-handed Phillis of a dairy maid instead of the grease fit only for cartwheels which one is dosed with by the pound (Sir Walter Scott).

> A little flattery will support a man through great fatigue (President Monroe, when he was asked if he were not worn out by attentions shown to him).

> I can live for two months on a good compliment. . . . When you cannot get a compliment in any other way, pay yourself one (Mark Twain).

> When a man makes a woman his wife, it's the highest compliment he can pay her, and it's usually the last (Helen Rowland).

Observation of everyday life proves conclusively that no flattering remark is too gross to swallow. The discrepancy between a person's intelligence and his ability to fall for the silliest flattery is amazing. The furlough given to the critical sense is so extensive that only desperate inner necessity can account for it. Although sages of all times and epochs have warned of the flatterer's hypocrisy, people on the receiving end of a compliment invariably take it at face value. These warnings are numerous:

> Their throat is an open sepulchre; they flatter with their tongue (Psalm V, 9).
>
> When flatterers meet, the Devil goes to dinner (John Ray).
>
> Compliments cost nothing, yet many pay dear for them (Thomas Fuller).
>
> Avoid flatterers, they are thieves in disguise (William Penn).
>
> Flatterers, like cats, lick and then scratch (German adage).
>
> Compliments are only lies in court clothes (Anonymous).
>
> Flatterers look like friends, as wolves like dogs (George Chapman).
>
> Compliment is taken literally only by the savage. The accuracy of compliment is not that of algebra (W. C. Brownell).
>
> Some people pay a compliment as if they expected a receipt (Kim Hubbard).

Despite these and similar warnings—"Flattery is like cologne water, to be smelt of, not swallowed," advised Josh Billings—people are taken in. Why?

The reason is intimately connected with the fact that each and every one of us is constantly under attack by his malicious *unconscious* conscience (superego). To counteract these avalanches of reproach, *"witnesses for the defense" are sought; they are found in flatterers. This accounts for the fact that there is no connection between intelligence per se and susceptibility to flattery.* Indeed, one would arrive at a very poor opinion of human intelligence if susceptibility to flattery were taken as the *sole* yardstick.

This inner necessity also explains why the phrase "I never thought of that" is typically used when one is confronted with an intellectual

Is Superego the Real Master of the Personality? 417

achievement on the part of someone else. Immediately the inner conscience launches a reproach accusing the listener of inefficiency and stupidity. The reproach is warded off with the bag of excuses included in the famous phrase.

There is a reason, too, for the comparative rarity of *sincere acknowledgment* rather than flattery. This form of recognition presupposes an ego strong enough not to be thrown off balance by someone else's achievement. Such an ego is seldom encountered. More frequently the weak ego attempts detraction and devaluation; at best, the narcissistic phrase "I never thought of that" is put in operation with its string of self-excuses.

I once asked a patient, a man of great achievement and high intelligence, how he explained his naivete in swallowing wholesale even the silliest compliments offered him by his "admirers." He laughed and replied that he did not really believe their nonsense but enjoyed the fact that he had achieved a position in which even hypocrites were obliged to flatter him. It was a good rationalization, omitting the unconscious reasons. The nearly identical rationalization was once offered by George Bernard Shaw, when he said, "What really flatters a man is that you think him worth flattering."

9. ERRORS IN JUDGMENT WHEN FACED WITH AN "AFFRONT" [73]

Some people admit it; some do not—but Boswell's dictum, "My favorite topic, myself," applies to everyone. Too much concentration on self has many disadvantages, but only one facet will be singled out here: the errors in judgment that invariably arise when a person is subjected to an "affront." The core of such errors consists of starting one's deliberations with the indignant question: "How can he do this to *me?*" Thus, one's own lovable self becomes the primum movens.

Placing the accent on oneself automatically renders these deliberations worthless. Doing so bypasses the fact that the other fellow (the offender) uses the identical priority list, and therefore places *himself* on top. A matter that should be explained in terms of the other fellow's needs and motivations is consequently twisted into a personal problem of self. This "little error" has far-reaching aftereffects: the entire deliberation ends with a faulty conclusion. It is as though a person worked on a complex mathematical problem, having started his calculation with the unobserved error: 1 plus 1 equals 27.

Mr. SS., a writer, made a luncheon appointment with his literary agent. The specific day, the specific hour, the specific restaurant had been set, and confirmed by letter. The agent did not appear. SS. waited one hour, getting more and more furious, and dwelling on the personal affront. He was so angry that he did not even call the agent's office; he preferred to indulge in self-pity and compensatory revenge fantasies. It was not until late in the afternoon that he telephoned the agent's office, only to learn that the agent was ill and at home in bed. Mr. SS. had the impression that the secretary at the other end of the line had been expecting his call; he thought her replies and regrets too pat to be true. He had asked why he had not been told of the agent's illness in the morning; he viewed with suspicion the secretary's apologetic explanation that she had forgotten to check the agent's appointments and therefore should be blamed. SS. was so furious that he did not even ask the obvious question: had the agent told her to check his appointments?

The next day he received a letter of apology in which the agent put the blame squarely on the inefficiency of his office staff. In discussing the incident during his analytic appointment, SS. complained bitterly of the affront and—probably with justification—declared that the "forgetting" was the agent's fault, not his secretary's. However, instead of shrugging his shoulders over the nuisance value of the incident, and simply asking himself whether he would be better off with another agent than with this one, he delivered a long, masochistic tirade on how meanly "poor little me" was being treated.

"He wouldn't dare if my books were selling like Hemingway or Mike Spillane!"

"Aren't you misusing the incident for self-reproaches over your moderate success?"

"Isn't that unavoidable?"

"Of course it's avoidable. Your inner conscience is on the warpath, and you're being a sucker, playing its game, instead of counteracting it."

"I still say it's a personal affront, a slap in the face!"

"Let's see. Is your agent antagonistic toward you?"

"That's the strange thing: he isn't. But unconsciously he must hate my guts. Otherwise he wouldn't have forgotten."

"Why do you overstress yourself in this incident? What appears like a personal affront may have reasons totally unrelated to you."

"Such as?"

"Not knowing the man, I can only speculate. Perhaps he was in a masochistic mood, unconsciously wanting to make trouble for himself. Perhaps he had to swallow too much nonsense from one of his best-selling clients, and in active repetition of a passively endured experience (a repetition in reverse) took it out on you. Or maybe he had a domestic conflict. Who knows?"

"But I am the injured party!"

"That is quite true. But it doesn't change the fact that the 'affront' may have reasons unconcerned with you. You committed not one but two cardinal errors: First, you began your train of thought with yourself, not the agent. Second, you misused the incident for a masochistic fiesta, thus shortchanging an attack of the inner conscience (superego). And the superego in its turn misused the situation to administer a severe beating to you."

Miss TT., an intelligent woman, was executive assistant to an industrialist. During one appointment she complained bitterly about her boss: all day, she declared, his behavior had been "impossible and insulting." Although the man was in general a rather pleasant and considerate person, she took his ill humor personally. I asked whether he had treated everyone badly or had singled her out as the target of his "impossible" behavior. She admitted that it had been a terrible day for everyone coming in contact with him; he had "kicked all of us around."

"Why do you take it personally?" I asked.

"What is that supposed to mean? He mistreated me, didn't he?"

"But if the reason for his extraordinary behavior—which affected everyone he came in contact with—had nothing to do with you, why not make allowances?"

Miss TT. then told of an incident that had added fuel to her indignation. She had overheard her boss speaking to his wife on the telephone during the morning. He had catered to his wife in the most humiliating manner. The theme song of his end of the conversation was, "Yes, darling; of course, darling." Miss TT. concluded: "At the same time, he was acting the big shot with me!" It seemed likely, from this evidence, that her boss had been through a severe domestic conflict the preceding night and had not cut a heroic figure in that crisis. To counteract his passivity at home, he exhibited aggression in the office.

Why didn't the intelligent patient see through that banality? Why did she start the "explanation" with herself? Why was she full of self-reproach—dictated by inner conscience? If she had understood the reasons for her employer's behavior, she would have deprived herself of a good case of injustice-collecting.

In short, an emotional situation such as that faced by a person who has met with an "affront" obscures factual thinking. If it did not, the starting point for the individual's subsequent attitude would be placed where it belongs: with the perpetrator of the injury. Equally typical is the fact that the inner conscience seizes the opportunity for a second installment of punishment and that the victim usually—unconsciously—misuses the attack for the purpose of injustice-collecting, hence psychic masochism.

One has to accept the dreary truth that people unconsciously misuse one another for the sake of solving their inner conflicts. The practical consequences that follow such misuse pose another—and again a practical—problem. But knowledge can help the individual who is not too severe a psychic masochist to escape the double pitfall described above.

10. "NOWHERE TO HIDE"—THE PROBLEM OF WEAK IDENTIFICATIONS

In all cases of unconscious identification the individual is in effect hiding behind someone else's broad shoulders. The preamble is an inner conflict which has been solved through acquisition of a "bodyguard." Typically the identification is performed in two layers, "leading" and "misleading." (This was first pointed out in my study, "The Leading and Misleading Basic Identifications," *The Psychoanalytic Review,* 32:263-295, 1945.) The *"leading"* identification pertains to the solution of the specific infantile conflict, secondarily bolstered through an identification; the stabilization is *permanent and unchangeable* during the individual's lifetime, except through clinical analysis. The *"misleading"* identification is more superficial, though still unconscious. It is performed under pressure from the superego, and its purpose is acquisition of a new shield to deflect or prevent the superego's attacks on the specific basic infantile conflict, which has been petrified in the "leading" identification. *Subsidiary and exchangeable* defenses are thus created and concretely expressed in changing identifications. This process frequently impresses the untrained observer as an indication of "changing" personality; in reality it proves only a specific defense has worn through and has had to be replaced.

For example, a promiscuous "wolf" has his "leading" identification with a masochistically mistreated person, whereas his "misleading" identification is with a hyper-he-man.

In the last few years I have frequently been confronted with patients who consulted me on the basis of my writings on psychic masochism. These patients were fascinated by that phenomenon. They had acquired a strange conviction (one could almost call it a seemingly unshakable conviction) of the universality of that inner scourge. In a rather self-flagellatory manner, they applied these principles to themselves.

When they came into analysis, it turned out that these patients were without exception of two types. Either they were severe psychic masochists, orally regressed neurotics, *or* they were schizoid personalities. The latter group was easier to understand than the former; schizoid people prefer to see themselves as neurotics rather than as half-psychotics.

The majority of these patients, however, were neurotic. In this group typical masochistic "injustice-collecting" predominated; inner passivity was combined with strong pseudoaggressive malice; bitter self-reproaches were in the forefront; irony was openly used in most of them, covertly in some.

One gathered the impression that the newly acquired book knowledge of the existence of psychic masochism procured them some kind of diminution of tension, as though personal responsibility had been lessened by the discovery that this was a universal phenomenon. At the same time, that very knowledge was used as added self-reproach and self-deprecation.

In the transference of neurosis the typical projections of the "bad, cruel mother" on the analyst were observable. Working through this transference and consecutive resistances had the usual beneficial effect.

Still, these patients differed in one respect from the run-of-the-mill patient of that type: they had difficulties in identification. What it amounted to, practically speaking, was that attempts to identify with the "corrected, good mother image" came into conflict with the defensive irony and malice already present. *These patients had established, early in life, their only "productive" technique of warding off reproaches of conscience: irony, debunking, deprecation of any authority.* (The debunking technique develops into the tendency to try to cut authority down to "proper size," as elaborated in my book LAUGHTER AND THE SENSE OF HUMOR.) The only *unproductive* technique of counteracting the constant stream of reproaches from the inner conscience known to them was psychic masochism.

In analysis, after a very short-lived enthusiasm for the newly and transitorily established ego ideal—the analyst—the latter was subjected to the identical ironic process of "debunking," which weakened his protective role in the "battle of the conscience." The result was unstable, and therefore ineffective "misleading identification."

The reason for this phenomenon became obvious the moment one clarified for oneself the fact that the newly established "analytic witness for the defense" could not be used as a weapon against the cruel, anachronistic, tyrannical part of the superego ("daimonion"). *The paradoxical fact emerged that the newly acquired ego ideal and the daimonion had one point in common: both brought into evidence the masochistic enjoyment in the patient's ego.* True, the daimonion did so maliciously and for punitive purposes, the analyst detachedly and for curative purposes. Presentation and purpose differed, but the *contents were identical.*

During this stage a specific factor became clear: Exchange of ego ideal in "misleading identifications" presupposes an inner helper whose face value fully corresponds to the opposite of the daimonion's accusation. Exactly that quality of total disparity was lacking.

Is Superego the Real Master of the Personality?

One could object that every analysis unearths facts corresponding to the superego's reproaches, so that this lack of disparity is typical. The argument is spurious. When partial identification with the analyst sets in, in typical cases the newly acquired "witness of defense" is not immediately demoted, as happens with the cases discussed here. Moreover, since the greatest of all mortal dangers, psychic masochism, is only rarely explained in present-day analyses, all possible (more superficial) interpretations are more acceptable, and therefore the analyst is usable as protective ego ideal.

Here is an example from the analysis of a patient of this type, a man who came to me for treatment because of his enthusiasm for my books THE BASIC NEUROSIS and THE SUPEREGO.

To describe the background of the situation: I had been asked to deliver a lecture in a course given at Columbia University. My talk was entitled "Seven Paradoxes in Shakespeare's HAMLET"; I was frankly proud of having been able to find, after studying the immortal play, seven points that had not yet been elaborated on in the analytic literature. My main point was that Hamlet had committed suicide by provocation and proxy, having decided his fate in the players' scene, which prompted the king to order Hamlet's death (the mission to England) and subsequently the poisoned rapier and poisoned drink. (Published in *The American Imago,* 16:379-405, 1959. Partly reproduced in ONE THOUSAND HOMOSEXUALS, Chapter XI.)

The clean copies of the manuscript reached me from the typist early one morning. I reread the talk and found that I was (perhaps childishly) proud of the title, so proud indeed that I repeated it to myself several times. In doing so I found that I had changed the figure; I had said "eight" instead of "seven." After catching myself on that "mistake," I began to laugh. The superego, being incapable of preventing subjectively enjoyed "success," devalued that success by ironically pointing out—after the "So what?" principle—that eight points would be more than seven. Through this ironic "overbidding," the "success" was nullified.

I used this incident as an example in two successive appointments that morning. In telling the story to the first patient, Mr. UU., a deeply depressed and analytically very ignorant person, I stopped short before telling him my reaction (laughter, which devalued the superego's attack), and asked him what his own reaction would have been in such a situation. Without hesitation he answered, "I would have run for Shakespeare's play to find out whether I had really missed something." I answered that he misunderstood the superego's intentions: these were not pedagogic but punitive.

My second appointment was with Mr. VV., the man who interests us in this connection. I related the incident, my reaction, and Mr. UU.'s reaction. My purpose was to demonstrate the thesis, just discussed in his analysis: "You cannot win against the superego; it either prevents success or—if that cannot be done—devalues it. The whole problem centers around the ego; one can reject the indictment (for example by laughing at it) or submit to it masochistically (Mr. UU.'s reaction)."

Some time later I delivered the lecture. Mr. VV. was in the audience. I used this identical example in explaining some of the techniques of the superego.

The next day Mr. VV. said to me ironically: "When you told me that story you said the title mentioned five paradoxes and you repeated it as having six. But in your lecture you mentioned the figures seven and eight. It seems that when the pinch came you acted just like that other patient and ran to the volume of Shakespeare's plays."

It could be proved that Mr. VV. had unconsciously on purpose "misheard" the figures. Since I acted out the little scene after receiving my manuscript from the typist and had not changed the typescript afterwards, it was obvious that it could not have been my mistake and had to be Mr. VV.'s.

The little incident made it possible to show again how Mr. VV. (and he is but a representative of a type) could live on the exclusive basis of disparagement, and how unstable his identifications were, though he still enthusiastically accepted the "basic neurosis."

The question arises: how are these people to be helped? Modified elaborations of a *new* ego ideal are typically observable in successful analyses; with these are coupled a strengthening of the ego. The former is poorly established in the patients under discussion, though the latter process may take place.

Before answering the question, it is necessary to clarify the fact that only a specific group of psychic masochists can be "convinced" by reading books on psychic masochism. The *typical* reaction is rejection of the whole deduction; the *exceptional* reaction is acceptance. Why does that small group react paradoxically?

It turns out that only "hyper-masochists" consciously accept the precept, and then only under the influence of the punitive superego and its telling accusation: "That's you!"

These hyper-masochists are extremely severe cases from the start. It seems that one has more difficulty with them in analysis than with the typical doubter.

The severity of these neuroses leads to one of two results, even in cases that are therapeutic half-successes. One result is that—years after conclusion of analysis—these people begin to doubt again whether "that damned masochism really exists"; hence continuation of treatment is advisable. The second possibility is that despite poor identification the ego has become strong enough to reject unjustifiable reproaches of conscience and to reject the masochistic preanalytical submission.

On the other hand, the real danger with orally, masochistically regressed neurotics lies in the possibility that they fall into the classification I have described earlier as the "empty bag" type. These patients cannot live without their pseudoaggressive defense, and therefore they adhere to their provocative techniques in spite of analysis. Building up that defense from early childhood on has sapped all their inner energy; the removal of the defense would leave them completely deflated. To avoid that specific danger, of which they are unconsciously aware, the defense is perpetuated, and any therapy defeated. At bottom, they are schizoid personalities (see Chapter 1).

The difficulty in establishing identifications without automatically corroding the new inner helper is one of the problems in treating severely masochistic neurotics. They are helpless and cannot find props for identification. They really have "nowhere to hide."

11. THE CLINICAL IMPORTANCE OF "RUMPELSTILTSKIN" AS ANTI-MALE MANIFESTO

Grimm's fairy tale "Rumpelstiltskin" contains a series of psychological fine points, so far overlooked. All of these pertain to one theme: the child's jealousy of woman's unique ability to produce children. In the fairy tale that purported superiority is coupled with a malicious and derogatory anti-male attitude. No less than five times in a tale covering two and a half pages is man described as despicable, "inferior," or ridiculous.

These are the five indictments of the male sex:

1. The story opens with the miller bragging that his beautiful daughter can weave straw into gold. He makes this boast to the king for the express purpose of self-aggrandizement ("um sich ein Ansehen zu geben," in the original).

2. The king puts the miller's daughter to work under penance of death; he marries her, not for love, but out of greed; "Even if she is but a miller's daughter, I cannot find a richer woman in the whole world."

3. Rumpelstiltskin, who comes to the girl's rescue, is described as an absurd dwarf ("ein kleines Maennchen"; note the diminutive!) propelled by greed. The girl must bribe him by offering three symbolically meant gifts: a necklace, a ring, and the promise to give him her first child.

4. Although Rumpelstiltskin can perform magic—he can weave straw into gold—he cannot magically conjure up a child; he depends on the girl for this. The suspicion arises that "the little man" symbolically represents the man's sex organ, made ridiculous. It is also likely that the act of making gold out of straw symbolically means that man can "make" money (feces) but not a child.

5. The suspicion also arises that the second part of the dwarf-magician's name, "Stilzchen," is an ironical diminutive of "Stelze," the German word for stilts. Thus man is again defined as one who puts on airs, elevates and elongates himself artificially (erection?), and is therefore to be ridiculed and regarded with contempt. So weak is his position that the mere revelation of his name becomes the denouement of the fairy tale: the dwarf must then pay the price of the discovery by giving up his claim to the queen's child. Her knowledge of his *name,* which means that she has seen through his bluff, so infuriates the dwarf that he stamps furiously on the floor, in the process losing both legs by pushing them into his body. He then

"tears himself apart." That symbolic castration also contains an allusion to two breasts: why doesn't Rumpelstiltskin choose an organ which has no partner, such as the nose, as the object of his anger with himself?

It seems to me that this fairy tale could have been invented by an ironic and malicious woman for the express purpose of deflating man. More likely, it contains the eternal jealousy of all children—both boys and girls—in their infantile competition with the mother. In addition to "owning" the father, the mother possesses two unachievable treasures: breasts and child-bearing powers. The girl consoles herself with hopes of future similarity and by equating the nipple and the clitoris; the boy consoles himself by unconsciously identifying penis and breast and by adopting the inflated he-man attitude which deflates woman. (See Chapter 7, Section I.) The well-known penis pride of the boy poorly covers his breast envy. It is at this point that the "complex of the small penis" has its emotional origin.

Recently I asked a woman patient, in her fourth week of analysis, whether she had dreamed in the nights since her last appointment. She answered: "No, I haven't any recollection of dreams. But I have been constantly thinking of Rumpelstiltskin. I cannot explain why. Can you make head or tail of this?"

The patient was young and a widow; her husband had been killed in an automobile accident some months earlier. Her depression after the accident had pushed her into continuing the analysis that had ended six years ago. Her first analysis had been with a colleague.

When she mentioned this well-known fairy tale, I asked her to tell me the story as she remembered it. She gave the essentials, leaving out all the fine points enumerated above but recording the final castration with a smile.

The "condensation word" Rumpelstiltskin contained her whole inner conflict in an unconscious innuendo.

She came from a family in which strife and unhappiness dominated. Her father had repeatedly been unfaithful to her mother; her mother had been a martyr who "hated" her money-making husband. When the child was about six years old, her mother told her that she would have left her husband if no child had been born. The girl loved her father, but by doing so acquired guilty feelings, as though she were being disloyal to her mother. She "just hoped" that her parents would remain united. As time went on, the open conflict between the parents became the order of the day. The girl was glad to escape into schools and jobs. At nineteen, half-promiscuous, she became so depressed that she entered a "highly sophisticated" sanitarium, where she received psychoanalytic treatment. The latter centered around oedipal explanations. In her half-promiscuity, she unconsciously identified herself partly with her father's girl friends, thus living out infantile wishes, and partly with her promiscuous father. In short, the analyst seemed to assume that he was dealing with a case of hysteria. In inner reality, the patient's conflict was *pre*-oedipal, centering around an unresolved masochistic attachment to the mother image. This was warded off with an oedipal blind.

The interpretation of oedipal superficial layers had a deteriorating effect. The patient became fully promiscuous, thus seeming to confirm the inaccurate diagnosis (why shouldn't she, since the analyst was falling into the trap of accepting her superficial, self-created defenses?). She began affairs with half-psychotic inmates of the sanitarium. She lived out two curious defenses: the more unimportant (emotionally) these men were, the more she insulated herself against her "real" feeling for the father (analyst); she hoped to become pregnant through one of these numerous premarital escapades "because then I can commit suicide."

Partially "improved" (though suspicious of her analyst), she left her analysis and shortly afterwards married a man many years her senior. The marriage was sometimes pleasant, sometimes a burst of conflict. In five years she produced three children. Her husband was then killed in an accident. After his death she changed her place of residence in order to be near her parents, although she always "felt worse" in the presence of her mother. Her rationalizations for moving were peculiar: the new location would provide "better educational opportunities for the children"—at that time aged four, three, and one. At first she took a furnished apartment. Among the books in this apartment were several written by me. She read these

Is Superego the Real Master of the Personality? 429

and decided that "psychic masochism permeated" her life. In this way, she came into analysis with me.

Her analysis clearly demonstrated that the patient had been desperately trying all her life to admit to her superego "the lesser intrapsychic crime" (oedipal) in order to cover up her "real crime" (psychic masochism centering around her mother). The proof of this was contained in a "paradox": Why had none of her numerous premarital affairs resulted in a pregnancy, though marital relations produced three children in quick succession?

The answer to this question emerged after some digging into the family history. The patient's paternal great-grandmother had borne two illegitimate children, refusing to marry their father although he was quite willing to marry her. The patient's own father had compensated for this family blemish by marrying a woman who came from "higher social circles." If the patient, as she had hoped, had become pregnant in one of her escapades, her mother's position vis-a-vis the father would have been strengthened, since the older woman could then accuse her husband of passing on a family failing to their daughter. Unconsciously the patient did not want to give her mother this satisfaction, and she probably created her infertility herself via spasm of the tubes, a well-known phenomenon in neurotic infertility. (See FERTILITY IN MARRIAGE, by Portnoy and Saltman, p. 160.)

At first glance this looked like hatred of her mother, not masochistic submission. That hatred, however, was defensive, and covered the patient's real aim, which was to keep the suffering mother in her position as the suffering model for identification. The patient's frantic attempts to keep her parents together represented more than guilt (arising from the wish that they separate); it was also a technique of preventing the mother from escaping from her impossible marriage.

What, then, was the mother's "crime," the crime to which the patient, as "innocent victim," became a party? It was *the mother's capacity to have children in the first place.* That crime was compounded by the mother's blunt statement that she would have left her husband except for the existence of their child.

When, in the sanitarium, the patient constructed the idea that she could commit suicide if she became pregnant, she was acting out an unconscious fantasy in which her mother was shown to be capable of killing her unborn child.

The patient's massive depressions did not pertain to being unloved or rejected, nor to her superficial oedipal guilt. The depressions were shifted to these deposits in order to cover up the real source: masochistic attachment to the mother.

Where does the "condensation word" Rumpelstiltskin come in? In the transference the patient demoted the analyst to a ridiculous figure—ridiculous as all men are. Seemingly the anti-male manifesto dominates the scene. But this is only an attempt at partially demoting, partially elevating, woman—the only being capable of producing children. The degradation of the miller's daughter in the fairy tale belongs to the demotion theme; the indispensability of woman in the child-bearing process represents the elevation theme.

Is this all? Experiences with such "condensation words" (or tunes, or visual pictures), published by me in a series of papers in previous years (starting in 1937; summarized in PRINCIPLES OF SELF-DAMAGE, 1959), prove with great regularity that these represent condensed and *highly malicious superego reproaches* (sometimes intermingled with some defensive efforts on the part of the battered unconscious ego) which are "arrested" by the ego and made incomprehensible, thus saving the ego pain. It is probable that in the condensation process under scrutiny, the original reproach reads: "You fool, you think you outgrew your masochistic attachment to your mother when you bore children yourself and acquired the right to disparage men. You are still the little misused girl, like the miller's daughter in the fairy tale. Nobody wants you for your own sake, but only because you can provide gold (parental wealth). *You* are still—Rumpelstiltskin!"

12. THE USE AND MISUSE OF YAWNING IN THE "BATTLE OF THE CONSCIENCE"

Nothing is known about the physiological or psychological reasons for yawning, besides the commonplace observation that this involuntary act appears in situations of drowsiness, boredom, dullness. Yawning is therefore taboo in company; this peculiar opening of the mouth is taken as proof positive of boredom with those present.

Is Superego the Real Master of the Personality?

And, since yawning is "infectious"—"one yawn makes two yawners," says a French proverb—it is also considered bad manners to seduce others to the thought of sleep—in company.

The unclarified problem is compounded with mystery when yawning appears in situations in which the yawner is neither sleepy nor bored. Yet he yawns and offends his companion. Such a case was presented to me by Mr. WW., a patient of forty-two, at the tail end of his analysis:

"Please explain this paradox to me. As you know, after living the promiscuous life of a wolf I decided to settle down and marry a beautiful young girl. We are very happy; everything fits and works out wonderfully. Yet if I'm with her for some length of time I am subjected to an involuntary attack of yawning. This may happen at twelve noon or at midnight. It has no connection with tiredness, nor am I bored. On the contrary, my fiancée's presence exhilarates me. These yawning attacks (something I have never experienced before) are embarrassing. Fortunately the girl has a sense of humor."

The patient's statements could be checked and verified. He had "never been so happy in his life." Why, then, the external paraphernalia of boredom in the girl's company?

WW.'s inner conscience acted in accordance with its "rules of torture": if possible it prevented success; if impossible (because of the analytical strengthening of the ego) it devaluated success. Even after his internal success had begun to match his external one his inner "torture machine," still operative (as in all human beings), voiced its scepticism: "Do you *really* want to give up the neurotic pleasure of your promiscuity? Confess that you still long for it!" WW.'s ego put in an unconscious disclaimer, *dramatizing his boredom with his previous way of life*. Hence the yawn was directed at his inner conscience ("My promiscuity has no allure for me—it bores me"). But since the dramatization was carried out before his fiancée he got at least some masochistic pleasure (the very thing he was trying to exorcise) in being "misunderstood" by the girl: whatever humor she could muster, she must also have been offended.

To the patient's surprise the interpretation was effective—his yawning "compulsion" disappeared.

It was amusing to observe that the scepticism with which Mr. WW. at first greeted the interpretation was based on his opinion that the explanation was "too simple." All psychic masochists have this difficulty: To reconcile their high-pitched narcissism with the wish to damage themselves.

13. PROOF OF BRILLIANCE BEFORE DEFEAT

A new version of "noblesse oblige" is encountered in some unusually gifted but masochistic people, who change the motto into "l'esprit oblige." This means that superiority in a particular field of endeavor does not prevent masochistic propensities from being lived out with disastrous effect. The undeniable gift makes the unconsciously sought downfall even more bitter.

To mention two examples:

In a written examination a student of mechanical engineering was the only one in a class of thirty who was able to solve a highly complex technical problem, but he substituted other figures for those given in the question. Since the papers were not marked by the "intelligent" professor (and the patient knew this) but by his "stupid" assistant, who simply looked at the answer without considering the working out of the problem, the young man failed the examination.

A brilliant foreign movie director was offered the job of directing the movie version of a worthless and offensive play written by an author in vogue at the time. His first impression was that this "piece of shit" should be "thrown in the ashcan." But he reconsidered and accepted the highly paid assignment because he believed that he could "do something" with the "impossible material." He did; he produced a work of magnificent technical achievement. What the wizard could not do was make the unacceptable acceptable. The result was that he became the scapegoat of stupid critics, who thus attacked the author in cowardly substitution. In the beginning the director had had two reasonable choices: to take the job cynically and consider the unavoidable adverse criticism as part of the payment *or* to refuse the impossible assignment. He did neither, being fooled by his self-confidence, and bitter depression came to the fore when the cacophony of critical rejection set in.

One gets the impression that the brilliance of some masochists imposes on them the necessity of first proving their great gifts to themselves and then descending into the wasteland of the average psychic masochist.

CHAPTER 9

IS THERE A BRIGHT OUTLOOK FOR THE FUTURE?

IT is customary to offset the scientific limitations of the present by envisioning bright, interminable vistas of "future research." Thus later generations of scientists are burdened with responsibilities that they will have difficulty living up to. Behind this compliment to unborn genius lies a not inconsiderable malice.

A few matters of fact in our human lot are unchangeable.

What must really be held accountable for human misery is that impersonal factor biology. Biology decrees both the long maturation time of the child and the endowment of the newborn, helpless human being with drives potentially as strong as those he will have at his disposal as an adult. The three inborn drives rebel vainly from the first moment of life: megalomania is offended, aggression rebounds against the ego, and libido, with saving grace, provides the unfortunate solution known as psychic masochism. In psychic masochism self-aggression is libidinized and megalomania artificially satisfied by provoking, and thus allegedly decreeing, punishment.

The majority of analysts avoid as unpalatable the fact that psychic masochism is universal; they show even more distaste for the fact behind the fact—the unremitting cruelty of the superego. But science cannot be converted to the program of happy endings persisted in by the slick magazines. Even distasteful facts must be swallowed when their accuracy has been demonstrated.

Biologically conditioned unfavorable depositions of rebounding aggression in earliest infancy result in the installation of the superego.

Is There a Bright Outlook for the Future?

Again in earliest infancy unplaceable megalomania, coupled with libido's rule of thumb, the pleasure principle, which tries to make the best of an impossible situation, results in the installation of the only possible defense against constant torture emanating from the superego—psychic masochism.

The future of psychoanalysis depends, in my opinion, on the speed (or lack of it) with which psychic masochism is made central in therapy. There is no reason to be especially optimistic on that score.

On the other hand, scientific progress is not merely a consoling phrase. More and more neurotic disease entities once considered hopeless, or unknown altogether, have been made therapeutically accessible. To name only one example: In 1930 Freud wrote:

> Another technique of fighting mental pain uses shifts of libido, which our psychic apparatus permits and which renders its function so much more elastic. The problem to be solved consists in shifting aims of drives in such a way that these cannot be hit by the outer world. The sublimation of drives lends its help in that endeavor. One achieves the most if one is capable of sufficiently increasing the pleasure stemming from psychic and intellectual work. In this case, fate can harm that person but little. Contentment of this type, like the *pleasure of the artist in creation* or in the personification of his fantasies, or that of the scientist in the solution of problems and finding of the truth, *carries with it a specific quality which—one day—we shall surely be capable of characterizing metapsychologically.* (GESAMMELTE SCHRIFTEN, XII, 45-46.)

Freud's hope that "one day" the "metapsychological" mystery of artistic creation would be unraveled and clinically put to use did actually materialize only ten years later when I presented the theory of artistic creativity, proving my contention with cured cases of "writer's block" (see pp. 276 ff.).

The old clinical and nosological entities in neurosis are too unprecise, especially since remnants of deeper layers infiltrate and are "reformulated" on higher developmental layers. The result is that, starting from different considerations, the distinguished dean of American psychoanalysts, Dr. Karl Menninger, suggested that neuroses should be described according to defenses used. I agree with this idea, provided psychic masochism—also an unconscious defense mechanism—is given its proper place.

Another hopeful sign is the growing cooperation between different branches of medicine and psychoanalytic psychiatry. Here I would like to single out two topics: a few psychiatric "pointers" for the diagnostician treating psychosomatic diseases and some other psychiatric hints for the gynecologist and obstetrician dealing with pregnant women.

In a recent study, "Psychiatric 'Pointers' for the General Practitioner and Internist Treating Psychosomatic Diseases," [74] I presented the following:

The most important single psychiatric fact that the G.P. and internist who treats psychosomatic diseases must know is that *there exists within the patient an unconscious wish to suffer, and that this unconscious desire counteracts his conscious wish to get well.* The unconscious longing for pain, or psychic masochism, accounts for the "incomprehensible" duration of some diseases, for equally "incomprehensible" relapses and recurrences, for illogical and inexplicable attitudes such as the failure to follow the doctor's orders, the constant flight from physician to physician, the failure to pay medical bills, and the generally provocative behavior displayed by some patients.

Too much stress cannot be put on the totally unconscious nature of the "wish to suffer," as opposed to the recovery wish. Consciously disease changes the patient—whatever his disguise—into a scared, complaining, sometimes whining child who wants help and reassurance. Unconsciously the patient also becomes a scared, complaining, whining child—but with a "plus." This "plus" comprises the unbelievable fact that he enjoys his suffering and wants to cling to it.

The objection is unavoidable: Assuming but not admitting that this is so, what can the G.P. and internist do? He cannot and should not "analyze" the patient. He cannot refer every patient to a psychiatrist. He cannot even mention his smattering of psychiatric knowledge to some patients lest they counter with the indignant question, "Do you

Is There a Bright Outlook for the Future? 437

think I'm crazy?" Why, then, bother the overburdened physician with "unusable fantasies"?

In defense of knowledge, let it be said that two quite powerful reasons justify informing the physician that the unconscious wish to suffer is at work in every patient.

First, there is no place in medicine for either therapeutic nihilism or overoptimism. But the G.P. will find it difficult to maintain even reasonable, cautious optimism when the favorable results presumably foreseeable and certainly expected from treatment fail to materialize, when the impatient patient blames the physician, when dissatisfaction and disgust—on the part of the patient for the physician, on the part of the physician for the patient—permeate the atmosphere. But if the physician knows that in a specific case the unknown factor consists of an overdose of psychic masochism, unreachable by a G.P.'s treatment, it may help his own "mental hygiene."

Second, although there is agreement that the G.P. and internist should not analyze the patient, *nothing prevents the physician from cautiously letting the patient know that every disease unconsciously "mobilizes" a specific amount of psychic masochism*. He can also—optimistically—add that the nuisance value of the disease may absorb this wish to suffer. But if the dose remains unabsorbed, additional—parallel—psychotherapy with a psychiatrist is indicated.

Now, what is the purpose of a statement stressing unconscious self-damage? It may benefit the patient. It may save the G.P. a good many reproaches from the patient and his family. How so?

The patient-physician relationship is more complex than meets the eye—or appears upon the bill. Once more, unconsciously, the patient projects upon the chance figure of the physician something peculiar: his own repressed fantasy of his own infantile omnipotence. This fantasy comprises feelings and illusions harbored by every child; in it the child can do whatever he fancies because he is all-powerful and all-knowing. Having unconsciously shifted this fantasy on to the physician—projection implies exactly that—the patient suddenly sees his doctor as a man with "X-ray eyes," an authority who is all-powerful and, more important, all-knowing and all-seeing. The physician who gives a general, though tangential "interpretation" concerning the "wish to suffer" (even if he does so with a smile and not too portentously) sets something in motion within the patient: inner fear. Paradoxically, this inner fear can prevent for at least a time the full emergence of the patient's lurking masochistic propensities.

Why should this be so? Many clinical examples in psychotherapy prove the point. Not all types of psychotherapy work with "deep interpretations" of the "uncovering type." Many operate with superficial suggestions of the "covering type"; many with blame-shifting, either social or cultural, or with interpretations so superficial that the deeper, dynamically decisive layers remain untouched. Nevertheless, all these therapies may result in temporary "successes." Some naive and not-too-smart observers erroneously conclude from such feats that the experience and emotional capacity of the psychiatrist outweigh in therapeutic importance the theories he carries in his head and the cards, attesting his membership in scientific societies, which he carries in his wallet, and the diplomas with which he adorns his walls.

Notwithstanding appearances, miracles do not happen, at least not in psychiatry. Specific reasons explain these temporary pseudo successes. They rest upon a mechanism for which I have suggested the name, "pseudo success because of unconscious fear" (see p. 54 ff.).

The alleged change makes for gratitude all around. The patient seemingly, is grateful to the physician for the "cure"; the physician, seemingly, is grateful to the patient for having provided confirmation of his power to heal. Unfortunately, the unconscious state of affairs is different. The patient is grateful for having been permitted to retain a part of his unconscious pleasures, while the physician is due for a deep disappointment—the patient's symptom will recur. If the patient has the "decency" to alter his symptoms, the therapist's ignorance and failure to connect facts will spare him even this disappointment: he will not realize that masochistic self-damage is a single tree with many branches.

Now, what happens so frequently and unintentionally in psychotherapy with the not-too-well trained or not-too-well informed psychiatrist (and admittedly this is a rather grotesque situation) can be seriously and intentionally put to use by the G.P. It is quite legitimate,

Is There a Bright Outlook for the Future?

I believe, for the internist and G.P. to apply as a palliative this not infrequent psychiatric error. The great mass of patients cannot afford psychiatric-psychoanalytic treatment. Aside from the question of cost, most of them are unwilling to seek it; if they were willing, there would not be enough trained psychiatrists available. Instead of shrugging one's shoulders and claiming the protection of the phrase "Nothing can be done," one can advocate the stopgap technique outlined here. A famous novelist, the late Charles Yale Harrison, once said: "The stopgap became a way of living, which is how it is with stopgaps."

In suggesting this "stopgap technique," it should be made clear that its purpose is by no means that of supplanting psychiatric-psychoanalytic treatment, treatment that goes to the root of the neurotic problem with all its masochistic ramifications. Quite the opposite: in severe cases only analysis of the masochistic regression can help. But the "stopgap technique" has its place as a trial balloon. It is harmless and may help in some cases.

To use a clinical example: A G.P. treats a man with ulcer of the stomach. Medication, diet, avoidance of alcohol, etc., help overcome the most acute symptoms. But in some cases these masochistically perceived sacrifices—who doesn't like to eat and take a drink?—do not suffice. Psychoanalysis should then be recommended to follow, or even better, parallel the internist's treatment. The psychoanalyst will typically find that the patient is a classical "injustice collector" who unconsciously plays this "game": To reduce the image of the "bad, refusing" mother to absurdity, he denies the inner accusation that he masochistically wants to be refused by demonstrating the opposite, "I want to get." To "document" his alleged wish to get he produces generous amounts of gastric acid as the preparatory act of digestion. The process is comparable to the flow of saliva resulting from thoughts of one's favorite food. But the gastric acid thus produced finds no food upon which to work; instead it "eats up" the mucosa of the stomach. In extreme cases the process ends in a neat hole.

Obviously, in severe cases, medication and diet alone cannot change the psychic structure. If the patient does not possess the means or the relative lack of resistance to therapy that would permit him to enter psychiatric treatment, or if he lives in a community lacking trained psychiatrists, the "stopgap technique" can be applied. It is also recommended in not-to-severe cases of neurotic personality structure.

The patient's personality structure, of course, supplies the cue to the entire problem. Let us clarify the fact that self-damage, the ominous unconscious "pleasure-in-displeasure pattern," is universal. A "masochistometer," if it could be invented, would undoubtedly show that people who possess up to a 49% deposit of that infantile scourge are those euphemistically called "normal," whereas the "higher brackets"—those registering above 51%—comprise the "neurotic." Only a quantitative difference separates the two. And even this separation would be fallacious. The imaginary scale could register only the masochistic deposit of the moment, and the distribution of the inner scourge of masochism is by no means static. At specific times, the score may increase under the impetus of certain disappointments, frustrations, or the collapse of cherished aims which are in reality defenses.

Today, people in general concede and accept the existence of inner conflicts, but—as is usual with new things—their acceptance rests more on misconceptions than on understanding. The G.P. confronted with psychosomatic manifestations often asks whether some emotional upset preceded the disease. When he hears of conflicts, mostly consisting of "anger" or "tensions" or "disappointments," he tends to jump to the conclusion that the patient suffers from "undischarged aggression" which has materialized against himself because of inner guilt. This is an everyday faulty diagnosis. Actually, what is visible at the high point of neurotic conflicts is never suppressed or repressed aggression, but psychic masochism covered by a thin layer of defensive fake aggression, scientifically designated as "pseudoaggression." The reason is simple. Nobody wants to admit, even to himself, to being a masochist. Anger and aggression, however, have the consoling connotation of being acceptable to the conscious ego; they are understandable, heroic and what not. Anyone who believes that repressed real aggression contributes to neurotic conflicts is as naive as the detective sidetracked by the criminal's fake clues.

"Pseudoaggression," covering psychic masochism, never fails to manifest itself in the behavior of the patient towards the physician. "Transference"—the repetition of repressed infantile conflicts in situations involving innocent outsiders—is not a prerogative of the analytic situation. It occurs on and off the analytic couch. The analyst, of course, uses it productively in dynamic interpretations. When transference occurs away from the analytic couch, no productive use follows; the outsider merely remains the victim of the repetition. When the repetition involves physician and patient, the G.P. should not be deceived by the patient's display of child-like helplessness and fright. Consciously, to be sure, the patient wants sympathy, understanding, and help. But unconsciously he wants suffering, and uses defensive aggression. This explains the double attitude of trust and mistrust, submission and rebellion, towards the objective, helpful physician.

This two-sided view of the physician also explains one of the least explored and most paradoxical of attitudes found in patients; the reluctance to pay medical bills. "Reluctance," it goes without saying, is a polite understatement. Patients explain their delinquency with a wealth of silly rationalizations, such as "A physician should be ashamed to think about money" or "Health is something so precious it should not be measured in money." Under these rationalizations lie two unconscious facts.

First: As far back as the patient can remember, his parents were the people who concerned themselves with his health. When, as an adult, he consults a physician who must be paid for his services, all his infantile resentment against "not being loved" enters the picture. Whoever heard of parents asking for money from their child when the child is sick? Once more, masochistic "injustice collecting" comes to the fore in the infantile adult.

Second: The projection of the patient's own infantile megalomania upon the chance figure of the physician has already been stressed. Here a basic difference between the physician and every other human being enters the picture. The physician alone, in his medical sphere, seems to have escaped the general fate of humankind; he, uniquely, has not had to relinquish that megalomania. He has some connection with this magic of infancy. His close link with life and death makes him—unconsciously—a bearer of magical powers. Hence, the reluctance to pay medical bills also has connections with emotional objections against one who still is clothed in the old but never outworn fantasy of childlike megalomania. The patient who puts off and puts off paying a medical bill is postponing what he unconsciously sees as a contribution to the support of a competitor who remained in the business while he himself was forced out of it.

There is only one exception to this form of behavior, and even then magic again plays a part. Strangely enough, these are patients who are overly prompt in paying medical bills. In most cases they do so because they are afraid of the doctor's magic power of revenge. They pay quickly in an unconscious attempt at appeasement, and in the unconscious hope that they can thus prevent his magical wrath. This is, by the way, the reason why physicians, and physicians alone, have achieved the unachievable: they cannot be openly shouted at. Nobody hesitates to shout at an engineer, an architect, lawyer, manufacturer, or even atomic scientist, but there exists the tacit agreement that shouting is entirely unacceptable in the patient-physician relationship.

Many questions of psychosomatics cannot be entered upon here because of space limitations; these include the meaning of "tensions," more recent evaluations of the role of sex life in the psychic economy, etc. One topic, however, can be covered briefly; it rates its priority because of its frequency and because of the widespread misunderstanding connected with it. This is the matter of psychosomatic diseases linked with man's "middle-age revolt." Although a good deal has been written about woman's climacteric complaints, little or nothing appears in the medical literature on man's difficulties in the late forties and middle fifties. Without discussing whether or not there exists a physiological substratum, I would like to stress the fact that every man goes through a period of crisis at some time during these decades. The "revolt" is not always full-fledged; sometimes it is abortive. It could be summed up as the stage when the man realizes that his youth has passed, and his inner conscience sits in judgment over hopes that have not materialized, illusions that have shattered, successes that have eluded the man's grasp. In other words, it is a masochistic field day. The battered ego fights back by attempting to achieve the irretrievably lost—and to do so in a hurry. Preceding

Is There a Bright Outlook for the Future?

this comes a phase in which the familiar becomes stale: office, work, social circle, hobbies, and especially his wife. She becomes the prime malefactor who holds the middle-aged man down. He thinks of divorce and a new start, of life begun again with a younger woman. This "middle-age revolt" is thus but an "emotional second adolescence" as I pointed out in my book THE REVOLT OF THE MIDDLE-AGED MAN.

Most of the time these "psychic measles" are harmless and the revolt collapses: masochism wins out. But one specific group of middle-aged pseudo rebels retires into psychosomatic diseases or hypochondria, in order to provide themselves with an inner excuse for abandoning their grandiose plans. These people are beyond medical treatment so long as the core—namely, the abortive "middle-age revolt"—remains unclarified. Actually, no treatment dispensed by an internist can have any effect upon personalities of that age group with a leaning towards hypochondria. The reason becomes clear if one thinks about the masochistic basis of the disease. Hypochondriacs elevate specific organs to the position of a self-appointed dictator; this leaves them self-appointed serfs. Masochism provides the cement which leaves this pattern impervious to any except psychiatric treatment.

To sum up: Among the many psychological complexities which face the G.P. and internist when treating patients with psychosomatic illnesses, one has been singled out for special consideration. This is the patient's hidden wish to suffer. The ancient Roman philosopher and dramatist Lucius Annaeus Seneca (5-65 A.D.) stated: "It is a part of the cure to wish to be cured." This conscious "wish to be cured" is impeded by the opposite unconscious tendency: the wish to suffer and continue to suffer. Since the G.P. cannot send every patient addicted to suffering into psychiatric treatment, the suggestion is made that he institute an automatic inner reaction in the patient, a reaction that will work in the direction of relinquishing symptoms. In a form of "stopgap technique," the physician would make the patient aware of the presence of these masochistic, self-defeating deposits. Although no physician can do what a wit described, "Some people think that doctors can put scrambled eggs back into the shell," he can help. All of today's progress in medicine can be judged when we compare the contemporary physician's admittedly still imperfect knowledge with Oliver Wendell Holmes's judgment of his own profession one hundred years ago. In an address delivered before the Massachusetts Medical Society on May 30, 1860, this leading physician declared: "I firmly believe that if the whole materia medica as now used could be sunk to the bottom of the sea, it would be all the better for mankind—and all the worse for the fishes." Today, perhaps, Holmes would retract this statement and not wish all the good things on the fishes.

An old G.P. of my acquaintance complained about the endless succession of "fads" he had encountered throughout his lifetime and bitterly recounted examples of "unlearning" he had been forced into by his patients, propelled in their turn by newspaper reports. He was especially indignant about the newest "unlearning" imposed upon him—psychsomatics. "Life is just one damn thing after another," he quoted. I consoled him by reminding him of the principle of shared responsibility. In the past every uncured case meant an offense to his fantasy of medical omnipotence. Today the G.P. can shrug his shoulders and gloatingly say, "It's a case for the psychiatrist."

The other example is the accessibility to control of after-birth blues, postpartum depression. In a lecture delivered before the Academy of Psychosomatic Medicine (Fourth Annual Meeting in Chicago, October 1957) [75] I said:

The psychoanalytic literature has repeatedly emphasized that the motives of postpartum depression are "numerous and not always clear" (H. Deutsch, THE PSYCHOLOGY OF WOMEN, II, page 249). Different phenomena have been adduced: fear of death, exhaustion, pain, absence of identification with the woman's mother, rebellion against the feminine role and motherhood, rejection of the child or husband, disturbance of the fantasies built up during pregnancy, separation and castration fears, inner guilt, the use of modern forms of anesthesia which exclude the woman from conscious participation in the birth and thus deprive her of the opportunity of placing masochistic depositions etc. Still, wisdom's last word is the statement that "there is an increasing number of women who, without being actually neurotic, nevertheless behave in an unusual fashion after a technically perfect painless delivery" (Deutsch, *loc. cit.,* page 251). This phenomenon is so typical that Deutsch suggested modifying the old saying *Omne animal post coitum triste est* to *Omnis mulier post partum tristis est,* though the joy of motherhood may appear after the "sad disappointment" (page 249).

In his valuable pioneer work, PSYCHOSOMATIC GYNECOLOGY William Kroger (in collaboration with Freed) collected the extensive literature on the topic, stressed the connection with frigidity, and correctly remarked that "pregnancy serves to bring into sharp relief these women's neurotic conflicts, even though these individuals were apparently well adjusted prior to pregnancy" (page 113).

In this discussion of the problem I am deliberately omitting the more complex phenomena of full-fledged postpartum neuroses and psychoses, in which a diseased personality uses the birth experience as a catalyst for aggravation of a state previously present but latent. These are extremely technical problems and belong in the realm of psychopathology. I am concentrating exclusively on women who are *not* neurotic, or not too neurotic, and who, despite a not too difficult delivery and a well-defined ability for maternal love, nevertheless go through a postpartum depression. In short, I am speaking about *normal women.*

The psychiatrist does not have an opportunity to observe transitory, "harmless" postpartum depression. If transitory, though painful, these depressions correct themselves in just a few days or a few weeks. Usually the psychiatrist is called on to treat only the longer-lasting neurotic and psychotic postpartum clinical pictures. On the other hand the obstetrician, with few exceptions, lacks psychiatric knowledge and is glad not to be bothered by these "unreasonable," seemingly hysterical phenomena or can offer reassurance only. But the women suffer none the less.

There is, however, one situation in which the psychiatrist has the opportunity to observe precursors of these fears and depressions *before* they fully materialize. This is when he happens to be treating a mildly neurotic woman during her pregnancy, the woman having come into analysis because of personality conflicts unrelated to the birth-giving situation. I have treated three women under these conditions. After interruption of treatment during their confinement, all three returned to analysis, and it was possible to check the results of the *preventive treatment* which I shall advocate. Postpartum depression did not develop in any of these three cases. Admittedly these women became pregnant under favorable conditions—after solving their neurotic conflicts with their husbands.

I have also had the opportunity of seeing in consultation, once or twice, two pregnant women who could not enter treatment at that time. The same preventive technique was applied in their cases. The results were favorable, they subsequently reported to me.

These five cases have given me the idea of suggesting, in simplified form, the preventive procedure to be outlined.

Pregnancy, and especially the act of giving birth, mobilizes (as all dangers do) repressed *infantile* fears present in everybody. These fears are unconscious and totally irrational. This "septet of baby fears," as I called it in THE BASIC NEUROSIS, comprises such fantastic entities as fears of being starved, devoured, poisoned, choked, drained, chopped to pieces, and castrated. All these fears have one common denominator: The fear-sufferer is on the *passive-masochistic* end—in short, he is the victim. It is true that later in life these fears disappear from consciousness and are transformed into more "rational" forms. Study of neuroses proves their presence. Whatever neurotic entity the psychiatrist touches, infantile fears come to the fore, under the analytic microscope. Of course, sceptics claim that these fears are only in the psychiatrist's mind and therefore he projects them onto the patient. This is a convenient joke, but facts are still facts. The older Huxley averred the ironic dictum: "Science is a beautiful theory killed by an ugly fact." This justifiably sceptical view of premature pet theories does not shut out the possibility that sometimes ugly facts are observed first, and secondarily elevated to a theory.

What fears, specifically, are thrown to the psychic surface in situations of danger, and then secondarily rationalized, will depend on the individual and the quantity and quality of his undigested baby fears. In these critical periods his "once upon a baby time" becomes his very real present.

It was Freud who stated that somewhere fear lurks behind all

Is There a Bright Outlook for the Future?

neurotic manifestations. In the specific fears connected with parturition the following fears of the past are activated: fears of being drained, choked, chopped to pieces, eviscerated (castrated). If one goes back to the baby situation and is familiar with the background of these fears, one can well understand why this should be so.

The fear of being drained stems, paradoxically, from the child's misconceptions of defecation and urination. The infant does not know that waste matter must be eliminated. As he sees it, parts of his body are taken away from him by a power stronger than himself, a mechanism that terrifies the child and offends his megalomania to boot. During birth, expulsion of the child is inwardly identified with anal mechanisms. It is well known that all children go though a phase in which the anal opening is considered the sexual aperture. Kroger (*loc. cit.*, pages 109 and 110) has correctly registered cries of distress uttered by such women before giving birth: "I feel like my bowels are going to move; I'll probably make a terrible mess! Please let me go to the toilet." This is not simply a transitory "anal regression" but is a regression to something deeper: a baby fear of more terrifying nature.

The fear of being chopped to pieces has a no less paradoxical humble beginning, namely, the handling of the baby during cleaning and washing procedures. The newcomer to this world finds the mother's purposes obscure. No matter how tender and careful the mother is, from the child's viewpoint the manipulations are terrifying. Later, all manipulations with surgical purposes are subsumed under this heading.

Fear of evisceration, later subsumed under castration fear, is the culmination of all baby fears. Numerous variations are encountered. Later these are also connected with lack of anatomic congruity between male and female genitalia.

One could go into additional detail and show how every infantile fear has a representation during pregnancy. For example, the vomiting during early pregnancy, although some authors believe there are toxic reasons, certainly has a psychic superstructure as well—the fear of being poisoned. The oral conception is nullified through oral expulsion. And breathing difficulties caused by ascension of the uterus during pregnancy activate old fantasies of being choked. Other examples could be adduced.

One should also mention that baby fears are later shifted to masturbation and guilt toward mother. Hence the spectacle of so many pregnant women afraid of giving birth to a crippled or moronic child. Added to all this are exhibitionistic fears. The girl's entire education emphasizes the idea of modesty. All at once, during pregnancy, and especially during the process of giving birth, the rules of "decency" are suspended. Not only physicians and nurses but even outsiders are involved, for during the last months pregnancy cannot be hidden.

To demonstrate the fantastic tricks the unconscious (the hidden child in the adult) can play, I am adducing the example of a business woman treated nearly thirty years ago. She sought analysis because of a bizarre phobia that a lion would attack her from behind in the dark. She could not remain alone at home evenings and was fearful of going out. "Don't tell me, please," she begged, "that there are no lions running around in apartments in this modern city. I know that my fears are stupid and irrational." She expressed preference for a treatment hour directly after lunch: "I suffer from an old stomach disorder and have cramps after every meal. Since I have to lie on a couch for analysis, I thought that to save time I could combine my midday rest with analysis." She was impatient with me when I tried to get some information about her "purely organic" stomach troubles. (This analysis took place before the advent of psychosomatic medicine.) She informed me that with every meal she had "peculiar" cramps in her bowels. Rest relieved distressing flatulence, and after her rest (ending with a "big flatus") she felt "like a newborn person."

Analysis disclosed her fear of being attacked by a lion to be a banal oedipal rape fantasy. When she was three years old her father, a Herculean man, had taken her to the zoo. She admired the lion. "He is nearly as big as you are," she told her flattered father. She wanted to feed the lions from her lunch box but her father warned her that this would be dangerous. The substitution of lion for father was easily established. An attack from behind corresponded to her infantile fantasy that the anus was the female sex organ.

Is There a Bright Outlook for the Future?

So far this is a commonplace anxiety hysteria. More interesting was the psychogenesis of her gastrointestinal symptoms. Eating proved to be a thinly disguised sexual fantasy. Each meal was an oral impregnation. The orally conceived baby developed in the bowels, and following labor pains (cramps) was delivered per anum (flatulence). It was psychologically quite appropriate that she felt "like a newborn person." This hysterical materialization of the typical childish fantasy of oral conception, intestinal pregnancy and anal birth (the genitalia were totally excluded) was consummated in one hour, three times daily. In addition to the complete disregard for the realities of time, and in addition to anatomic absurdities, other evidences of infantile omnipotence were the multitude of "children" she "produced" (no less than 1,095 in the course of a year). In this way she won the "competition" with her mother, who was able to produce no more than a single child a year.

Now, all these apprehensions, normally dormant in repression, were "once upon a baby time" connected with some uncanny unconscious pleasure—the pleasure in fear, psychic masochism. Hence when these apprehensions come alive (one can adduce Homer's poetic simile of the Greek heroes in Hades who were resuscitated when they drank blood) the defense sets in too. Thus, at bottom, all fear is directed against the masochistic inner danger and allure; it is only later that the fear is rationalized (because the origin is not conscious) in terms of reality dangers confronting the woman during birth-giving.

This also explains the omission from the list of baby fears of the most logical one, the fear of death. Freud's opinion that fear of death is not represented in the unconscious has been confirmed time and again. In the unconscious, death means suffering, loneliness, being left helpless in the cold, immobility—once more the paraphernalia of psychic masochism.

The preventive technique advocated here consists of two parts:

1. *Familiarizing pregnant women beforehand (during the last months of pregnancy) with the unavoidable resuscitation of repressed infantile fears during pregnancy and parturition,* contrasting these with the harmless reality situation. Reassuring statements that "everything will be all right" are quite insufficient. The obstetrician or

general practitioner who will assist the woman during the birth-giving process can mention the baby fears previously enumerated. Only in severe and unmanageable cases should the woman be sent to a psychiatrist.

2. Familiarizing pregnant women with the fact that in refusing to admit their fears to themselves *they are mortgaging their happiness in the period after birth of the child and will pay the price of postpartum depression.* Once inner fears, covering psychic masochism, have been mobilized, they cannot be dismissed, they inundate the personality. This is a new discovery, first stated in my book THE SUPEREGO, published in 1952.

The latter statement requires elaboration. If one takes a vacation or pleasure trip and allots x dollars to cover expenses, and returns from the trip having spent less than expected, the surplus funds are generally returned to the savings account. The money was prepared, not spent, and saved. The situation is quite different with psychic energy. Once prepared, it *must* be spent, though in different disguises. This peculiar fact applies also to masochistic deposits and can be demonstrated in the phenomenon called "crying because of happiness." [72] Nothing is more paradoxical than a person shedding tears when joy is expected. Viewed psychiatrically the story is less grotesque. A happy event, or even a conspicuously felicitous event calling for the comment "I am overjoyed," does not enter the life of the individual as *deus ex machina*. It is preceded by long periods of dreary expectations and long barren stretches when success is absent from the circumscribed area of activity. If this were not so, the reaction to the happy event would be mere complacency: The expected outcome has materialized.

Both dreary expectations and periods when success is not forthcoming unconsciously mobilize a good dose of psychic masochism in the form of inner fears. Once psychic masochism—the unconscious pleasure-in-displeasure pattern—is activated, it cannot be dismissed without discharging its accumulated and "ready to jump" store of energy. If the outcome of dreary expectations is a flat failure, the ensuing depression absorbs the masochistic discharge. But if, unexpectedly, the outcome is favorable, a new deposition is inwardly sought and found. Despite the happy event, *the beneficiary behaves as if he were bemoaning the suffering that preceded the fortunate result.*

This mechanism can be illustrated by an old gag. A passenger in a train moans audibly. His neighbor, unable to concentrate on his magazine, asks if he is in pain. The afflicted one explains that he is suffering from excruciating intestinal cramps. The neighbor, a good Samaritan, offers some pills, which are accepted. Immediate relief follows the taking of the medicine. The good Samaritan returns eagerly to his magazine, but his peace is again disturbed by a second performance of moans and groans. "Are you in pain again?" he asks. "No," is the reply, "but I'm thinking of the pain I had before." Substitute for the conscious irony of the witticism an unconscious technique and the simile fits.

One could conclude that the more pain is subsumed in the actual process of giving birth the less postpartum depression is to be expected. The conclusion is erroneous. The yardstick is not the *actual* pain and discomfort experienced but the *"psychic amount" prepared for the event*. If the fear was overdimensional, even a painful birth will not absorb all the expected suffering. The "leftover" will be materialized in the ensuing depression.

This depression is really a "depression because of missed masochistic opportunities," as I would call it. (Further elaboration in my study, "Depression as Aftereffect of Missed Masochistic Opportunities," *Psychiatric Quarterly,* 31:36-41, 1957.) This is a new and, so far, never-stressed element in depression, although the principle of discharging accumulated psychic energy (cathexis) is a basic psychoanalytic principle that views psychic phenomena as dynamic, not static.

One should not be deceived by the fact that these masochistically tinged depressions (using as vehicle infantile repressed fears, later rationalized) are frequently cloaked in guilt because of "aggressive" thought. That "aggression" is but spurious aggression (pseudo-aggression), hiding the real masochistic substratum. Then, guilt is accepted for the "lesser intrapsychic crime" (aggression). It should also be stated that guilt and psychic masochism are not identical.

Punishment and guilt are precursors, and they are later changed into some *inner* pleasure—the pleasure in displeasure.

It is obvious that the clinical material presented—five cases—is not sufficient to draw on for very far-reaching conclusions. I am therefore presenting these findings in a tentative manner and suggesting further research. If the obstetrician and general practitioner apply the preventive technique advocated, there is no danger of damaging the patient. At worst, if the physician is unsuccessful in preventing postpartum depression, he has at least given the patient something to hold on to. It is a lot better for the woman to bear in mind, after the child is born, that her depression corresponds to the discrepancy between prepared and used-up fears than for her to believe, in her depression, that her whole life is collapsing.

Personally, I am expressing the cautious conviction that the avoidance technique outlined here, although it amounts to no more than a stopgap, will be of benefit to suffering women and at the same time initiate a better understanding between psychiatrist and general practitioner, gynecologist and obstetrician.

The joker who devised the slogan "Time marches on," an optimistic pronouncement, would not have been so wrong if he had considered the other side of the coin: progress is by no means an automatic process always going in the same direction.

In the ideas of the last part of the nineteenth century and the first decade of the twentieth, a *direct* development of the human genus to better and higher levels of culture and humanity was frequently forecast. In the last five decades this "from better to better" philosophy has been rudely upset by successive waves of barbarism, enforced by successive waves of dictatorship from the right *and* the left. Goethe's words have proved sadly prophetic, "Progress has not followed a straight ascending line, but a spiral with rhythms of progression and retrogression, of evolution and dissolution." What consequences this will have in the atomic age it is difficult to foresee.

Too much emphasis is put on technical progress, disregarding the fact that the human mind, burdened with deep-seated masochism, is poorly equipped to face the staggering novelty of hydrogen weapons capable of laying waste whole continents. Too little study has been devoted to the psychological element, meaning the masochistic propensities. Without these, the fact that nearly half the population of this globe has submitted to the rule of megalomaniacal dictators is incomprehensible. True, this masochistic submission is counterbalanced in some of the slaves by inner rebellion. Alone against these forces of dictatorship are the democracies, with dignity of the individual as their central tenet—and they are preparing to fight for their very lives.

Appeal to self-interest is a weak bargaining point when unconscious self-damage is in the driver's seat. And criminal psychopaths draped in ideologies and puffed up with power and dreams of world domination are unpredictable. The very technical progress we are so proud of may lead to the graveyard of civilized life as we know it today.

Since the future—even the immediate future—is unforeseeable and the scientist who, outside his own circumscribed field where he knows at least something, ventures to clothe his ignorance in the prophet's mantle is rather ridiculous, the psychiatrist does well to abstain from predictions. It is better to concentrate on the job in hand: to find out more and more about the unconscious and to give help to those in mental distress. That is exactly what we are trying to do.

Although it is an exaggeration nowadays to maintain, as Oliver Wendell Holmes did (MEDICAL ESSAYS, 1883), that "science is the topography of ignorance," it must be admitted that we still have a great deal to learn about the unconscious mind. And only naive people say that their learning days are over.

NOTES

1. For the psychology of love and the division of the superego into daimonion and ego ideal, see the Jekels-Bergler theory expounded in "Transference and Love" (*Imago*, 1934), partly reproduced in *The Psychoanalytic Quarterly*, 18:325-350, 1949.

2. For the decisive role of the superego in connection with this indispensable process, see "'Working Through' in Psychoanalysis," *The Psychoanalytic Review*, 32:449-480, 1945. Partly reprinted in THE BASIC NEUROSIS (Grune & Stratton, N. Y., 1949), pp. 110-136.

3. For elaboration, see THE SUPEREGO (Grune & Stratton, N. Y., 1952), pp. 283-286.

4. Elaborated in THE SUPEREGO, Chapter X.

5. The parallel development in the little girl is described in COUNTERFEIT-SEX (second, enlarged edition, Grune & Stratton, N. Y., 1958).

6. "The 'Empty Bag' Type of Neurotic," *The Psychiatric Quarterly*, 25:613-617, 1950. Summarized in THE SUPEREGO, pp. 327-330.

7. THE REVOLT OF THE MIDDLE-AGED MAN (second, enlarged edition, Hill & Wang, N. Y., 1957), case 1.

8. E.g., I have been repeatedly censured (or made fun of) for dividing every psychic phenomenon I described into numerous types, representing subdivisions. Without going into the naivete of the objectors, I should like to state that each subdivision represents a self-made objection to the completeness of the formulation. These self-made objections are of two types: conscious ones referring to clinical cases seemingly not fitting the general statement or, more frequently, unconscious superego objections begrudging every new evaluation. The latter can be productively used because—though the intent of the superego is not clinical correctness but personal torture exclusively—they are identical with the objections of enemies. All this shows how many safeguards are built in against "exaggerated claims."

9. See my books, COUNTERFEIT-SEX (l.c.); HOMOSEXUALITY: DISEASE OR WAY OF LIFE? (Hill & Wang, N. Y., 1956); ONE THOUSAND HOMOSEXUALS (Pageant Books, Inc., Paterson, N. J., 1959).

10. For elaboration, COUNTERFEIT-SEX (l.c.) Ch. IX.

11. "Eight Prerequisites for the Psychoanalytic Treatment of Homosexuality." Published in *The Psychoanalytic Review,* 31:253-286, 1944.

12. Attempts at reconstruction of the patient's infantile situation revealed a weak, ineffective father and a strong, rather domineering mother. Consciously the patient rejected this domineering trait in women; still, he fell for it twice—in his wife and, years later, in his present girl friend. Asked how he could explain the contradiction, he stated that at first, in both cases, he did not have the impression that these two women were domineering. Their attitudes of "strength" rather gave him an amused feeling of being a joke he "could handle." This camouflage (covering the masochistic wish to be again a victim) served his self-deception well: he became the victim, just as he unconsciously wanted to do. In his own estimation what he always wanted was a "kind, loving woman"—a conscious illusion typical of every psychic masochist. Superfluous to mention that the patient's voyeuristic and defensively exhibitionistic traits (partly sublimated in his profession) were discussed.

13. First reported in ONE THOUSAND HOMOSEXUALS (l.c.).

14. The case is described at length in COUNTERFEIT-SEX, Chapter III.

15. Details in ONE THOUSAND HOMOSEXUALS (Mr. Y., pp. 92ff).

16. "Psychoanalysis of a Case of Agoraphobia." *The Psychoanalytic Review,* 22:392-408, 1935.

17. The case is described at length in ONE THOUSAND HOMOSEXUALS (l.c.), pp. 75ff.

18. First reported in *Samiksa* (Calcutta), 9:81-92, 1955.

19. To speak of "masochistic wishes" is, in itself, a simplification. Psychic masochism is a complex defense mechanism of the unconscious ego (see Chapter 1). But, after its establishment as the leading personality pattern, it acquires, for practical purposes, the valency of an unconscious wish.

20. For the role intuition plays in clinical discoveries, see the author's PRINCIPLES OF SELF-DAMAGE (Philosophical Library, N. Y., 1959), Chapter IX ("On Intuition").

21. Patients who "give in" only a little are generally suspected of holding on to their "repressed wishes." I believe this to be a fallacy; in my opinion they are holding on to their basic masochistic solution, hiding out behind their camouflaging symptoms.

22. For the psychology of Lesbianism, see pp. 74f, and COUNTERFEIT-SEX, Ch. IX.

23. One could, of course, suspect that ironically demolishing the competence of their husbands' authority, the analyst, was of some unconscious pleasure to ladies 2 and 3. This was not true in Case 1 (I was Mrs. N.'s choice), nor in Cases 4 and 5. My impression is that

the *singleness of purpose* visible in "grand design" neuroses works with a self-propelling force.

24. Paper presented at the International Psychoanalytic Convention in Wiesbaden, 1922.

25. "The Mechanism of Depersonalization," *Int. Zeitschr. f. Psychoan.* (Vienna), 21:258-285, 1935.

26. Theodor Reik once correctly, though purely descriptively, observed that depersonalized people change into a "psychic observatory."

27. That paper specifically excluded psychotic cases.

28. "A New Approach to the Theory and Therapy of Erythrophobia." Paper read at the XV International Psychoanalytic Convention, Paris, 1938. Printed in *The Psychoanalytic Quarterly*, 13:43-59, 1944.

29. "Psychoanalysis of a Case of Agoraphobia." *The Psychoanalytic Review*, 22:392-408, 1935. The convincing material is presented for both parts of the visual orbit without my clearly showing the interconnections in the form of mutual and multiple defenses. See pp. 244ff.

30. "Fear of Heights," *The Psychoanalytic Review*, 44:447-551, 1957.

31. "On the Disease Entity Boredom ('Alysosis') and Its Psychopathology," *The Psychiatric Quarterly*, 19:38-51, 1945.

32. Twenty-some studies, summarized in my book THE WRITER AND PSYCHOANALYSIS (Doubleday, 1950; second, enlarged edition, Robert Brunner's Psychiatric Books, N. Y., 1954).

33. *The Psychiatric Quarterly*, 24:268-277, 1950.

34. The objection could be made that the first object of visual interest in the baby is his own body; everyone has observed babies staring with fascination at their fingers or big toe. What is overlooked in this objection is the fact that these self-inspections are later forcibly "discouraged" by educators because of their connection with masturbation and "self-centeredness." Thus the child's interest is diverted *outward*. Here also is one of the reasons for the change of "pleasurable" into "unpleasurable" self-observation, described in 1935 for depersonalization (see above). Education so thoroughly inhibits self-inspection that the only way to smuggle it in is—illness. In illness self-observation, masochistically tinged, *is* allowed.

35. Elaboration in COUNTERFEIT-SEX.

36. The little girl has two other grievances against her mother which are, in general, passed over lightly: her mother's ability to have children and her own sibling rivalry. Both are subsumed as "jealousy." There is more to it. See "Psychology of Jealousy," *Internationale Zeitschrift fuer Psychoanalyse und Imago* (London), 24:4, 1939.

37. I prefer the term "repetition in reverse" to Freud's cumbersome and confusing "unconscious repetition compulsion," confusing because

of its linguistic vicinity to "unconscious repetitions." Every neurotic is an unconscious repeating machine; but his repetitions of stabilized inner defenses are under the influence of the pleasure principle, whereas in "repetitions in reverse" experiences are *actively* repeated to which one was once *passively* subjected, regardless of whether the experiences were pleasurable (they are, according to Freud, "beyond the pleasure principle")—the only purpose being the eradication of a narcissistic wound sustained in the passive act. To repeat: it is only Freud's term that is objectionable; his observation of the phenomenon is brilliant and of greater clinical importance than the creator of psychoanalysis suspected. The first practical application to the psychology of intercourse was suggested by me (in collaboration with L. Eidelberg) in "The Breast Complex in the Male," *Int. Zeitschr. f. Psychoan.* (Vienna), 19:547-583, 1933. Later, it was enlarged (in DIVORCE WON'T HELP NEUROTICS, Harper & Bros., N. Y., 1948) to subsume the psychology of the "he-man."

38. In the neurotic part of his personality our scientist did not do so well. His masochistic conflict with his wife was the remnant of his infantile masochism.

39. For a fuller account, see the author's book TALLEYRAND-NAPOLEON-STENDHAL-GRABBE (Int. Psychoan. Verlag., Vienna, 1935). Partial summary in HOMOSEXUALITY: DISEASE OR WAY OF LIFE, l.c.

40. See LAUGHTER AND THE SENSE OF HUMOR (Grune & Stratton, N. Y., 1956).

41. See COUNTERFEIT-SEX. Also: "Psychology of the Uncanny," *International Journal of Psycho Analysis* (London), 1934. This study is a continuation of Freud's famous paper "The Uncanny," COLLECTED PAPERS, IV.

42. Elaboration in: DIVORCE WON'T HELP NEUROTICS; CONFLICT IN MARRIAGE (Harper & Bros., N. Y., 1948 and 1949, respectively).

43. For a fuller account, see FASHION AND THE UNCONSCIOUS (Brunner's Psychiatric Books, N. Y., 1953).

44. "A New Approach to the Therapy of Erythrophobia," *The Psychoanalytic Quarterly*, 13:43-59, 1944.

45. In the original publication the literature is collected; twenty-nine references are adduced, p. 58f.

46. "Preliminary Phases of the Masculine Beating Fantasy," *The Psychoanalytic Quarterly*, 7:514-536, 1938. "Further Studies on Beating Fantasies," *The Psychiatric Quarterly*, 22:480-486, 1948.

47. Starting with different assumptions, B. Lewin came—independently—to similar conclusions.

48. "Psychoanalysis of a Case of Agoraphobia." *The Psychoanalytic Review*, 22:392-408, 1935. The reason for the delayed publication was Hitler and—Jung. The paper was accepted in 1932 by the *Zentralblatt*

fuer Psychotherapie in Berlin under the editorship of Dr. Kronfeld. In January 1933 Hitler came to power; the *Zentralblatt* suspended publication till the Fall, when it came out under the editorship of Jung, proclaiming the Aryan psychotherapy and denouncing Freud's "Jewish" approach. The "scientific" journal also had in its first issue an editorial written by an obscure nephew of Goering's declaring that Hitler's MEIN KAMPF was the new Bible of psychotherapy. The galleys of my paper (the paper was already in print) were returned, the first page crossed out with the remark "Geht nicht [idiomatic: won't do, cannot be done, impossible]. C. G. J. [Jung's initials]." I also received a letter from the Secretary of the "new" Society informing me that my paper contradicted the "heldische Weltanschauung" (heroic outlook on life) of the Nazi movement.

49. First stated in "Fear of Heights," *The Psychoanalytic Review*, 44:447-451, 1957.

50. See E. Hitschmann's well-known paper on Keller, *Imago*, 1915.

51. "Plagiarism." Psychoanalytische Bewegung. 1932. Partly reproduced in THE WRITER AND PSYCHOANALYSIS (l.c.).

52. See "On a Five-Layer Structure in Sublimation," *The Psychoanalytic Quarterly*, 14:76-97, 1945.

53. For elaboration, see THE BASIC NEUROSIS, Ch. 3 ("The Nine-Point Basis of Every Neurosis") and Ch. 7, pp. 87-97.

54. This was a polite statement; the patient was schizoid.

55. "On Negative Exhibitionism," *The Psychoanalytic Review*, 43:454-457, 1956.

56. Described in MONEY AND EMOTIONAL CONFLICTS (second, enlarged edition, Pageant Books, Inc., Paterson, N. J., 1959).

57. First published in "Psychology of Gambling," *Imago*, (Vienna), 1936.

58. Some of these manifold fears have previously been investigated in the author's books, e.g., FASHION AND THE UNCONSCIOUS (1953), MONEY AND EMOTIONAL CONFLICTS (1954). (Problems of criminosis, excluded in this study, in THE BATTLE OF THE CONSCIENCE, 1948.) Other elements play an important role in these fears: castration fears (in deeper regressions covering "baby fears"), the discrepancy between ego and ego ideal, etc.

59. Shortened version of my study, "Voyeurism," *Archives of Criminal Psychodynamics*, 2:211-225, 1957.

60. Summary from "Suppositions about the 'Mechanism of Criminosis' ", *Journal of Criminal Psychopathology*, V:2, 1943.

61. I once had the opportunity of observing an exhibitionistic act in statu nascendi: the journalist mentioned on p. 322.

62. See also pages 151f., and 263f. The Jekels-Bergler theory of love

as an episode in the "battle of the conscience" was first published under the title "Transference and Love," *Imago,* 20:5-32, 1934. Further elaboration in DIVORCE WON'T HELP NEUROTICS, THE BATTLE OF THE CONSCIENCE, and FASHION AND THE UNCONSCIOUS.

63. Lecture delivered before the Vienna Psychoanalytic Society, November 8, 1933. Printed in *Imago* (Vienna), XX:5-31, 1934, and *The Psychoanalytic Quarterly* (New York), XVIII:325-350, 1949.

64. First published in *Internationale Zeitschrift fuer Psychoanalyse,* XX:252-260, 1934; translated in 1935 in *International Journal of Psycho-Analysis,* XVI:89-95.

65. Eleven years later the topic of defensive camouflage in masturbation fantasies was taken up by L. Eidelberg in "A Contribution to the Study of the Masturbation Fantasy," *Int. Journal of Psycho-Analysis,* XXVI, 1945, Parts 3 and 4.

66. For elaboration: KINSEY'S MYTH OF FEMALE SEXUALITY, by Bergler-Kroger, Grune & Stratton, N. Y., 1954.

67. "Further Studies on Depersonalization," *The Psychiatric Quarterly,* 24:268-277, 1950.

68. "A Contribution to the Multiple Meaning of Psychogenic Phenomena," *The Psychoanalytic Review,* 42:168-171, 1955.

69. THE REVOLT OF THE MIDDLE-AGED MAN (l.c.).

70. Many neurotic marriages are held together on that basis. For clarification, see the author's books DIVORCE WON'T HELP NEUROTICS and CONFLICT IN MARRIAGE (Harper & Bros., N. Y., 1948 and 1949).

71. First stated in THE SUPEREGO (1952).

72. Why crying should have been the specific defense used is a problem discussed in my study "Paradoxical Tears—'Tears of Happiness,'" *Diseases of the Nervous System,* 13:337-338, 1952.

73. Printed in *Diseases of the Nervous System,* 20:39-42, 1959.

74. Printed in *Diseases of the Nervous System,* 20:420-424, 1959.

75. This study was requested by Dr. Charles W. Mayo for *Postgraduate Medicine,* of which he is editor-in-chief, and was printed in Vol. 25, No. 2, Feb., 1959.

INDEX

A

Acrophobia, 246f
Active repetition of passively endured experiences (repetition in reverse), 194, 205, note 37/457
Activity vs. passivity, 196f
Admission of the lesser intrapsychic crime, 39, 65, 79, 152, 218, 254, 334
Aggression
  all neurotic aggression but pseudoaggression, 59
  confused with pseudoaggression, 59
  equal partner with libido, 57
  infantile, divided into four parts, 41
  inexpressibility in infants, 30
  itinerary of the opposites, 339
  normal and neurotic, differentiation between, 41
  passive defeats and aggressive countermeasures on all three genetic levels, 44
  and pseudoaggression, 41
  pseudoaggression in clinical picture of psychic masochism already a defense in schizoids, 46
  and pseudomoral connotation, 130ff
  and psychic masochism, see: Psychic masochism
  recoiling of, against the ego, see: Superego
  retrieving of, from the neurotic masochistic amalgam, 81
  See also: Pseudoaggression, Psychic masochism, Superego

Agoraphobia, 244ff
Anal regression, 43
Anticipation tendency in punishment, 238ff, 410
Aspermia, psychogenic, 406
Autarchic fiction
  in baby, 26
  in psychic masochism, 115
  in uncanny, 232ff
  See also: Megalomania

B

Baby fears, see: Septet of baby fears
Basic fallacy, 139, 403
Basic neurosis, 15ff
Beating fantasies, 201, 242, 259f, 381
  unexpected importance of, 381ff
Blushing, 237ff
Boasting, infantile, and consequences in ego ideal, 34
Boredom, 306ff
Breast complex, see: Orality
Breast-envy vs. penis-pride vs. penis-exhibitionism, 112
Breast and penis, unconsciously identified, 37, 110
Bychowski, Gustav, 47

C

Caricaturistic relationships, 407ff
Case histories, excerpts, 48ff, 68, 82-95, 95-105, 105-121, 133ff, 146ff,

462   INDEX

Case histories (*Cont'd*)
    153ff, 158, 159-164, 164, 169-173, 173f, 175, 178f, 181-185, 185-188, 189-190, 190-192, 208-213, 222, 239f, 240, 244f, 251f, 255f, 257f, 273, 278, 288f, 293-299, 312-316, 320, 322, 332, 341f, 403, 408, 411, 418f, 419, 427f, 431
Castration, 43
    anal, 43; see also: being drained, fear of
    oral, see: Septet of baby fears
    phallic, 29
Child, alleged happiness of, 25
Choking, fear of being, 29
Chopped to pieces, fear of being, 29
Clinical picture in psychic masochism, see: Psychic masochism
Clinical picture in visual drive, see: Visual drive
Clothes, psychology of, 235
Complex of small penis, 202f, 213f
Condensation words, 430
Condition of the forbidden, 235
Confusion between:
    aggression and pseudoaggression, 59, 334f
    analytic geology and actual development of the child, 56
    conscious and unconscious conscience, 34
    criminosis and neurosis, 356ff
    cultural standards and severity of superego, 36
    essentials and "also present," 398
    feminine identification and homosexuality, 73
    genetic and clinical pictures in psychic masochism, 31ff, 253
    genetic and clinical pictures in visual instinct, 195, 207
    guilt and psychic masochism, 57
    guilt and shame, 348f
    leading and misleading identifications, 420f
    legitimate and illegitimate silence in analysis, 136ff
    libidinous and megalomaniacal frustrations, see: Septet of baby fears
    masochistic and pseudoaggressive basis of fear, 249f
    masturbation with pre-Oedipal masochistic content and exclusive Oedipal strivings, 376ff
    Oedipal regression and Oedipality as defense against deeper layers, 54; see also: Case histories
    oral and phallic regression, 54
    parasitic tendencies and defensive misuse of those in neurosis, see: Orality
    psychic masochism and "love surrogate," see: Psychic masochism ("pet theories")
    real love and counterfeit-love, 151f
    real therapeutic successes and spurious ones, 55f, 150, 283
    "suffering" in analysis and masochistic misuse in the analytic situation, 136ff
    thinking and "rearranging of prejudices," 323ff
    three and five layer structure in neurosis, 61ff
    wish to get and be refused, 140, 405
Conservatism in science, 16ff, 125
Conscience, see: Superego
Coprophemia, 340
Counterfeit sex, 205f
Criminosis, mechanism of, 356ff
Curiosity, 252

D

Daimonion, see: Superego
Darwin, Charles, 291f
Defense mechanisms
    created by the unconscious ego, 374
    defense against the defense, 61ff
    irrevocability, when prepared, 39
    only defense against the defense visible in neurotic symptoms, see: Neurosis
    psychic masochism holds first priority among all inner defenses, see: Psychic masochism
    and superego, see: Superego
Depersonalization, 199f, 292ff
Depression
    anticipation type, 410
    created by unconscious ego, 374f
    post partum, 444ff
    preventive, 410

INDEX

Depression (*Cont'd*)
  regret depression because of missed masochistic opportunities, 142, 398, 451
  three major sources of, see: Case histories, Superego
Devoured, fear of being, 29
Differences of opinions concerning three- or five-layer structure in neurotic manifestations, 61f
Discrepancy between ego and ego ideal, see: Superego
Drained, fear of being, 29
Dreams
  interpretation of, as part of analytic technique, 58, 80
  of devaluating success, 36ff
  refutation dreams, 38
  of schizoid people, 27ff
  unconscious wishfulfillment plus refutation of superego's reproaches, as dream formula, 368

E

Ego ideal
  boasting, infantile, and consequences, 34
  genesis of, 32f
  and love, 150f, 263f, 368ff
  technique of daimonion using ego ideal as weapon, 34
  See also: Superego
Ego, unconscious
  creates all defense mechanisms, 374f
  function in making superego's reproaches incomprehensible to conscious ego, thus saving the latter pain, 430
  and fear, 268f
  forced by superego to supply cathexis for its own torture, 28
  mediation role of, 374f
  temporary collapse of dual function: changing unconscious wishes into defenses acceptable to superego, and shortchanging superego's punishment into masochistic pleasure, see: Case histories
  See also: Defense mechanisms, Depression, Fear, Psychic masochism

Eidelberg, Ludwig, 196, 199, 353, note 37/457, note 65/460
"Empty bag" type of neurotic, 48
Endresult of infantile conflict, see: Psychic masochism.
Errors in clinical psychoanalysis, 127f
Errors in judgment when confronted with an "affront," 417f
Escapism in treatment
  "acting out" by misuse of transference, 176f
  flight into "love" with an outsider, 150f
  giving up some trimmings, while maintaining neurosis, 150
  intellectualization, 165
  interruption of treatment, 147f
  lies about the analyst, 165ff
  naive transference improvements, 149f
  post-analytic misuse of pre-analytic symptoms, 153f
  premature resignation, 159f
  pseudo-success because of unconscious fear, 55f, 150, 283
  reopening of insoluble problems, 158f
  shifting of psychic masochism to points unrecognizable to the patient, 164
"Exaggerated claims," 61, note 8/455
Exhibitionism, see: Visual instinct

F

Fantasy of "passive victim," traced through oral, anal, phallic phases, 42f
Fear
  of confined places, 243f
  loss of beneficial effects of protective fear in schizoids, 51
  predominant in every neurosis, see: Neurosis
  pseudoaggressive camouflage of basic masochistic conflict, 249
  pseudo-success because of unconscious fear, 55f, 150, 283
  progression of infantile fears, 30f
  septet of baby fears, 28f
  theory of, 214, 249f, 268f
  "uncanny," the, 232f

Federn, Paul, 141f
Fenichel, Otto, 311
Frank, Jerome, and Frank, Barbara, 337ff
Free associations
    alleged suffering derived from waiting for, 136
    masochistic misuse of, 136f
    and oral regression, 138f
    and technique in orally regressed cases, 138
Freud, Sigmund, 16, 23, 24, 26, 31, 32, 53, 56, 57, 62, 125, 141, 193, 199, 340, 435
Frustration
    danger of confusing libidinal and megalomaniacal components in, see: Septet of baby fears
    See also: Megalomania, Psychic masochism, Superego

G

"Grand design" type of neurosis, 180ff
Greatest compliment, "I never thought of that," 413f
Guilt
    acceptance of, for lesser intrapsychic crime, 39, 65, 152, 218, 254, 334; see also: Case histories
    and psychic masochism not identical, 57f
    and shame, 348f
    sources of, see: Superego
    See also: Neurosis, Superego, Aggression

H

Happiness, alleged, of child, 25
Hoch, Paul, and Catell, James, 51f
Homosexuality
    baby-mother relationship, masochistically elaborated on, repeated in, 70
    basic problem in, 66f
    bisexuality, a popular misnomer, contrasted with biological meaning of term, 72
    clinical pictures in, 70f
    curability, recent, of, 65ff
    genetically, no connection with negative Oedipus, 73
    personality traits in, 67f
    psychic masochism, plus:
        1) handing over "power to torture" from mother-image to man, 66
        2) "reduplication of one's own defense mechanism," 66
    spurious type in, 73
    statistically induced type, 72f
    tension in, not sexual, but masochistic, 76
Hysteria, neurosis, see: Phallic regression

I

Identifications, unconscious
    breast-buttocks, 387
    breast-penis, 66, 206
    leading and misleading, 420f
    milk-urine-sperm, 205
    weak, corroded by irony, 420
    See also: Beating fantasies, Superego
Identity of refusing and giving under impossible conditions, 404f
Injustice collecting, see: Psychic masochism
Intercourse, superstructure of, 205
Intuition, 329

J

Jealousy, 252ff
Jekels, Ludwig, 141f, 376f

K

Karpman, Ben, 352, 356

L

Lesbianism, 185f
Lewin, Bertram, 368, note 47/458
Libido
    inborn, 56f
    "itinerary of the opposites," 339
    libidinized selfaggression, see: Psychic masochism
    used as defense, 311
    See also: Aggression, Psychic masochism, Superego
Logorrhea, 269f

INDEX

Love
  automaticity of, in adults, disputed and psychological reasons adduced, 150
  child's need for love as counteraction against fear, see: Septet of baby fears
  counterfeit-love, 151
  and fear, see: Tender love
  neurotics incapable of, 151
  powerful weapon against guilt, 51
  tender (romantic) love, 150f, 263f, 368f
  and transference, 151

M

Magic gesture
  negative, 361ff
  positive, 71, 361f
  structure of, 361f
Malice, neurotic
  used as defense, see: Pseudoaggression
Masturbation, 376ff
  allure of, 379, 380
  beating fantasies, in, camouflaging the inexpressible terror from the septet of baby fears, 384
  game quality in, 377
  modified inner defenses in, 377
  passivity as basis of, 378f
  sanctuary of masochistic passivity, 379
  septet of baby fears in, 378
Megalomania, infantile, 25ff, 63, 253
  constant reformulations of, see: Septet of baby fears
  desperate attempts at retaining it, in psychic masochism, 253
  and ego ideal, 34
  misconceptions concerning food intake, 27
  offense to, 26f
  remnants present in everyone, see: Psychic masochism
  safeguards, megalomaniacal, in psychic masochism, 253
  and "the uncanny," 232f
  See also: Frustration, Ego ideal, Narcissism, Psychic masochism

Menninger, Karl, 435f
"Middle-age revolt," 48ff
Modesty, theories on, 228ff; see also: Shyness
Mortgaging one's future through indignant reproaches, 402f
Mother
  demotion of pre-Oedipal, 43
  dichotomy of, 42ff, 62f
  Oedipal-and pre-Oedipal, 42, 62f
  See also: Ambivalence, Oral regression
Multiple meaning of psychogenic phenomena, 397

N

Narcissism
  attenuation of infantile megalomania, see: Megalomania
  in love, see: Love
  "unification tendency," see: Writers
Negative (inverted) Oedipus complex, 43, 44, 173
  confusion with anal regression, see: Anal regression
  connection with oral conflicts, 62
  contents of, 44
  neurotic results if miscarried: "Milktoast" and "Super-He-man," 73
Neurosis
  acceptance of inner guilt for substitute crime, see: Admission of lesser intrapsychic crime
  admission of lesser intrapsychic crime, 39, 65, 79, 152, 218, 254, 334
  all neurotic aggression but pseudoaggression, 59
  basic masochistic conflict, covered by libidinous-pseudoaggressive camouflages, 18f, 81
  consequences of misunderstanding of neurotic structure, 54
  conspicuous "first line of defense" vs. inconspicuous "inner fortress," 18ff, 63
  core of neurotic conflict, 18f, 81
  counterfeit sex in, 205f
  deep masochistic pleasures in, 17f
  defense against the defense in, 61f

Neurosis (Cont'd)
   difference between neurotic and not-too-neurotic people, 15f
   disease of the dynamic unconscious, 15, 23
   dramatizes a libidinous and/or pseudoaggressive denial of the masochistic attachment, 63f
   "empty bag" type of, 48
   every neurotic has lost his individual "battle of the conscience," See: Superego
   fear in, see Fear, Superego
   "grand design" type of, 180ff
   "gratitude" of uncured neurotics, 17f
   guilt in, see: Guilt
   identifications in, two types, 420
   incurable neurotics mostly schizoid personalities detected too late, 19f
   infantile debacle in, 17
   "itinerary of the opposites" in, 311
   libidinous and pseudoaggressive camouflages, covering basic masochistic conflict, 63f
   manageable and unmanageable neurotic traits in, 15
   manifestations in, 23
   Oedipality, according to Freud's later statements, 62
   progressive, not selflimiting, disease, 40f
   pseudo-moral connotation in, 126, 132
   psychic masochism indispensable for understanding of, 63
   rescue station from unsolved oral-masochistic conflicts, 17, 63
   schizoid cases confused with neurosis, 19
   shifting defenses in, see: Superego
   shortchanging of torture, emanating from superego, into masochistic pleasure, 79
   six factors influencing curability of, 126
   superego paramount in, see: Superego
   three layers vs. five layer structure in, 61f
   transference only emotional attachment in, see: Transference
   twice filtered innuendos in, 61f
   two types of repetitiveness in, note 37/457
   two way "immobilization trick" in, 131f
   unchangeability of, without analysis of oral-masochistic basis, 126
   unconsciously, neurotics in analytic treatment, want to improve their neurotic pleasures, 17
   unconscious "exchange rate": one ounce of unconscious pleasure paid for with tons of conscious unhappiness, 80
   unproductivity of neurotic solution in, 79
   victory of superego in, see: Superego

Neurotic symptom
   compared with sublimation, 88f
   defense against a defense, 61f
   five layer structure in, 61f
   "pseudo-moral connotation" in, 126, 132ff
   spurious disappearance without destruction of genetic basis, see: "Success because of unconscious fear"
   structural basis, see: Neurosis
   substitute for twice filtered substitute gratifications, 61f
   "volcanic eruption" of id-strivings disputed, 61f

Nunberg, Herman, 377

O

Oedipus complex
   and ambivalence, 43
   as blind, hiding deeper layers, 54, 62f
   enlargement of term by Freud, 62
   inverted (negative), 43ff
   positive, 43
   prehistory of, 62f
   rescue station from oral danger, 62f
   and septet of baby fears, see: Septet of baby fears
   transition from pre-Oedipal to Oedipal phase, 43, 62ff

Omnipotence, fantasy of, see: Megalomania

INDEX 467

Optimism, 135
Oral regression
  ambivalence and, 43
  analytic technique in, 138f
  defined as basic neurosis, 18
  genetic and clinical pictures in, see: Psychic masochism
  mechanism of orality, 41; see also: Clinical picture in psychic masochism
  and patient's wish to get, as defense against the wish to be refused, 140, 405f
  reformulation of contents, on higher developmental levels, 44f
  remnants, degrees of, determining health or neurosis, 15
  and septet of baby fears, 28ff
  therapeutic chances of destroying it, see: Psychic masochism
  unchangeability without deeper analysis of, see: Psychic masochism
"Overdetermination," 397f

P

Passive defeats and aggressive countermeasures at three genetic levels, 44
Penis exhibitionism, 224f
Perversions, psychodynamics of, 353f
Phallic regression
  confused with deeper layers, see: Orality
  rescue station from oral-anal dangers, see: Orality
Pierced, fantasy of being, 27
"Pointers" for G.P. and internist treating psychosomatic diseases, 436ff
Poisoned, fear of being, 29
Post-analytic misuse of pre-analytic symptoms, 153f
Post-partum depression, 444ff
Pre-Oedipality, see: Oral regression
Privacy, battle for, 197
Pseudoaggression, see: Agression
Pseudo-moral connotation in neurosis, 132ff, 136
"Psychic apparatus," 25
Psychic "bookkeeping" of infant, 26

Psychic masochism
  aggression, boomeranging because of inexpressibility and guilt, secondarily libidinized, as genetic basis (Freud), 31
  analysis of, does not invalidate accepted principles of psychoanalysis, 58f
  analyst's prerequisites for analysis of, 57
  and anxiety, see: Fear
  argument of "exaggerated claims," 61, note 8/455
  basic neurosis, 15f
  "crime of crimes," 80
  decisive importance of, 15ff
  deepest of all dangers, 80
  defense mechanism, not id-wish, see: genetic and clinical pictures in
  depression as "aftereffect of missed masochistic opportunities," 142ff
  differentiation between neurotic and malignant types of, 19, 44ff
  emotional resistance to analysis of, 57
  end result of infantile conflict, 15ff
  extent of, underestimated, 15ff
  first priority among unconscious defense mechanisms, 80
  "fourth narcissistic hurt," 142
  genesis of, 31f
  genetic picture of, 31f, 41, 253
  indispensable for understanding neurosis, see: Neurosis
  "injustice collector," see: Clinical picture in,
  inner obstacles to understanding of, 57
  irrevocability of cathexis in, 39
  lifeblood of neurosis, 20
  "love surrogate," theory of, disputed, 58; see also: Pet theories, below
  and "magic gesture," see: Magic gesture
  malice, as secondary defense against, See: Pseudoaggression
  malignant and neurotic forms of, 19, 44ff
  megalomaniacal safeguards in, 253
  neutralization of superego's power in, 80

Psychic masochism (*Cont'd*)
"pet theories" on, 58
preserves infantile megalomania, 115, 253
present in everybody, 32
proof of brilliance before defeat, 432
provocation, as technique of, see: Clinical picture in psychosomatics, 436f
"ratrace" in, to prove to superego non enjoyment in, 42
regret depression of missed masochistic opportunities, 142
"the only pleasure one can derive from displeasure is to make pleasure from displeasure," 31
two types of, 44
unproductiveness in, 29f
See also: Oral regression, Pseudo-aggression, Superego

Psychoanalysis
affective understanding in, 80
confusion in analytic "geology," 56
conservatism in, unjustified, 16ff, 125
crucial question in: neurotic or malignant psychic masochism, 23ff
cure in, definition of, 15
difficulties in accepting deeper layers in, 57
dreary consequences of misunderstanding of neurotic structure, 54
errors in, 127f
"footnote attitude" towards deeper layers, 156
fourteen technical errors in our transitional period in, 127f
"fourth narcissistic hurt," 142
free associations in, 136f
Freudian, deepest and most successful tool in helping neurotics, 20
future of, 435
handling of "regret depression because of missed masochistic opportunities," 142
"improvement of neurotic trade balance," 16
incomplete without thorough analysis of psychic masochism, 58
legitimate differences of opinions, 16

medical applicability to neuroses exclusively, 19, 125
minimum and maximum program in, 157
no cure all, 125
objection against concentrating on superficial layers, 127
obstacles to analysis of psychic masochism in, 57
poor therapeutic results traced to overlooking psychic masochism in, 58
post-analytic misuse of pre-analytic symptoms, 153
provides patient with new energy to fight superego's torture, avoiding the "masochistic solution," 81
pseudo-successes because of unconscious fear, 55f, 150, 283
pseudo-moral connotation as resistance in, 130ff
resistance in, see: case histories
scale of therapeutic successes and failures in: excellent, 143; half-losers, 144f; middle of the road improvements, 143f; failures, 145
schizoid cases in, 44ff
"self-analysis" defined as fancy word for arriving at wrong conclusions about one's wonderful self, 24
silence in, see: Free associations
six factors influencing the patient's analysis, 126f
source of new energy put at the patient's disposal in, corresponding to retrieving original aggression from masochistic amalgam, 81
"success because of unconscious fear," 55f, 150, 283
summary of changes in:
demasochization, 122
humanization of ego ideal, 122
technique in orally regressed cases, 138f
"throwing a monkey wrench in the machinery of neurosis" in, 79
transference in, 61; see: Case histories
transference "improvements," 149
unconscious pseudo-moral connota-

INDEX

Psychoanalysis (*Cont'd*)
  tion, a dangerous prop in neurosis, 130f
  "working through" in, 80
Psychogenic oral aspermia, 406
Psychotherapy, two types of, 17

R

Rationalization, 136
Reformulation of oral-megalomaniacal material on higher developmental levels, see: Septet of baby fears
"Refusing giver," 406
Resistance, see: Case histories

S

Schizoid personalities, 23ff
  clinical examples of, 48ff
  confused with neurotics, 52
  dread of being manipulated by mother-image in complete helplessness, 46
  early and late diagnosis, 47
  loss of beneficial effects of protective fear, 51
  malignant masochism in, 45f
  neurotic psychic masochism already an inner defense in, 46
  neurotic vs. schizoid cases, 123
  phenomenological types in, 47
  problems of advisability of analytic treatment in, 53
  reasons for therapeutic inaccessibility, 47
  transference in, 47
  two dreams of, 28f
Selfdamage, see: Psychic masochism
Septet of baby fears, 28
Sex
  counterfeit sex, 205f
  normal, 205
  precursors of, see: Oral regression
  psychological superstructure in, 205
Sham-shame and shame, 344ff
Shyness, 223ff
Silence
  legitimate and illegitimate in treatment, 141f
Simmel, Ernst, 197, 208

Starvation, fear of, 28
Stendhal, 216ff
"Stroke," progression from noun to verb, 387ff
"Stupidity," psychological basis of some cases, 24, 271
Sublimation
  collapse of, process of, 94; see also: Stagefright, Writers
  compared with neurotic symptom, 88ff, 301f
  defined as defense against a defense, originating historically on an id-wish, 88f, 301f
  five-layer structure in, 88ff, 301ff
  limited victory of unconscious ego over superego, 88f
  opposite of masochistic solution, 88f
  See also: Stagefright, Writers
Success and failure, guideposts, 331f
Success hunter, 327
"Suffering" in analysis
  fallacies of, 127ff
  technical mistake of the analyst, 127ff
Superego
  acceptance of ruse of damaging pseudo-crime by, 39
  accumulation of recoiling aggression, 32
  antihedonistic principle of, 35
  beneficiary of inexpressible baby aggression, 33
  both, failure and success, used as torture material, 36
  confusion between conscious and unconscious conscience, 34
  cruelty of, 34
  cultural standards uses as blind, 36
  daimonion part of, 33
  deed and wish equated by, 35
  defenses built for its benefit, 374f
  delayed punishment, 38
  devaluation of success, 38
  discrepancy between ego and ego ideal used as weapon by, 34
  and dreams, 36, 368
  ego ideal part of, 32f
  encouragement of repetitive mistakes by, 40
  enlargement of current mistakes used as torture material, 39

INDEX

Superego (*Cont'd*)
  formalism of, 35
  genesis of, 32
  immediacy of torture by, 36
  introjected aggression in, 33
  and intuition, 329
  killjoy treatment of happiness after success, by, 38
  mutual interaction of both "departments," 32
  mock rules of procedure of, 35
  origin of, 32
  psychic masochism as counteraction against torture by, 80
  psychic masochism as proof of superego's mastery of the total personality, 374ff
  real master of personality, 374
  responsible for progressive deterioration of neurosis (if untreated), 40
  selfcreated torture bribes, 79
  simplicity of trapping ego, enjoyed by, 39f
  "taking the blame for lesser intrapsychic crime," partly accepted by, 39
  torture for torture's sake, 34
  two parts of, 34
  two way immobilization trick, 131
  twenty one "rules" of torture by, 34f
  and work, 309

T

Tears
  of anticipation, 410f
  of happiness, 39
Technique of treatment in orally regressed cases, 138f
Temper tantrums, 334f
Transference
  acting out by misuse of, 176ff
  confusion of contents, 61; see: Case histories
  deciphering of inner attitudes by observing inner repetitions in, see Case histories
  and love, 150f
  and neurotic's inability to love, 151
  in schizoids, 47
  and patient's masochistic misuse of, 61
  positive and negative, 61
  and "suffering" in, 136, 152
Truth fanatics for others, 260f

U

Uncanny, psychology of, 232ff
Unconscious as dynamic force, 23
Unconscious fear, pseudo-successes because of, 55f, 150, 283
Unconscious repetitions, note 37/451f; see also: Case histories, Transference
Unconscious repetition compulsion (repetitions in reverse), 194, 205, note 37/451f

V

Visual drive, 193-373
  basic problem: voyeurism original drive, exhibitionism but defense, 193ff
  "battle of the breast," 201
  beating fantasies plus, see: Depersonalization, Blushing
  bidding up of educational interdictions in, 197
  both ingredients can be used as defense against each other—after endresult of infantile conflict established, 200f
  clinical vs. genetic picture in, 207f
  clinical pictures in neurotic elaboration of:
  acrophobia, 246ff
  agoraphobia, 244ff
  alysosis, 306ff
  block in scientific, photographic, journalistic endeavors, 340f
  coprohemia, 340f
  demonstration character of neurotic and psychosomatic manifestations, 344
  depersonalization, 199, 292ff
  erythrophobia, 237ff
  fear of confined places, 243f
  fear of examination, 251

INDEX

Visual drive (*Cont'd*)
  general inability to reproduce, verbally or graphically, what has been seen or heard, 337
  jealousy, 250ff
  lack of imagination in perceiving external phenomena and lack of "business acumen," 327ff
  logorrhea, 269ff
  negative exhibitionism, 318ff
  pathological curiosity, 252ff
  perversion exhibitionism, 361ff
  perversion voyeurism, 352ff
  sham-shame and fear of being found out, 345ff
  shyness, 223ff
  stage fright, 300ff
  temper tantrums, 334f
  thinking block, 323ff
  writer's block (painter's, sculptor's, composer's block), 276ff
  "confessional elements" in exhibitionism, serving as guilt diminisher, plus invitation to punishment, 193
  confusion between genetic and clinical pictures in, 196, 207
  connection between "battle of the breast" and visual factors, 201
  exaggerated caricature executed on one's own substitutive organs, 193f
  exhibitionism as defense: admission that one has actually passively seen (or wished to have seen) what one now, in active repetition, exhibitionistically repeats, 194
  imagination as flight from dilemma of visual dependence, 195
  imagination of disaster, 195
  incognito exhibitionism, 213f
  looking as "proof" of having been denied sight, masochistically exploited, 194; see also: Perversion voyeurism
  magic gesture in, 361f
  mechanism of stubborn reparation, 213
  meeting ground with infiltrating psychic masochism, 194
  parity between voyeurism and exhibitionism spurious, 193
  and privacy, 197
  psychic masochism in, 194
  reparative attempts in, 202f
  specific features (eleven) in, 206ff
  Stendhal's visual problem, 216ff
  terminological difficulties, 193
  therapeutic dangers in neglecting that psychic orbit, 198
  two basic elaborations of peeping interdictions in infancy: exhibitionistic defense (normal, half-neurotic, masochistic solutions), 203; imagination as flight from the dilemma of voyeuristic dependence (subjectively creative fantasies, objectively creative fantasies, imagination of disaster, 193
  two types of defense in, 222
  "visual imperative," 253f
  voyeuristic-exhibitionistic exchange mechanism, 200, 248, 281

W

Wish to be refused, see: Superego
Words
  giving and refusing in analysis, 137f
  "senseless" words, tunes images, 430
Work, psychology of, 309
Working through, see: Case histories
Writer's block, 276ff
Writing, creative, 276ff

Y

Yawning, 430

Z

Zilboorg, Gregori, 47